Mosby

London   Philadelphia   St Louis   Sydney   Tokyo

FUNDAMENTALS OF

Obstetrics and Gynaecology

DEREK LLEWELLYN-JONES

OBE, MD, MAO, FRCOG, FRACOG

in collaboration with
SUZANNE ABRAHAM AND JEREMY OATS

Mosby

London Philadelphia St Louis Sydney Tokyo

Publisher	Richard Furn
Development Editor	Erica Vowles
Project Manager	Claire Brewer
Designer	Paul Phillips
Layout	Jim Evoy
Illustration	Jenni Miller
	Amanda Williams
	Debra Woodward
Cover design	Paul Phillips
Cover illustration	Deborah Gyan
Copyeditor	Joanna Billing
Proofreader	Roderick Crews
Production	Andrea Ford
Index	Anita Reid

Cataloging-in-Publication Data:
Catalogue records for this book are available from the US Library of Congress and the British Library

For full details of Mosby titles please write to:
Mosby International Ltd
Lynton House
7–12 Tavistock Square
London WC1H 9LB
UK

Contents

Foreword

Before his death on the 28th November 1997, Derek Llewellyn-Jones had essentially completed the preparation of this Seventh Edition of *Fundamentals of Obstetrics and Gynaecology*.

Medical students are exposed to an almost limitless amount of information. The first task for those charged with introducing them to Obstetrics and Gynaecology is therefore to ensure that their core knowledge has a sound foundation. From this base they should then be able to pursue the detail and depth that they require for their medical practice. The second is to present a balanced account especially of new developments; one of Derek Llewellyn-Jones' gifts was his foresight that could predict where the pendulum would ultimately rest.

One of the major changes in this edition has been the upgrading to colour of many of the original clinical photographs and microphotographs. We are indebted to our colleagues for generously giving us access to their archives. Derek Llewellyn-Jones made numerous revisions throughout this edition especially in the medical aspects of Obstetrics and Gynaecology. As previously, he consulted widely with his colleagues to ensure that all changes were clinically and scientifically justified.

Even with electronic exchange of data, producing a text book when the editors and the publishers are at opposite ends of the globe remains a challenge and we are grateful to the production team at Mosby for their patience and perseverance.

The daunting challenge that Derek Llewellyn-Jones left to his successors is to maintain the standard that he set, so that *Fundamentals of Obstetrics and Gynaecology* will continue to provide students of Obstetrics and Gynaecology with the information, and we hope the inspiration, which will ensure that women throughout the world receive the quality of care to which they are entitled.

Jeremy Oats and Suzanne Abraham

Preface

This Preface was written, by Derek Llewellyn-Jones, for the sixth edition of *Fundamentals of Obstetrics and Gynaecology*. Derek intended to update and modify this for each new edition of the book. We, Suzanne Abraham and Jeremy Oats, wish to retain it in its original form as it was written by Derek, as inherent in this Preface is the philosophy and approach to the teaching of obstetrics and gynaecology to medical students of Derek Llewellyn-Jones. This Preface will provide the foundations for future editions of this book. For this edition we wish to thank our collegues who are listed in the acknowledgements for providing pictures, photographs and figures to enable this edition to be published in colour.

Suzanne Abraham and Jeremy Oats

THE CONTENT OF OBSTETRICS AND GYNAECOLOGY

The expansion of medical knowledge over the past 20 years and its increasing complexity makes it difficult for medical students and interns to know what they need to know to be competent doctors and to pass the examinations set at the end of their assignments in various medical disciplines. This has led in the words of the General Medical Council to a situation in which 'it is distressing to see the progressive disenchantment [of many students] as they work their way through the course. Imagination and curiosity are soon dulled'. This opinion is echoed by the Dean of St. Bartholomew's Hospital Medical School who was horrified at the transformation of eager, bright school leavers into dull, demoralised doctors in the space of five years.

The question is: 'What has occurred to change the best and brightest into unhappy, disillusioned doctors, particularly in the intern year?'. In part, the change is due to the enormous collection of facts that students and interns appear to have to learn: in other words there is too much rote learning and too little encouragement of curiosity and of inquiry. In part it is because teachers in a discipline appear to believe that it is essential for students and interns to learn a great deal about the discipline and resent having to curtail the information they provide in the interests of the medical curriculum as a whole.

If teachers insist that students remember facts and gear their teaching sessions to encompass this, if teachers fail to inspire students to seek further, the situation will not change. If teachers 'put down' students in tutorials and fail to respect the patients during bedside teaching, the situation will not change.

Students are realists and if they know that they will be examined on matters they have memorised they will continue to rote learn facts and to forget most of the material as soon as they have passed the examinations. During the pre-registration year interns learn that to progress it is best to adopt the attitudes of their consultants towards patients, particularly when interns' working conditions often are appalling and not conducive to continued learning.

The difficult of each of the medical disciplines is to determine what is the essential knowledge medical students and interns should acquire (and, equally importantly, what they do not need to know), and how to encourage them to retain their curiosity as well as to memorise facts.

This leads to further question: 'Should women's health issues, that is, obstetrics and gynaecology (or, as I prefer, 'gyniatry') be a core subject or an optional subject?'. The General Medical Council considers that understanding of the human reproductive cycle and the understanding of human relationships are essential aspects of the undergraduate medical curriculum, which suggests that women's health issues should remain a core subject.

Fundamentals of Obstetrics and Gynaecology was first published over 25 years ago in two volumes. The contraction of the assignment in obstetrics and gynaecology in the undergraduate curriculum to 10 weeks or less means that the size of a text book should also be reduced. It is for this reason that the books, which have sold over 100,000 copies, have been completely rewritten as a single volume. In undertaking this task I have discussed the content with some of my colleagues and although we have not always agreed, there has been sufficient consensus for the book to be written. However, the published opinions are mine and are based on the literature and on the discussions. If teachers do not agree with some of them I hope that students will be encouraged to find out why there is disagreement and to evaluate the information critically and creatively.

In the evolution of new medical curricula I believe that there will be a mix of teacher-centred information transfer and self-directed problem-based learning. I hope that this text book will serve as a source book for both approaches, supplemented by literature searches and evaluation of chosen topics. This is the reason why I have limited the bibliography mainly to reference books.

Readers will note that some of the material may seem to be irrelevant for many students. Does a student need to know, for example, the steps required to perform a forceps delivery or a caesarean section? These topics have been included, largely as illustrations with captions, as the book is used in several developing countries where this information has a practical value.

I have tried to describe the effect of a chosen procedure on the woman (and in many cases on her partner) as it appears that some teachers are brilliant diagnosticians and skilled surgeons, but are poor communicators. Modern medicine increasingly involves the patient in the treatment process, and the patient's fears, anxieties and psychosocial values need to be addressed.

It is my hope that *Fundamentals of Obstetrics and Gynaecology* will meet the needs of today's medical students and interns and will encourage self-learning skills whilst providing essential information in a readable manner.

Derek Llewellyn-Jones

Sydney, 1994

Acknowledgments

We wish to thank Dr John Anderson, Dr John Bell, John Gocking, Dr Jenny King, Dr Roger Livsey, Gwen Moody, Dr Diane Paynton, Dr Peter Scally, Professor Brian Trudinger, Fetal Welfare Westmead Hospital, Sydney, and Down Syndrome Association of NSW, Australia for generously providing ultrasound, pathology and clinical photographs.

Figure credits

Figure 3.3 redrawn from Patten. *Tend Act Gynecol et Obstet* 1959, Montreal: Beauchemin.

Figure 3.5 redrawn from Hertig AJ and Rock. *J Contrib Embry Carnegie Inst* 1941, 29:127.

Figure 3.7 redrawn from Hamilton, Boyd and Mossman. *Human Embryology*, Cambridge: Heffer; 1962.

Figure 7.9 redrawn from Danforth DN and Ivy AC. *Amer J Obstet Gynecol* 1949, 57:831.

Figure. 7.22, 7.23, 7,24, 23.3, 23.4, 23.5 redrawn from Caldeyro-Barcia R and Poseiro JJ. *Trans Cong Int Gynecol et Obstet* 1958. Montreal: Librairie Beauchemin; 1959.

Figure 9.2 redrawn from J Studd.

Figure 9.4 redrawn from Greenhill. *Obstetrics*, 13th ed. Saunders; 1965.

Figure 27.3 redrawn from Moya, James, Burnard and Hanks. *Anaesthesiology* 1961, 22:644.

Figure 42.2 reproduced with permission from Taylor S, Raffles A. *Diagnosis in Colour: Pediatrics*, London: Mosby; 1997: 239.

Figure 43.6 reproduced with permission from Sambrook PN, Dequeker J and Rasp HH, Metabolic bone diseases. In: Klippel JH, Dieppe PA eds. *Rheumatology*, 2nd ed. London: Mosby; 1998: 8.36.1.

Data

Fig 2.2 data from Aptar D et al. *Acta Paediatr Scand* 1978, 67:417.

Fig 3.11 data from Dawes GS. *Am J Obstet Gynecol* 1962, 84:1643.

Fig 5.5 data from Hytten and Leitch, *The Physiology of Human Pregnancy*, 2nd ed. Oxford: Blackwell; 1971.

Fig 27.6 data from Cuckle et al. *Br Med J* 1987, 94:387–402.

Fig 23.7 data from Cardozo LD et al. *BJ Obstet Gynaecol* 1982, 89:33–8.

CHAPTER 1

Gyniatric history and examination

Examining a woman who presents with gynaecological problems

It is generally accepted that most gynaecological problems are medical or psychological, rather than surgical. For this reason it is crucial that a careful history of the woman's complaints is obtained.

HISTORY

Doctors must be aware of the reluctance of many women to discuss gynaecological and sexual matters. The medical practitioner must be sensitive to this, tactful, communicative, courteous, gentle and unhurried. The history of the patient's complaints should be recorded sequentially.

The manner in which the woman answers questions may give a clue to the origin of the complaint. This is important as studies in Britain and Australia show that 10% of women have psychiatric morbidity (measured by the Present State Examination). Other studies have noted a significant relationship between gynaecological symptoms, adverse life events and psychiatric morbidity. The doctor should exclude depression by inquiring about sadness, irritability, fatigue and so on.

The questions should seek information about the woman's:
- *Menstrual history.* Age at menarche; duration of the menstrual cycle; menstrual pain; and the duration and severity of menstruation. This may cause some confusion. For example, if the woman says that she bleeds for 5 days every 20 days, the doctor may believe that her periods are occurring too frequently. The doctor may need to explain that the menstrual cycle starts on day 1 of bleeding and includes the menstrual phase as well as the interval between menstrual bleeds. The woman in the example given in this designation, would bleed for 5 days every 25 days, which is normal. This designation is conveniently recorded as 5/25.
- *Obstetric history (if any).* The number of pregnancies and the outcome; that is, spontaneous miscarriages or induced abortions; ectopic gestation; children born, their birth-weights and the year of the birth of each; complications occurring during pregnancy, labour or the puerperium (the end of the third stage of labour until involution of the uterus is complete, approximately 6 weeks).
- *Previous medical history (past illnesses and operations) and family history.*
- *Psychological history.*
- *Sexual history.* This needs to be obtained with great sensitivity, and should be left until late in the interview.
- *History of the main complaint.*

EXAMINATION

Unless the patient has been seen before, a general examination should be made, as the gynaecological complaint may only be a local manifestation of a general disorder. This examination, which can be performed quite quickly, should include inspection of the head and neck, palpation of the supraclavicular areas for enlarged lymph nodes, auscultation of the heart and determination of the pulse rate and blood pressure.

The gynaecological portion of the examination should include:
- A breast examination.
- An abdominal examination.
- An inspection of the external genitalia.
- A pelvic examination, by speculum, and then digitally as a bimanual vagino-abdominal examination.
- A rectal examination in certain instances.

Breast examination

With the patient sitting facing the examiner, the breasts are inspected, first with the patient's arms at her sides and then with her arms raised above her head (*Fig. 1.1*). The shape, contour and size of the breasts, their height on the chest wall, and the position of the nipples are compared, any nipple retraction being noted. The supraclavicular regions and axillae are next palpated. The latter can only be palpated satisfactorily if the pectoral muscles are relaxed. This relaxation can be obtained if the physician supports the patient's arms whilst palpating the axillae. Palpation is then performed with the patient lying supine, her shoulders elevated on a small pillow. Palpation should be gentle and orderly, using the flat of the fingers of one hand. Each portion of the breast should be palpated systematically beginning at the upper, inner quadrant, followed by palpation of each portion sequentially until the upper, outer quadrant is finally examined.

The breast self-examination that many doctors recommend to women is similar to the breast examination made by the doctor, except that the woman usually does not palpate the axillary area. *Figure 1.1* demonstrates how a woman should examine her breasts. The technique can be taught to her easily by her doctor.

Abdominal examination

The examination is conducted with the patient lying comfortably on her back, *having emptied her bladder immediately before*. Inspection of the abdomen will show its contour, and the presence of striae and scars or of dilated veins. If the patient raises her head and coughs, hernias and divarication of the recti abdominis muscles will be evident.

Palpation of the viscera is performed systematically, the liver, the gall bladder, the spleen and the kidneys being palpated in turn. The caecum and colon are next palpated, the hand pressing down gently as the patient breathes out. Percussion may be required if the presence of free fluid is suspected.

Pelvic examination

The pelvic examination should follow the abdominal examination, and never be omitted unless the patient is a virgin. The external genitalia are first inspected under a good light with the patient in the dorsal position, the hips flexed and abducted, and knees flexed. If she or the doctor prefers, she may lie in the left lateral position. Some women are more comfortable and feel less exposed in the latter position. The patient must have voided just before the examination (unless she is complaining of stress incontinence), and should preferably have defaecated that morning. If urinary infection is suspected, a mid-stream specimen of urine may be obtained at this time.

The patient is asked to strain down, to enable detection of any evidence of prolapse, after which a bivalve speculum is inserted and the cervix visualized. For the woman's comfort the speculum should be warmed and the doctor's approach sensitive and communicative. If the physician intends to take a cervical smear to examine the exfoliated cells, *no lubricant apart from water* should be used on the speculum. The vagina and cervix are inspected by opening the bivalve speculum (*Fig. 1.2*). If the patient has a prolapse, the degree of the vaginal wall or uterine descent can best be assessed if a Sims speculum is used with the patient in the left lateral position (*Fig. 1.3*).

Digital examination follows, one or two fingers of the gloved hand being introduced. In most countries, apart from the USA, it is usual to use the right hand as the fingers of this hand in a right-handed person are more 'educated'. After the labia minora have been separated with the left hand to expose the vestibule, the fingers are introduced passing *upwards and backwards* to palpate the cervix. The left hand palpates the pelvis through the abdominal wall simultaneously so that the uterus and ovaries may be palpated. Normal oviducts are never palpable. As the intravaginal fingers push the cervix backwards, the abdominally located hand is placed just below the umbilicus and the fingers reach down into the pelvis, slowly and smoothly, until the fundus is caught between them and the fingers of the right hand in the anterior vaginal fornix (*Fig. 1.4*).

The information obtained by bimanual examination includes:

- *By palpation of the uterus*. Position, size, shape, consistency, mobility, tenderness, attachments. The normal uterus is either in the anterior or posterior position, and is about 9cm long. It is pear-shaped and of firm consistency, and can be moved in all directions. It is normally tender when squeezed between the two hands.

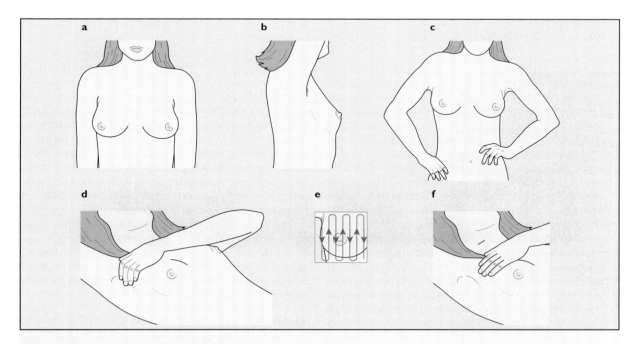

Fig. 1.1 Breast self-examination. (a) Inspection of the breasts – the patient's arms at her side. (b) Inspection of the breasts – the patient's arms raised above her head. During the inspection, the contour of the breasts, the size and shape of the areolae and the condition of the nipples are examined. An indentation or a bulge in the contour may indicate a lesion. (c) Placing hand on hip tenses the pectoralis major accentuating any tethering from an infiltrating neoplasm. (d) Axillary palpation. (e) Systematic examination of four quadrants of the breast. (f) Palpation of the upper outer quadrant of the breast.

- *By palpation of the ovaries and oviducts (Fallopian tubes).* The tips of the vaginally located fingers are placed in each lateral fornix in turn and then pushed backwards and upwards as far as possible without causing pain. The abdominally located fingers simultaneously press backwards about 5cm medial and parallel to the superior iliac spine (*Fig. 1.5*). The normal oviduct cannot be palpated, and the normal ovary may or may not be felt. If the latter is palpable, it is extremely tender on bimanual pressure.

Rectal examination

A rectal examination, or a recto-abdominal bimanual examination, may replace a vaginal examination in children and in virgin adults, but the examination is less efficient and more painful than the vaginal examination. A rectal examination is a useful adjunct to a vaginal examination, when either the outer parts of the broad ligaments or the uterosacral ligaments require to be palpated. On occasion, a rectovaginal examination, with the index finger in the vagina and the middle finger in the rectum, may help to determine if a lesion is in the bowel or between the rectum and the vagina.

TESTS

Appropriate tests may be required. For example if the woman complains of a vaginal discharge, swabs should be taken to determine the cause (see page 248). Urinary symptoms may require a specimen of mid-stream urine to reach a diagnosis.

Medical practitioners have a crucial role in encouraging sexually active women to have a cervical smear (Pap smear) taken at regular intervals, to detect abnormal cells. At present fewer than one-third the number of women over the age of 40 years, who are at greatest risk of developing cervical carcinoma, have regular Pap smears.

ANCILLARY GYNAECOLOGICAL INVESTIGATIONS
Pelvic ultrasound

The development of pelvic ultrasound scanning enables doctors to identify many disorders in the genital tract with greater accuracy than with clinical examination. Ultrasound is particularly helpful in defining cystic benign and malignant tumours of the internal genital organs. The examination may be made transabdominally through a full bladder, or transvaginally when the bladder is empty.

Colposcopy

The colposcope is a low-powered microscope for inspecting the cervix and vagina in some cases where abnormal cells have been detected in a Pap smear. The cervix and vagina are exposed by introducing a bivalve vaginal speculum. The colposcope is placed in front of the vagina and its focal length is adjusted to examine the suspect part of the lower genital tract (see page 290).

Computed tomography and magnetic resonance imaging

These technologies have a role in assessing the nature and spread of malignant disease of the genital organs, but both are expensive and should only be used when they are likely to confer a real benefit.

Fig. 1.2 Introducing the bivalve speculum. Care should be taken to avoid applying painful pressure on the urethra by inserting the speculum initially obliquely.

Fig. 1.3 The patient in the left lateral position; a Sims speculum has been inserted into the vagina.

Fig. 1.4 Bimanual examination of the uterus. Note that the bladder is empty, the patient having voided just before the pelvic examination. (a) The vaginal fingers push the cervix back and upwards so that the fundus can be reached by the abdominally located fingers; (b) The vaginally located fingers now palpate the anterior surface of the uterus, which is held in position by the abdominally located fingers.

Fig. 1.5 Bimanual palpation of the adnexal area. Note the position of the fingers; normally the ovary cannot be felt. In this case a cystic mass lying in the position of the ovary can be identified.

Laparoscopy

Inspection of the pelvic organs with a laparoscope inserted into the peritoneal cavity through a small subumbilical incision, may give valuable information about the state of the pelvic organs, particularly in cases of infertility, chronic pelvic pain and probable ectopic gestation. Techniques have been developed which enable operations to be conducted through a laparoscope, avoiding long hospital inpatient stay.

Hysterosalpingography

The injection through the cervix of a radiopaque substance and following its progress on a screen as it fills the uterus and Fallopian tubes provides information in cases of infertility.

Hysteroscopy

A small fibre-optic telescope is inserted through the cervix into the uterine cavity, which is inspected. The procedure may help the doctor to reach a diagnosis in cases of menstrual disorders. Endometrial polyps can be removed and the endometrium ablated (see page 224) using this technique.

Endometrial biopsy

This technique is used to obtain a sample of endometrium for histological examination, by introducing a small curette through the cervix without anaesthesia. Endometrial biopsy has a role in the investigation of infertility and in helping to reach a diagnosis in cases of postmenopausal bleeding.

The obstetric patient

Most women consulting a medical practitioner have a good idea that they are pregnant. The woman may have:
• Missed a menstrual period (has amenorrhoea).
• Noticed that her breasts are fuller and may be tender.
• Nausea and perhaps may have vomited.
• Frequency of micturition.
• Purchased a 'Home Pregnancy Test' or have had the test taken by their pharmacist.

The woman visits the doctor to confirm that she is pregnant and either to seek antenatal care from the doctor or to be referred to an obstetrician or to a hospital clinic.

HISTORY

At this first visit the doctor should take a history in the manner described earlier. The information includes more than that described for gynaecological examination. The history of previous pregnancies should be detailed and include information about:
• Spontaneous and induced abortions.
• Complications during pregnancy.
• The gestation period at delivery.
• The method of delivery (spontaneous vaginal birth, forceps, ventouse delivery, caesarean section).
• Complications in the puerperium.

The medical practitioner should enquire about any problems in the current (presumed) pregnancy.

CLINICAL EXAMINATION

Having taken a history the doctor should examine the woman as described earlier. The vaginal examination should include taking a Pap smear if this has not been taken in the previous 12 months. The vaginal examination will usually reveal that the uterus is enlarged. If the woman first attends the doctor between 6 and 10 weeks after her last menstrual period (LMP), the uterus may feel as if it is separate from the cervix. This is because the cervix has softened, and the examiner's fingers seem to meet below the ball-shaped uterus (Hegar's sign) as shown in *Figure 1.6*.

In most cases the doctor will confirm the pregnancy either clinically or by an immunological pregnancy test. The test depends on the fact that human chorionic gonadotrophin (hCG) is secreted into the circulation within 10 days of conception. Using a sensitive monoclonal antibody test, small amounts of the beta fraction of hCG can be detected if the woman is pregnant.

Once the pregnancy has been diagnosed the medical practitioner should ask if any close family member has hypertension or diabetes mellitus, as these may be pointers to the development of the condition in the pregnancy.

A question invariably asked by the patient when the pregnancy has been confirmed is 'When can I expect my baby to be born?'. This can be determined by asking the woman if the length of her menstrual cycle falls into the normal range (22–35 days). The calculation is to add one year and 10 days to the first day of her LMP and then to subtract 3 months. This gives the estimated date of confinement (EDC). Thus if her LMP began on 14 November 1998 she

Fig. 1.6 Hegar's sign.

may expect to give birth on 24 August 1999 (±14 days). Most doctors do not need to do the calculations as obstetric calculation discs are readily available.

The calculation has to be altered if the woman's menstrual cycle is prolonged, or if she was taking oral contraceptives during the cycle before she became pregnant, as ovulation may have been delayed and conception may have occurred up to 14 days later than expected. In these two circumstances, the EDC will be later than calculated, and to obtain greater accuracy of predicting the EDC an ultrasound examination at the 18th to 20th week of pregnancy may be needed. Many obstetricians have an ultrasound of the fetus performed routinely at this time, to firmly establish the gestation and the presence of some fetal abnormalities.

Most women seek to have the pregnancy confirmed in the first 10 weeks of pregnancy. Some women delay until later in the pregnancy. In the second quarter the uterus becomes palpable on abdominal examination (Fig. 1.7) and fetal heart sounds can be heard using an ultrasonic heart detector at this time. The woman feels her fetus moving from about 18 weeks' gestation.

Once pregnancy has been diagnosed further investigations should be made. These are discussed in Chapter 6, Antenatal care.

EVIDENCE OF A PREVIOUS PREGNANCY

In a few cases the woman may deny that she has been pregnant previously but the doctor is suspicious. This suspicion can grow stronger if:
- The breasts show pigmentation of the areolae.
- The abdominal wall has silver-grey longitudinal lines (striae gravidarum).
- On inspection of the vulva, the perineum shows evidence of damage and repair.

However, a firm diagnosis cannot be given as these signs can be produced by other disorders.

PSEUDOCYESIS

Emotional disturbance such as an intense desire to have a baby or fear of losing a lover, may lead some women to believe that they are pregnant, when they are not. The emotions stop the release of gonadotrophic hormones with resulting amenorrhoea. The woman's emotions cause her to complain of the symptoms of pregnancy, often in a bizarre order. The breasts become full and may secrete a cloudy fluid; the abdomen becomes enlarged because of fat or flatus. On superficial examination the woman appears to be pregnant; however, vaginal examination shows the uterus to be normal in size. It may be necessary to have an ultrasound examination to convince the woman that she is not pregnant. Once the absence of pregnancy has been confirmed, the woman should be given sympathetic psychiatric attention.

Medicolegal aspects

In the past few years increasing numbers of patients have been complaining that their diagnosis and treatment has been inadequate and that the doctor has been medically negligent. This trend has been most apparent in the USA and Canada but has spread to the developed countries in Europe, Australasia and South Africa. Obstetricians and gynaecologists are seemingly particularly vulnerable to patients' complaints and the reasons for the increase in litigation appear to be:
1. The obstetric patient's expectation that she will give birth to a perfect baby.
2. The gynaecological patient's expectation that her diagnosis, treatment and operation, if needed, will have a perfect result.

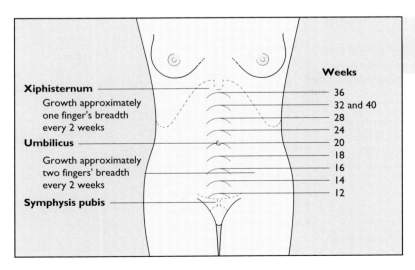

Fig. 1.7 The abdominal markings of uterine growth related to the number of weeks after the last menstrual period.

Weeks

Xiphisternum —— 36
Growth approximately one finger's breadth every 2 weeks —— 32 and 40
—— 28
—— 24
Umbilicus —— 20
—— 18
Growth approximately two fingers' breadth every 2 weeks —— 16
—— 14
—— 12
Symphysis pubis

3. The trend of some lawyers using contingency litigation in medicolegal claims.
4. The large amounts of compensation determined by some judges and juries.

The effect of these issues has forced medical insurance indemnity organisations to raise the annual premiums considerably and has induced many obstetricians to cease to practise obstetrics, confining their practice to an obstetric subspeciality or to gynaecology.

WHAT CAN BE DONE?
The Government
The Government could pass legislation limiting the amount of compensation claimable, and could institute a process whereby a senior specialist advised the judge and jury on contentious medical issues raised by the expert witnesses selected by the barristers for the plaintiff and defendant.

The doctor
The doctor should take the following measures to reduce litigation:

First consultation
The doctor should listen carefully to what the patient says and should seek clarification of the issues. The patient (and her partner if she wishes) should be given ample opportunity to ask questions, which the doctor should answer in clear English, if necessary through an appropriate interpreter. He should outline the treatment he intends to follow, stating the benefits and disadvantages (if any) of his proposal. When possible he should not institute treatment or surgery precipitously, giving the patient time to reflect and ask further questions. He should record the conversations in his notes and date and sign them.

Follow-up visits
At each visit the doctor should follow the procedure outlined above, giving more time for the patient to ask questions to clarify issues which she may find obscure. Again the doctor's notes should be completed meticulously, dated and signed, pathology and ultrasound reports should be seen, evaluated and signed off before they are filed.

Operative procedures in obstetrics and gynaecological surgery
When a consultant or a trainee undertakes an operative procedure, the record of the procedure should be recorded in some detail in the operation notes, preferably by the operating surgeon himself, signed and dated. The alternative is for him to ask his assistant or trainee to complete the notes, which he dictates and signs, immediately after the procedure has been completed. When he visits the patient after childbirth or after an operative procedure he should give her time and opportunity to ask questions, give her clear answers and record and sign his own observations.

Ultimately, a reduction in litigation will occur if the doctor can communicate well with the patient, being sensitive to her concerns and answering her questions without showing any haste or arrogance (*Fig. 1.8*).

Fig. 1.8 Doctor–patient communication

Good communication is essential to patient assessment, treatment and the avoidance of subsequent medicolegal problems.

To achieve this:

- The doctor should listen attentively and with empathy to what the patient is saying.

- He or she should listen more and talk less, only interrupting the patient to clarify a point.

- He or she should avoid being confrontational, condescending, overbearing or judgemental, particularly in sensitive matters such as sexual preferences and practices.

- When responding, the doctor should avoid using medical jargon and answer in simple, clear understandable English and make sure that the patient understands the explanation of the obstetrical, gynaecological, medical or surgical procedures proposed. This may be helped if the doctor provides an appropriate pamphlet.

- The doctor should avoid creating the appearance that he or she wants to conclude the consultation prematurely.

- The doctor should make a follow-up appointment if any doubt exists that the patient has not understood clearly, so that the issues can be discussed further with the woman and, if she wishes, her partner.

CHAPTER 2

Ovulation and the menstrual cycle

The endocrinological changes which take place to transform a female child into an adolescent who menstruates and ovulates and is capable of conceiving a child, begin several years before puberty, but the most marked changes occur in the 2 years before the girl's first menstrual period (menarche).

Psychosomatic disturbances occurring during the menstrual cycle are discussed in Chapter 30, Psychosomatic and physical disorders of the menstrual cycle.

Menarche

The underlying major endocrinological change is that the hypothalamus begins to secrete releasing hormones. These lead to the release into the circulation of adrenal androgens and pituitary human growth hormone (hGH). It is hGH which causes the growth spurt which begins 3–4 years before the menarche, and is maximal in the first 2 years (*Fig. 2.1*). The physical growth slows down as the first menstruation (menarche) approaches. This is because increasing quantities of oestrogen are secreted by the ovaries and feed back negatively, reducing hGH secretion. Shortly after the secretion of hGH starts, the hypothalamus begins to release gonadotrophin-releasing hormone (GnRH) in an episodic

pulsed manner. At first, the pulses are greater in amplitude during sleep, but after 2 years they occur by day and night at about 2-hour intervals. GnRH induces the release of follicle-stimulating hormone (FSH) and luteinizing hormone (LH) from the pituitary gland, which in turn bind to receptors in the ovaries and induce the secretion and release of oestrogen and progesterone into the circulation. The quantity of FSH and LH increases as the girl matures.

Until the age of 8 years, only small quantities of oestrogen are secreted (and less of progesterone). After that age, oestrogen secretion begins to rise, slowly at first, but, after the age of about 11 years, the rise is quite rapid. The FSH levels reach a plateau when the girl is aged about 13 years. LH levels rise more slowly until 1 year before menarche, at which time a rapid rise occurs (*Fig. 2.2*). By this time, the GnRH pulses occur every 90 minutes. These hormonal changes persist until after the age of 40, when changes presaging the menopause begin (see Chapter 43, A woman's middle years: menopause).

It is thought that the rapid rise of LH induces onset of the menarche, but other factors are also involved. These include an increase in the fat:lean ratio of body composition, which in turn is related to good nutrition and the absence of debilitating diseases.

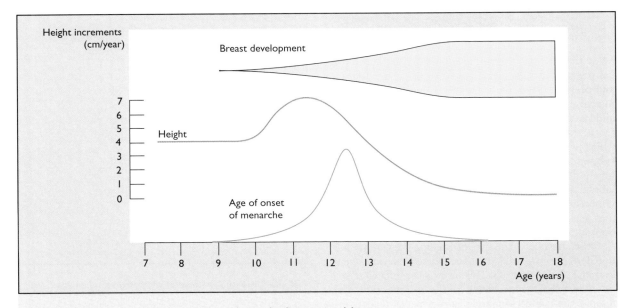

Fig. 2.1 The menarche in relation to growth and breast development in adolescence.

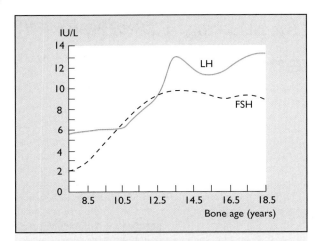

Fig. 2.2 *Pubertal changes in levels of FSH and LH in girls.*

nuclear gene activation, oestradiol is rapidly converted to the relatively inactive oestriol, which is transported to the liver where it is conjugated with glucuronic acid. The conjugate is then excreted, mostly in the urine. This leaves the cell receptors free to bind more oestradiol.

Oestradiol stimulates the growth of the vulva and the vagina after the menarche, the hormone causing proliferation of both the epithelial and muscular layers. This oestrogen also stimulates the formation of more blood vessels which supply the organs. The uterus is particularly stimulated by oestradiol, which increases the vascularity of the organ. Oestradiol causes endometrial proliferation, stimulating the growth of the glands and stroma as well as the growth of the muscular layers of the uterus, so that the uterus grows from its prepubertal size to its adult size in the perimenarchal years (*Fig. 2.3*). The great increase in circulating oestrogen in pregnancy causes the rapid growth of the uterus, and the lack of this hormone after the menopause leads to uterine atrophy.

A century ago, the menarche began at about age 15 years, but it has fallen to the age of 12 and a half years today. This reduction is believed to be due to better childhood nutrition. It is hypothesized that the greater amount of body fat in girls today, permits the greater aromatization of androgens to oestrogens. Rapidly rising levels of oestrogens feed back positively to the hypothalamus and pituitary gland leading to the LH surge, which precedes the menarche.

The menarche may be delayed among women who are of low body weight such as ballet dancers, women who have anorexia nervosa or those who are compulsive exercisers.

Effects of oestrogen and progesterone on body tissues

More than 20 oestrogens have been isolated; the three considered the most important being oestrone, oestradiol and oestriol. Oestrone is a relatively weak oestrogen and interconverts with 17-β oestradiol, which is the most active and the predominant oestrogen in the reproductive years. Oestradiol is rapidly transported in the blood to tissues which have oestrogen-binding receptors. In the blood, 60% is bound to albumen, 37% to sex-hormone-binding globulin and 3% is free. The tissues of the genital tract and the lobular elements of the breasts have the highest concentration of cells containing specific oestrogen-binding receptors and consequently are most affected by circulating oestradiol.

Once attached to the specific binding sites, oestradiol is transferred to the cell's nucleus, where it activates genes, leading to RNA synthesis. This process is regulated to some extent by progesterone, which blocks the formation of new receptors and induces intracellular enzyme production; these enzymes also regulate oestrogen metabolism. Following

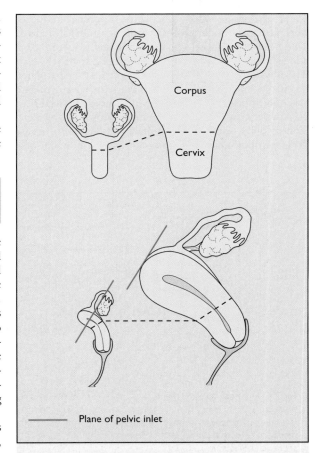

Fig. 2.3 *The prepubertal uterus compared with the adult uterus. Note particularly the change in ratio of the corpus and cervix.*

Progesterone acts on tissues which have oestrogen receptors but only if they are first sensitized by oestrogen. Progesterone hinders the maturation of the vaginal epithelial cells and renders the cervical mucus viscous while also increasing the thickness and succulence of an oestrogen-primed endometrium, preparing it to accept a fertilized egg. Progesterone aids in fat deposition and is thermogenic, raising the body temperature by 0.2–0.5°C.

Menstruation and ovulation

At puberty each ovary contains about 200,000 oogonia surrounded by mantles of theca lutein cells, many of which have developed fluid-filled cavities (antra) to become primary follicles.

From now on until their disappearance at the time of the menopause, and in the absence of pregnancy, severe

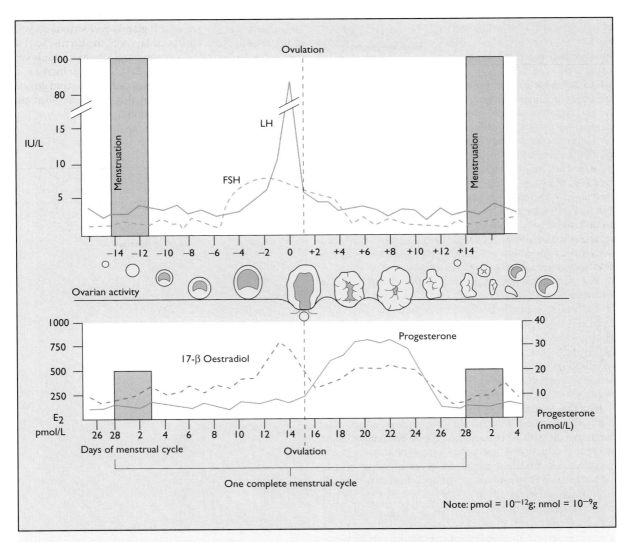

Fig. 2.4 Hormone levels in the normal menstrual cycle – considerable variations are compatible, however, with normal menstrual function. Here, the inter-relationship of ovarian steroids and hypothalamic–pituitary gonadotrophins is shown. After menstruation, rising levels of oestrogen exert a negative feedback, reducing FSH release. Towards midcycle still higher oestrogen levels exert a positive feedback causing a sudden peak release of LH which induces ovulation. An increased release in FSH also occurs. Failure of this sequence will lead to anovulation and irregular cycles. In the luteal phase, LH levels must be sufficiently high to maintain the corpus luteum until the conceptus has implanted and commenced hCG secretion, which then maintains corpus luteum function. If conception fails to occur, the corpus luteum deteriorates after about 7 days, with the resulting falling levels of progesterone and oestrogen. As a consequence menstruation occurs, and FSH levels rise, initiating a new menstrual cycle.

weight loss or of certain other conditions, between 15 and 20 of these follicles are stimulated to grow each month by FSH and LH secreted by the anterior pituitary gland. One (occasionally more) of the follicles grows more rapidly than the others, and, reaching the ovarian surface, causes the release of an ovum. If an ovum is released and pregnancy does not occur, menstruation follows.

The control of this system is complex and reciprocating. The initial stimulus originates in the hypothalamus with the release of GnRH into the hypophyseal portal vessels. As mentioned, GnRH released in a pulsatile manner, reaches the pituitary gland where it stimulates the growth and maturation of gonadotrophs which secrete FSH and LH. FSH acts on 10–20 'selected' primary follicles, by binding on to the theca granulosa cells which surround them. The effect of the rising amounts of FSH is to cause fluid to be secreted into the cavity of the follicles, one of which grows more rapidly than the remainder. Simultaneously the theca granulosa cells which surround the selected follicles secrete increasing amounts of oestradiol, which enters the circulation.

The endocrinological effect of the rising levels of oestradiol is that it exerts a negative feedback on the anterior pituitary and the hypothalamus, with the result that the secretion of FSH falls whilst that of oestradiol rises to a peak (see Fig. 2.4). Some 24 hours later a sudden large surge of LH and a smaller surge of FSH occurs. This positive feedback leads to the release of an ovum from the largest follicle. Ovulation has occurred. (If large amounts of FSH are produced by the anterior pituitary gland, or usually if FSH injections are given, superovulation occurs, seven or more follicles reaching maturity, a technique used in in-vitro fertilization.)

The collapse of the follicle from which the ovum has been released leads to a change in its nature. The theca granulosa cells proliferate, become yellow in colour (luteinized) and are referred to as theca-lutein cells. The collapsed follicle becomes a corpus luteum. The lutein cells of the corpus luteum secrete progesterone as well as oestrogen. Progesterone secretion reaches a plateau about 4 days after ovulation and then rises progressively should the fertilized ovum implant into the endometrium. The trophoblastic cells of the implanted embryo immediately

secrete hCG which maintains the corpus luteum so that the secretion of oestradiol and progesterone continues. On the other hand if pregnancy fails to occur, the theca-lutein cells degenerate and produce less oestradiol and progesterone. This reduces the negative feedback on the gonadotrophs with a rise in the secretion of FSH. The falling circulating levels of oestradiol (Fig. 2.5) and progesterone cause changes in the endometrium (see page 15) which leads to menstruation.

Endometrial cycle

Menstruation is the periodic discharge from the uterus of blood, tissue fluid and endometrial cellular debris, in varying amounts. The quantity of tissue fluid is the greatest variable. This means that some women who complain of heavy periods do not become anaemic as might be expected (see Chapter 29, Disorders of menstruation). The mean blood loss during menstruation is 30ml (range 10–80ml). Menstruation normally occurs at intervals of 22–35 days (counted from day 1 of the menstrual flow to day 1 of the next) and the menstrual discharge lasts from 1 to 8 days.

Fig. 2.6 Endometrium – early proliferative phase. Note that the glands are straight, short and narrow. The surface epithelium is thin.

Fig. 2.5 Plasma oestradiol levels during the menstrual cycle	
	Plasma oestradiol (pg/ml)
• Early follicular phase	40–80
• Mid-follicular phase	60–150
• Late follicular phase	80–300
• Periovulatory peak	300–800
• Early and mid-luteal phase	100–150
• Late luteal phase	80–400

A convenient way to describe the endometrial menstrual cycle is to start just after menstruation ceases and follow the cycle to the next menstruation as it passes through the proliferative and secretory (luteal) phases.

PROLIFERATIVE PHASE

As each area of the endometrium is shed during menstruation, regenerative repairs begin, the endometrial surface being reformed by the metaplasia of stromal cells and by an outgrowth of epithelial cells of the endometrial glands. Within 3 days of menstruation ceasing, the repair of the entire endometrium is complete.

The endometrium, in the early proliferative phase, is thin, the glands few, narrow, straight and lined with cuboidal cells, and the stroma is compact (see *Fig. 2.6*). The early regenerative phase lasts from day 3 of the menstrual cycle to day 7, when proliferation speeds up. The epithelial glands increase in size and grow down perpendicular to the surface. Their cells become columnar with basal nuclei. The stromal cells proliferate, remaining compact and spindle shaped (*Fig. 2.7*). Mitoses are common in glands and stroma. The endometrium is supplied by basal arteries in the myometrium which send off branches at right angles to supply the endometrium. At first, as each artery penetrates the basal endometrium, it is straight but, in the middle and superficial layers, it becomes spiral. The coiling permits the artery to supply the growing endometrium by becoming uncoiled. Each spiral artery supplies a defined area of endometrium.

LUTEAL PHASE

If ovulation occurs, as is usual, except at the extremes of the reproductive years, the endometrium undergoes marked changes. The changes start in the last 2 days of the proliferative phase, but increase dramatically after ovulation. Secretory vacuoles, rich in glycogen, appear in the cells lining the endometrial glycogen. At first the vacuoles are basal and displace the cell's nucleus superficially (*Fig. 2.8*). They rapidly increase in number and the glands become tortuous. By the 6th day after ovulation, the secretory phase is at its peak. The vacuoles have streamed past the nucleus. Some have discharged mucus into the cavity of the gland; others are full of mucus, leading to a saw-toothed appearance (*Fig. 2.9*). The spiral arteries increase in length by uncoiling (*Fig. 2.10*).

In the absence of pregnancy, the secretion of oestrogen and progesterone fall as the corpus luteum ages. The fall

Fig. 2.7 Endometrium – late proliferative phase. The glands have become longer and tortuous, and in a few, early secretory changes may be observed. The stroma remains dense.

Fig. 2.8 Endometrium – early luteal phase. The tortuosity of the glands, and the subnuclear vacuoles, can be seen.

leads to an increase in endometrial free arachidonic acid and endoperoxidases. These enzymes induce stromal cell lysosomes to synthesize and secrete prostaglandins ($PGF_{2\alpha}$ and PGE_2) and prostacyclin. $PGF_{2\alpha}$ is a powerful vasoconstrictor and causes uterine contractions; PGE_2 causes uterine contractions and some vasodilatation; prostacyclin is a vasodilator, causes muscle relaxation and inhibits platelet aggregation. During menstruation the ratio of $PGF_{2\alpha}$ to the other two prostaglandins increases. This change reduces the blood flow through the endometrial capillaries and leads to a shift of fluid from the endometrial tissues into the capillaries, with a resulting decrease in endometrial thickness. This leads to increased coiling of the spiral arteries with a further decrease in blood flow. The area of endometrium supplied by the spiral artery becomes hypoxic, and ischaemic necrosis occurs. The vasoconstriction occurs in different spiral arteries at different times, alternating with vasodilatation. The necrotic area of the endometrium is shed into the uterine cavity accompanied by blood and tissue fluid. Menstruation has begun.

In the past decade molecular biology has identified at least 50 proteins secreted by the endometrium which may be involved in controlling menstruation. For example,

Fig. 2.9 Endometrium – day 6 after ovulation. The glands are now very tortuous with secretion in the lumen and increasing fluid separating the stromal cells. In a fertile cycle day 6 is the day the ovum reaches the uterine cavity.

Fig. 2.10 Endometrial vascular patterns.

endothelin causes marked vasoconstriction of the spiral arteries and consequently reduced blood flow in them. Other proteins promote cell division, which could help in repairing the endometrium.

MENSTRUAL PHASE

During menstruation the superficial and middle layers of the endometrium are shed, the deep basal layer being spared (*Fig. 2.11*). The shedding occurs in an irregular, haphazard manner, some areas being unaffected, others undergoing repair, whilst simultaneously other areas are being shed. The shed endometrium, with tissue fluid and blood, forms a coagulum in the uterine cavity. It is immediately liquefied by fibrinolysins and the liquid, which does not coagulate, is discharged through the cervix by uterine contractions. If the quantity of blood lost in the process is considerable, there may be insufficient fibrinolysins and the woman expels clots through the cervix.

The blood vessels supplying the area beneath the shed endometrium are sealed with a haemostatic plug consisting of aggregated platelets and by fibrin fibres which infiltrate the platelet aggregations to form a stable occlusive plug. In addition vasconstriction occurs. The basal layer of the endometrium regenerates and new epithelium covers the denuded area. When regeneration exceeds necrosis and repair is complete or nearly complete, menstruation ceases and a new menstrual cycle begins.

Cervical cycle

During the follicular phase the glands lining the clefts of the cervical canal proliferate and secrete a thick mucus, which forms a complex mesh in the cervical canal. Just before ovulation, the sudden surge of oestrogen changes the character of the cervical mucus, which becomes thin and forms long strands through which helical channels appear. Following ovulation, progesterone alters the nature of the cervical mucus which again becomes thick and impenetrable.

Vaginal cycle

Cyclic changes occur in the vaginal epithelium, which are dependent on the ratio between oestrogen and progesterone. In the follicular phase, superficial and large intermediate cells predominate. As ovulation approaches, the proportion of superficial cells increases and few leucocytes can be seen (see *Fig. 2.12*). Following ovulation a marked change occurs as progesterone is secreted. The superficial cells are replaced by intermediate cells, and leucocytes increase in number causing the smear to look dirty (see *Fig. 2.13*).

Fig. 2.11 Endometrium – early menstrual phase. The section shows the beginning of focal necrosis in the superficial zone of the endometrium with small areas of haemorrhage into the stroma and infiltration with neutrophils.

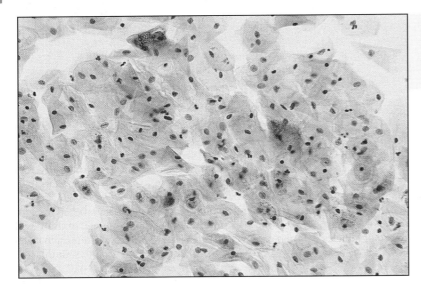

Fig. 2.12 Vaginal exfoliative cytology – late proliferative phase. Note the discrete cells with small nuclei and the clear background.

Fig. 2.13 Vaginal exfoliative cytology – luteal phase. The cells have clumped and the background infiltration of leucocytes has begun.

CHAPTER 3

Conception and placental development

By the time a woman reaches puberty each of her ovaries contains about 200,000 primary oocytes, enclosed in primordial follicles. Each oocyte is separated from the cellular primordial follicle by a clear area, the perivitelline space and a thickened 'shell', the zona pellucida. Each primordial follicle is capable of growing under the influence of follicle-stimulating hormone (FSH) to form a mature follicle. Each month from about the age of 15 years to the age of 45 years, some 20 of the primordial follicles grow through the stage of vesicular follicles to become mature antral follicles.

In contrast to other body cells, the oocyte has only 23 chromosomes. At some stage of its growth the oocyte undergoes a meiotic division of its nucleus and an unequal division of its cytoplasm, to become a secondary oocyte. The smaller cell is expelled into the perivitelline space, and is termed a polar body (*Fig. 3.1b*). The oocyte and its polar body both contain 23 chromosomes.

One of the 20 follicles (occasionally 2 or more, particularly if the ovaries are hyperstimulated in an in-vitro fertilization programme) outstrips the others, developing a large fluid-filled antrum and migrating to bulge through the thickened surface of the ovary (*Fig. 3.2*). With the release of the luteinizing hormone (LH) surge by the pituitary, at mid-cycle, the follicle bursts expelling the ovum, which is gathered into the Fallopian tube by the fimbriae which project from its proximal end. The ovum, surrounded by the perivitelline is contained in a condensed opaque substance 5–10μm thick, called the zona pellucida.

Adherent to the zona pellucida are theca granulosa cells derived from the mature follicle.

Once the ovum has been expelled, the follicle collapses and turns yellow, forming the corpus luteum (see *Fig. 3.2*). The ovum is now ready to be fertilized should it be reached by a sperm.

Of the 60–100 million sperm ejaculated into a woman's vagina at the time she ovulates, several million will negotiate the helical channels in the cervical mucus to reach the uterine cavity. Several hundred sperm will pass through the narrow entrance to the Fallopian tubes, and a few will survive to reach the ovum in the fimbrial end of the Fallopian tube. One sperm may penetrate the zona pellucida of the ovum, its head entering the substance of the ovary. When this occurs a chemical reaction prevents the entry of any other sperm. At the same time the oocyte undergoes another division of its chromosomes and a second polar body is formed (see *Fig. 3.1d*).

Once inside the cytoplasm of the ovum, the sperm's nuclear membrane dissolves, leaving a naked male pronucleus. The ovum, having divided to produce a second polar body, also loses its nuclear membrane. The two naked nuclei approach each other and fuse (see *Fig. 3.1e*). Fertilization and conception have occurred.

Within a few hours of fertilization, the fused nuclei divide to form two cells. (see *Fig. 3.2e*). Once this event has occurred, further cell division proceeds rapidly until, within 3–4 days, a solid mass of cells (the morula) has formed (see *Fig. 3.2g, h*).

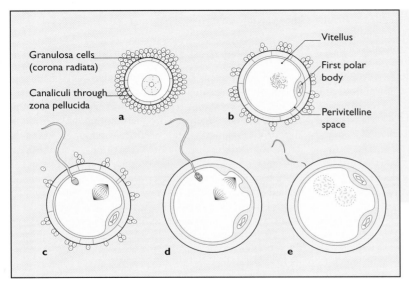

Granulosa cells (corona radiata)

Canaliculi through zona pellucida

Vitellus

First polar body

Perivitelline space

Fig. 3.1 Formation of the ootid and fertilization: (a) primary oocyte; (b) secondary oocyte formed after first maturation division, first polar body pinched off; both oocyte and polar body have undergone reduction division and now each has a haploid number of chromosomes (b, c); (c) second maturation division stimulated by sperm penetrating into vitellus; (d) second polar body forming. The first polar body may also undergo a reduction division; (e) male and female pronuclei formed.

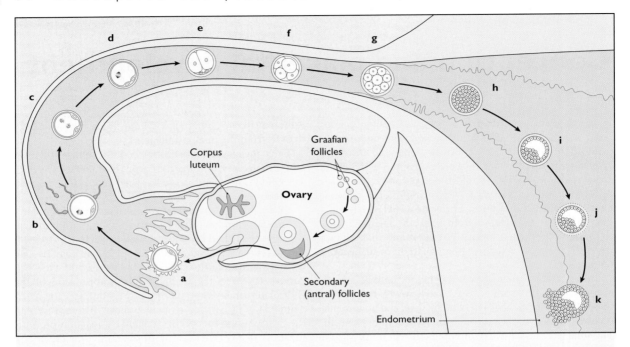

Fig. 3.2 Development of the ovum and its passage through the Fallopian tube into the cavity of the uterus: (a) unsegmented oocyte; (b) fertilization; (c) pronuclei formed; (d) first spindle division; (e) two cell stage; (f) four cell stage; (g) eight cell stage; (h) morula; (i) and (j) blastocyst formation; (k) zona pellucida lost and implantation occurs.

Implantation

The morula is rapidly propelled along the Fallopian tube to enter the uterine cavity. During its passage, fluid passes through canaliculae in the zona pellucida to create a central fluid-filled cavity in the morula, forming a blastocyst (see *Fig. 3.2i*). On reaching the uterine cavity the zona pellucida becomes distended and thin. It soon disappears leaving the surface cells of the blastocyst in contact with the endometrial stroma. About 50% of blastocysts adhere to the endometrium. The surface trophoblastic cells of the adhering blastocyst differentiate into an inner cellular layer, the cytotrophoblast, and an outer syncytiotrophoblast.

Knobs of trophoblast rapidly form, which invade the endometrial stroma in a controlled manner (*Fig. 3.3*). By the 10th day after fertilization, the knobs of trophoblastic tissue have developed a mesodermal core and have pushed deeply into the endometrial stroma (*Fig. 3.4*). The stromal cells react to the invasion by becoming polyhedral in shape and filled with glycogen and lipid, converting into a decidua, which supplies the energy needed by the invading trophoblast. At the same time a number of deep cells at one pole of the blastocyst differentiate to become an inner cell mass, from which the embryo will develop.

By the 9th to 10th day after fertilization, the inner cell mass has differentiated into an ectodermal layer, a mesodermal layer and an endodermal layer in which a small fluid-filled cavity, the amniotic sac, has formed (*Fig. 3.5*).

The further development of the amniotic sac, in which the fetus will float relatively weightless until it is born, is shown in *Figure 3.6*.

The inner cell mass projects into the original blastocystic cavity, the walls of which are formed from cytotrophoblast, and the cavity is filled with mesoderm (*Fig. 3.7*). Quickly, the surface layer of ectoderm divides to surround a fluid-filled cavity in the mesoderm – the yolk sac (see *Fig. 3.6a–c*).

With further development the yolk sac shrinks in size and a second fluid-filled cavity, the amniotic sac, surrounds the growing embryo (see *Fig. 3.6d, e*).

Formation of the placenta

Meanwhile the trophoblastic syncytium has penetrated more deeply into the decidua. As well as invading the endometrial stroma, the syncytium secretes human chorionic gonadotrophin (hCG), which aids in maintaining the function of the corpus luteum to secrete oestrogen and progesterone. In some areas of the decidua the syncytium has surrounded and invaded the walls of the interdecidual portions of the uterine spiral arteries to convert them from relatively thick-walled arteries to thin-walled vessels, permitting a greater flow of blood. These vessels are fragile and break to form small blood lakes, or lacunae. In normal pregnancies the process is complete by 20–22 weeks' gestation. Failure of the process to occur normally may be a factor in the development of pregnancy-induced hypertension.

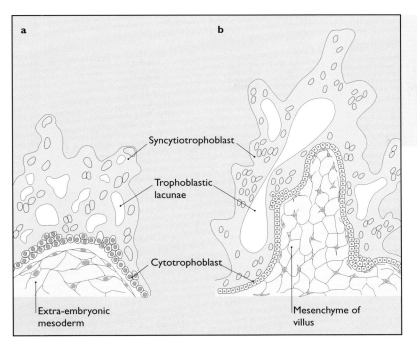

a
b

Syncytiotrophoblast

Trophoblastic
lacunae

Cytotrophoblast

Extra-embryonic
mesoderm

Mesenchyme of
villus

Fig. 3.3 Early stage in development of chorionic villi. (a) Trophoblast projection has occurred with the development of lacunae, and much intermingling with maternal tissue, which for clarity is not shown. No mesoblastic core has yet entered the villus. (b) The mesoblastic core is now developing within the villus.

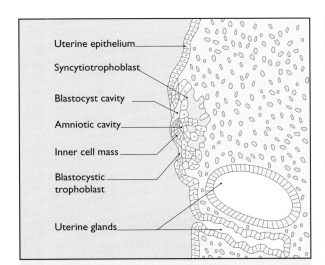

Uterine epithelium

Syncytiotrophoblast

Blastocyst cavity

Amniotic cavity

Inner cell mass

Blastocystic
trophoblast

Uterine glands

Fig. 3.4 Section of a 7½ day human ovum partially implanted in secretory endometrium (× 100). The embryo is represented by the inner cell mass; the blastocyst has collapsed.

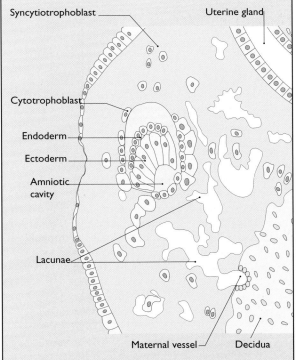

Syncytiotrophoblast

Uterine gland

Cytotrophoblast

Endoderm

Ectoderm

Amniotic
cavity

Lacunae

Maternal vessel

Decidua

Fig. 3.5 A section through the middle of the Hertig–Rock 9-day embryo.

19

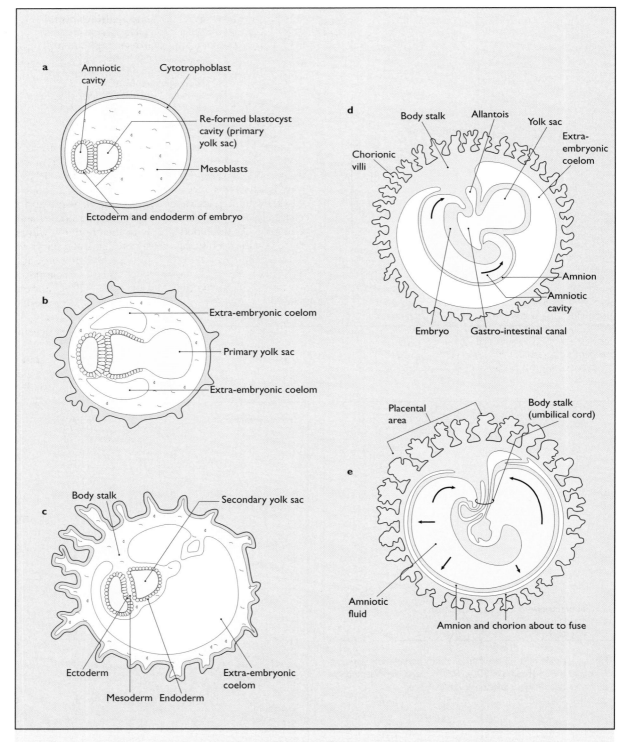

Fig. 3.6 Formation of the amniotic cavity. (a) Formation of the inner cell mass, and the development of the amniotic cavity and the primary yolk sac. (b) Spaces appear in the mesoblast to form the extra-embryonic coelom. (c) The primary yolk sac diminishes in size as the extra-embryonic coelom enlarges. (d) The amniotic sac develops and begins to occupy the extra-embryonic coelom. (e) By the 45th day, the amniotic sac has surrounded the embryo, which is suspended in the protective liquor amnii.

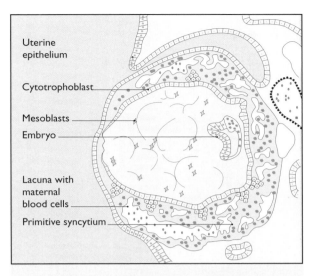

Uterine
epithelium

Cytotrophoblast

Mesoblasts

Embryo

Lacuna with
maternal
blood cells

Primitive syncytium

Fig. 3.7 Section of an 11½ day human embryo (Barnes embryo). The blastocystic trophoblast has differentiated into primitive syncytium and cytotrophoblast. Mesoblast has differentiated from the inner surface of the latter and almost fills the original blastocyst cavity. Lacunae have appeared in the actively growing syncytium, and maternal blood cells have seeped into several of them. Buds appear at intervals on the syncytium; these are the forerunners of chorionic villi.

With further proliferation the knobs of trophoblast become finger-like and blood vessels appear in their mesodermal core. These vessels will soon link up with blood vessels forming in the embryonic mesoderm. The finger-like projections are termed chorionic villi. The chorionic villi proliferate and erode more vessels so that the lacunae increase in size. Blood flows under pressure into them to create large blood-filled spaces in which the proliferating chorionic villi float.

By the 19th day after fertilizaton, the entire conceptus is covered by growing chorionic villi, some attached to the decidua (anchoring villi) but most floating freely in the blood lakes. At this stage further penetration of the decidua ceases, by immunological or chemical mechanisms, and a collagen layer appears through which the spiral arteries and veins pass. As the blood supply to the chorionic villi is greatest on the deep surface of the conceptus, the villi grow profusely here, resembling leafy trees (chorion frondosum). The chorionic villi covering the remainder of the conceptus degenerate, forming the chorion laeve. The chorion frondosum forms the placenta, which is the functional union between the conceptus and the maternal tissues. By the 70th day after fertilization the placental development is complete (Fig. 3.8).

The placenta is composed of about 200 trunks, some large, some of medium size but most small, which divide into limbs, branches and twigs, covered with chorionic villi.

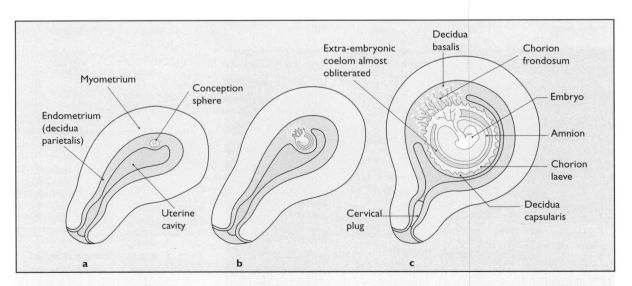

Fig. 3.8 The relationship of the chorionic sac, amnion and developing embryo to the endometrium and uterine cavity at successive stages in early pregnancy. (a) 3 weeks, (b) 5 weeks and (c) 10 weeks after the last menstrual period.

Each of the main trunks forms a cotyledon, 10 being large, 40 medium and the rest small and of little functional significance.

As the blood lakes coalesce, a large blood-filled space is created in which the villi covering each fetal cotyledon float, moved by the motion of the blood. The roof of the space is formed by chorion (the chorionic plate) and its base by trophoblast and decidua (the decidual plate). Septa of varying heights and sizes grow from the decidual plate to separate each fetal cotyledon, each forming an intervillous space. Each intervillous space is supplied by a number of separate arteries, which enter the space at the base of the septa. During maternal systole, arterial blood spurts into the space, like a fountain, at a pressure of 80mmHg. The pressure of the blood pushes the villi aside and the blood hits the chorionic plate and then flows laterally and down-wards, bathing the villi, to escape slowly through the veins in the decidual plate (Figs 3.9 and 3.10).

It has been estimated that the maternal blood flow through the placenta increases from 300ml per minute at 20 weeks' gestation to 600ml per minute at 40 weeks. The total surface area of the villi has been estimated to be 11m², and the placenta at 40 weeks weighs one-seventh of the weight of the baby.

Each villus has a complex anastomosis of capillaries (Fig. 3.10), so there is ample opportunity for exchange of gases and nutrients. The exchange is enhanced by the vascular resistance in the vessels of the chorionic villi (Fig. 3.11).

The increasing blood flow as pregnancy advances compensates for ageing changes which occur in the placenta, and for the development of placental infarcts.

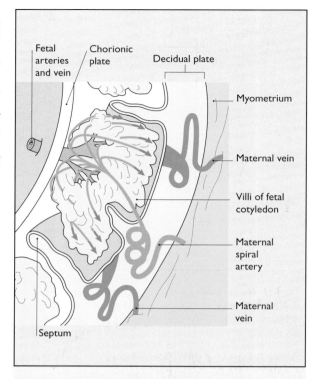

Fig. 3.9 An intervillous space. A fetal cotyledon can be seen, in which the fountain effect of the maternal arterial blood is demonstrated. The blood cascades over the tree-like villi to escape through the maternal veins.

Fig. 3.10 Cast of placental vasculature showing the branching of the vessels.

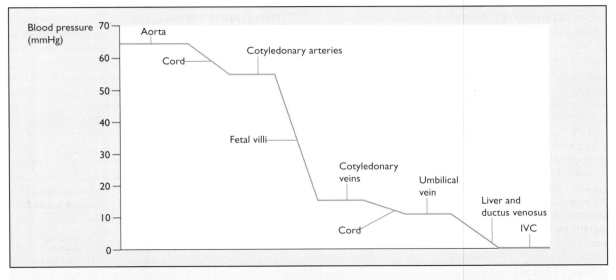

Fig. 3.11 *The fall in blood pressure from the aorta through the umbilical circulation and liver to the inferior vena cava (IVC) in the mature fetal lamb.*

Function of the placenta

The placenta acts for the fetus as:
- An organ of respiration.
- An organ of nutrient transfer and excretion.
- An organ of hormone synthesis.

It might act as an immunological barrier protecting the fetus (formed from paternal as well as maternal genes) from rejection by the mother's immune system.

TRANSPORT MECHANISMS THROUGH THE PLACENTA

Transport of substances through the placenta takes place by:
- Passive transport   simple diffusion
                                    facilitated diffusion
- Active transport   enzymatic reaction
                                    pinocytosis

These mechanisms require the expenditure of energy and the rate of placental metabolism has been calculated as comparable to that of the liver or kidney. The transfer of substances is shown in *Figure 3.12*.

RESPIRATORY FUNCTIONS

The extensive vasculature in the villi and the relatively slow passage of maternal blood through the intervillous space permits a good exchange of oxygen and carbon dioxide between the fetal and the maternal blood by passive diffusion. The exchange is further enhanced by the maternal blood entering the intervillous space having a 90–100% saturation and a PO_2 of 90–100mmHg. After the metabolic needs of the placenta have been met, the fetal erythrocytes take up the oxygen, which is 70% saturated and has a PO_2 of 30–40mmHg, sufficient to meet all fetal needs. Carbon dioxide, like oxygen, passively diffuses across the placenta (*Fig. 3.13*).

Hydrogen ions, bicarbonate and lactic acid diffuse across the placenta, the acid–base status of mother and fetus thus being closely related. As the transfer takes place slowly, the fetus is able to buffer any additional acidity from its reserves, unless maternal acidosis is aggravated by dehydration or ketoacidosis, as may occur in late labour, when fetal acidosis may result.

The efficiency of these exchanges depends on a good maternal blood supply to the spiral arteries and a well-functioning placenta. Should the maternal blood supply to the arteries be reduced, as may occur in severe hypertensive states (see Chapter 15, Hypertensive diseases in pregnancy), placental ageing (see Chapter 20, Variations in the duration of pregnancy), uterine hyperactivity or cord compression (see Chapter 21, The at-risk fetus), fetal ketoacidosis may occur independently of maternal acidosis.

NUTRIENT TRANSFER

Most nutrients are transferred from mother to fetus by active transfer methods, involving enzyme processes. Complex nutrients are broken down into simple components before transfer and are reconstituted in the fetal chorionic villi. Glucose is particularly important as it is the major source of energy for the growing fetus, supplying over 90% of its requirements (10% deriving from amino acids). The quantity of glucose transferred increases after the 30th gestational week. Towards the end of pregnancy about 10g of glucose per kilogram weight is retained daily and the excess over metabolic requirements is converted into glycogen and fat. The glycogen is stored in the liver and the fat is deposited around the heart and behind the scapula. In the last quarter of pregnancy, 2g of fat are synthesized daily, and thus by 40 weeks' gestation, 15% of the fetal body weight is fat. This provides an energy store of 21,000kJ and provides for the metabolic functions and the regulation of body temperature in the days after birth. In preterm and dysmature babies, the energy stores are lower, which may cause problems (see Chapter 20, Variations in the duration of pregnancy).

Oddly, lipids, as free fatty acids, are poorly transferred. Those transferred are resynthesized into phospho- and other lipids and are stored in fetal adipose stores until the 30th gestational week. After this time the fetal liver becomes capable of synthesizing lipids and now takes over.

DRUG TRANSFER

The transfer of drugs through the placenta is no different from that of nutrients and all pass through to some extent. The rate is governed by the solubility of the ionized molecules in fat and the thickness of the trophoblast. In the second half of pregnancy the trophoblast becomes thinner, whilst the placental area increases in size; drugs therefore pass through more rapidly.

Illegal drugs (narcotics, cocaine and marijuana) taken by the mother pass through the placenta and may affect fetal development. The extent of their effect is difficult to determine as most drug abusers also smoke and drink alcohol. The fetus tends to be growth restricted, may have congenital abnormality, and is likely to be born preterm and, if the mother takes narcotics, the infant may have withdrawal symptoms.

HORMONE SYNTHESIS

The placenta synthesizes a number of hormones, the function of which, in many cases, is not understood. The main hormones produced are human chorionic gonadotrophin, human placental lactogen, oestrogen and progesterone.

Human chorionic gonadotrophin

Human chorionic gonadotrophin is synthesized from the early days of placentation. Its blood level reaches a peak between the 60th and 80th days of pregnancy when 500,000–1,000,000IU of hCG are secreted each day. The amount secreted then falls to between 80,000 and 120,000IU a day, a level which is maintained to term (Fig 3.14). The peak is higher and lasts longer in multiple pregnancy and in gestational trophoblastic disease. After childbirth the level falls rapidly. Initially the function of hCG is to maintain the corpus luteum's secretion of progesterone and oestrogen. Once the placenta takes over this function, the level of hCG declines. Human chorionic gonadotrophin may also regulate oestrogen production by the placenta and suppress maternal immunological reactions directed against the fetus.

Oestrogen

In pregnancy the main source of oestrogen is the placenta. The synthesis of oestrogen requires the intervention of the fetus, as the placenta lacks specific enzymes (C17, 20-desmolase and 16-hydroxylase) which are required in the synthesis of oestrogen from acetate and cholesterol. Of the three classic oestrogens, oestriol (E_3), oestradiol (E_2) and oestrone (E_1), the placenta produces more oestriol and retains it selectively. The result is that compared to a non-pregnant circulating E_3:E_2:E_1 ratio of 3:2:1, in pregnancy the ratio of E_3:E_2:E_1 is 30:2:1. This

Maternal blood	Intervillous space	Placental transfer methods		
		Passive	**Active**	**Pinocytosis**
H_2O, O_2, CO_2, urea, Na, K	⟶	+		
Glucose	Facilitated by carrier molecule		+	
Polysaccharides	Mono- and disaccharides		+	
Protein ⟶	Amino acids		+	
Fat ⟶	Free fatty acids		+	
Vitamin A ⟶	Carotene	+		
Vitamin B complex, vitamin C	⟶		+	
Iron, phosphorus	⟶		+	
Antibodies	Only IgG	+		+
Erythrocytes	⟶	±		+

Fig. 3.12 Transfer of substances through the placenta

means that over 90% of the oestrogen secreted in pregnancy is oestriol and the level rises progressively throughout pregnancy (*Fig. 3.14*).

Actions of oestrogen

At the cellular level, oestrogen, mainly in the form of oestradiol, enhances RNA and protein synthesis. Oestrogen alters the polymerization of acid mucopolysaccharides, which has the effect of increasing the hygroscopic properties and reducing the adherence of collagen fibres in connective tissue. This effect is most marked in the cervix, which becomes swollen and soft in pregnancy. Oestrogen also aids the growth of uterine muscle both by its enzymatic action on the muscle fibres and by increasing the blood flow.

In the breast, oestrogen increases the size and mobility of the nipple and causes duct and alveolar development. It may also play a part in causing water retention in pregnancy.

Progesterone

In pregnancy, progesterone is secreted initially by the corpus luteum but, by the 35th gestational day, the placental cytotrophoblast takes over all significant production from maternally supplied precursors, mainly cholesterol. At this stage of pregnancy the plasma progesterone level is 50ng/ml. From now on the level rises in a linear manner to reach 150ng/ml by term (see *Fig. 3.14*).

Actions of progesterone

In pregnancy the main action of progesterone is to cause muscle relaxation and, because the uterus has a large number of progesterone receptors, its effect is most marked on the myometrium. Progesterone also relaxes the lower oesophageal sphincter, the stomach muscles, the intestines and the ureters. These effects account for some minor disturbances of pregnancy, for example, heartburn, delay in stomach emptying, ureteric dilatation and reduced peristaltic activity leading to constipation.

Progesterone regulates the storage of body fat to some extent and is hyperthermic, leading to a rise in body temperature of 0.5–1.0°C. It may have a hypnotic effect on brain cells and may be responsible for the placidity experienced by many pregnant women. Progesterone is implicated in the hyperventilation some women experience.

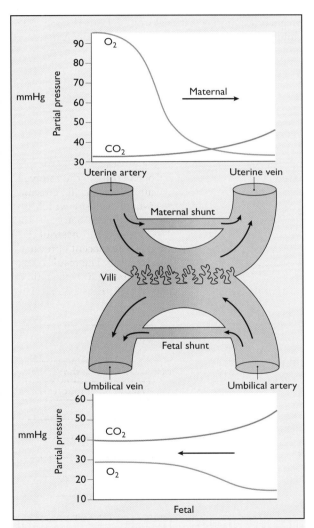

Fig. 3.13 *A schematic representation of placental gas exchange. It can be seen that fetal blood has a much lower partial pressure of oxygen than adult blood; the fetus in utero has been described as living in conditions of oxygenation resembling those at the top of Mount Everest.*

Fig. 3.14 *Oestriol, progesterone, hCG and hPL (human placental lactogen) plasma levels in pregnancy.*

Protein hormones

The placenta secretes a number of pregnancy specific hormones, of which human placental lactogen (hPL), or human chorionic somatomammmotropin is the best understood. Its secretion is the reverse of that of hCG: when hCG falls from its peak, hPL continues to rise (see *Fig. 3.14*). The most important pregnancy-preserving function of hPL is to mobilize free fatty acids from maternal body stores. This lipolytic effect reduces utilization of maternal glucose, which is then diverted for fetal energy needs. Human placental lactogen also stimulates insulin secretion, but inhibits its effects at peripheral sites, and aids in the transfer of amino acids to the fetus.

Immunology of the trophoblast

The fetus is an allograft, but paradoxically is not rejected by the maternal immune system. The explanation for this is unclear. One hypothesis is that the trophoblast secretes antigens which bind to sites on the trophoblast. Bound to these sites it induces the production of fetal immuno-suppressor cells. A further mechanism may be that hCG partially blocks maternal immunological responses. These mechanisms prevent the 'foreign' cells of the conceptus from being recognized and rejected.

CHAPTER 4

Embryo and fetus

The embryo develops rapidly once implantation has occurred. A neural primitive streak develops in the 2nd week after fertilization; during the 3rd week the fetal heart develops and links up with a primitive vascular system; during the 4th week the gut has formed; and by the 6th week a urogenital sinus has formed.

By the 7th week after fertilization, most of the organs have formed and the embryo becomes a fetus. The early growth of the fetus is shown in *Figure 4.1*.

Nutrition

Fetal growth is determined by many factors, both genetic and environmental. Of the latter, adequate placental perfusion and placental function are crucial. Maternal nutrition is not a limiting factor except in cases of extreme starvation, although chronic undernutrition may be associated with anaemia and may lead to a low-birth-weight baby.

The fetus, insulated in its protective amniotic sac and relatively weightless, has most of the energy supplied to it directed to growth. The energy is derived mainly from glucose. Only small amounts of lipids, as free fatty acids, cross the placenta until the fourth quarter of pregnancy. Any excess carbohydrate, after the growth and metabolic energy needs of the fetus have been met, is converted into lipids, and this conversion increases as term approaches.

From the 30th gestational week the fetal liver becomes increasingly efficient and converts glucose into glycogen, which is stored in the fetal heart muscle, the skeletal muscle and the placenta. Should fetal hypoxia occur the

Period of gestation (weeks from the 1st day of the last period)	Period of gestation (weeks from fertilizaton)	Length of fetus (crown to rump [cm])	Characteristics
8	6	2.3	Nose, external ears, fingers and toes are identifiable but featureless, head is flexed on the thorax
12	10	6.0	External ears show main features, eyelids fused, neck has formed, external genitals formed but undifferentiated
16	14	12.0	External genitals can be differentiated, skin transparent red
20	18	15.0	Skin becoming opaque, fine hair (lanugo) covers body
24	22	21.0	Eyelids separated, eyebrows, eyelashes and fingernails present, skin wrinkled due to lack of subcutaneous fat
28	26	25.0	Eyes open, scalp hair growing

Fig. 4.1 *Characteristics indicating maturity of the fetus*

fetus is able to obtain energy from the heart muscle and placenta for anaerobic glycolysis (see Chapter 21, The at-risk fetus).

Free fatty acids are formed and stored in brown and white adipose tissue. Brown fat is deposited around the fetal neck and behind the scapulae and the sternum and around the kidneys. It is metabolized to provide energy to maintain the infant's body temperature after birth. White adipose tissue forms the subcutaneous cover of the body of a term fetus, but in preterm babies the layer may be thin. It acts as an insulator and as a lipid store.

The fat stores of an 800g fetus (24–26 weeks' gestation) constitute 1% of its body weight; by the 35th week fat constitutes 15% of fetal body weight.

As the placenta clears the blood of bilirubin and other metabolic products which require a transferase activity, the fetal (and neonatal) liver is deficient in certain transferases. The result is that unless the deficiencies are corrected in the early neonatal period, bilirubin may accumulate in the neonate's blood, which is of some consequence in haemolytic disease of the newborn (see page 133).

Amino acids cross the placenta by active transfer and are converted into protein. Protein synthesis exceeds protein breakdown, and the fetus uses some of the breakdown amino acids for resynthesis.

The fetus also synthesizes a specific protein, alphafetoprotein (AFP) in its liver. The peak of AFP is reached between the 12th and 16th gestational week, after which a decline occurs to term. The protein is secreted in the fetal urine and swallowed by the fetus to be degraded in its gut. If the fetus is unable to swallow, as in cases of anencephaly, the level of AFP in the amniotic fluid rises.

Cardiovascular system

The circulatory pattern of the fetus is shown in *Figure 4.2*. It should be noted that over 50% of the cardiac output passes through the umbilical arteries to perfuse the placenta. The cardiac output increases to term, at which time about 200ml/kg per minute is usual. The heart rate lies between 110 and 150bpm to maintain this output. The fetal blood pressure also increases through the pregnancy and, after the 36th week, has a mean of 75mmHg systolic, 55mmHg diastolic.

The red cell count, the haemoglobin level and the packed cell volume increase as pregnancy advances. Most of the erythrocytes contain fetal haemoglobin (HbF). At 15 weeks' gestation all the cells contain HbF; by the 36th week 70% of the erythrocytes contain HbF, and 30% adult haemoglobin, but there are wide variations. Cells containing HbF are able to absorb more oxygen at a given PO_2. They are more resistant to haemolysis but less resistant to trauma than cells containing adult haemoglobin.

Lungs

In the early embryo the lungs are made up of epithelial tubes surrounded by mesoderm. With further development the epithelium becomes folded and glandular to form primitive alveoli. By the 22nd gestational week a capillary system has developed and the lungs are capable of gas exchange. By term, three or four generations of alveoli have developed and been replaced. Their epithelium, which has a cuboidal appearance, becomes flattened with the first breath. By the 24th week, fluid fills the alveoli and the passages. By this stage the lungs begin to secrete a surface-active lipoprotein, surfactant, which facilitates lung expansion at birth and helps the air-containing lung to maintain its normal volume. However, until the 35th week the amount of surfactant may be insufficient for some babies to expand their lungs after birth and hyaline membrane disease may develop.

The fetus makes respiratory movements (breathing) from early in pregnancy. At first, they are sporadic, but by mid-pregnancy the movements become regular and increase in frequency as the pregnancy advances. Respiratory activity results in the inspiration of amniotic fluid into the bronchioles but no further, as the fluid secreted into the alveoli is under higher pressure. Episodes of hypoxia in late pregnancy or during the birth may stimulate gasping and amniotic fluid, often meconium-contaminated, is inhaled deeper into the lungs.

Gastrointestinal tract

In the uterus the intestinal tract is relatively quiet. Some of the swallowed amniotic fluid, and the cellular material it contains, enters the gut, where it is acted upon by the enzymes and bacteria to produce meconium. The meconium remains in the gut unless an episode of severe hypoxia leads to contractions of the gut, at which time the meconium is expelled to mix with the amniotic fluid.

Renal system

The fetal kidney develops from the metanephros, and new glomeruli continue to be formed until the 36th gestational week. Urine is secreted and expelled into the amniotic fluid from the 16th week and probably earlier. Its rate of flow increases as term approaches.

Immune system

In early pregnancy the fetus has a poor capacity to produce antibodies in response to invasion by maternal antigens or by bacteria. From the 20th week (perhaps earlier) it becomes able to mount an immune response to a challenge.

The fetal response is supplemented by the transfer of maternal antibody molecules (provided that they are not too large in size) to the fetus which provide it with passive protection which may persist for some weeks after birth.

Muscular system

Almost weightless in its amniotic capsule, the fetus makes movements from an early age. As the pregnancy advances the fetal movements become stronger, and occur more often. Bouts of activity are followed by periods when the fetus seems to be sleeping. These movements strengthen the fetal muscles and a count of them gives an indication of fetal well-being (see page 156).

Endocrine activity

As noted earlier, the fetus is involved in the production of oestrogen. In addition, the fetus produces thyroid-stimulating hormone (TSH) from about the 14th week of pregnancy, which leads to the release of T_3 and T_4. The quantity of T_3 is secreted. Immediately after birth a surge of TSH is released, causing a surge in T_3 and T_4 and a fall in reverse T_3.

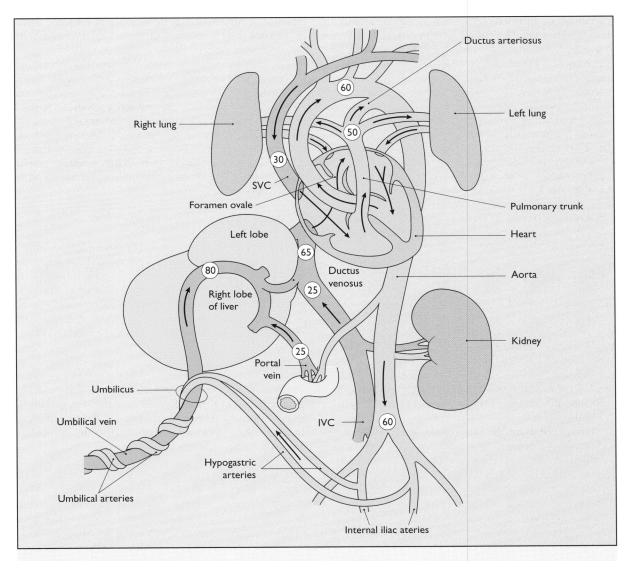

Fig. 4.2 Normal circulation in the fetus in utero. IVC, inferior vena cava; SVC, superior vena cava. The figures give the approximate oxygen saturation of the blood at given points in the circulatory system.

CHAPTER 5

Physiological and anatomical changes in pregnancy

Hormonal changes

Most of the anatomical changes which occur in pregnancy are due to the hormones secreted by the placenta. These hormones and their effects on the woman's body are described in Chapter 3, Conception and placental development. In addition, other endocrine glands synthesize hormones, in different quantities during pregnancy compared with the non-pregnant state. These changes are briefly described below.

PITUITARY GLAND

In pregnancy the secretion of follicle-stimulating hormone (FSH) and luteinizing hormone (LH) falls to low levels, whilst the secretion of adrenocorticotrophic hormone (ACTH), thyrotrophin, melanocyte hormone and prolactin increases. Prolactin levels, for example, increase to the 30th gestational week and then more slowly to term. Prolactin may be a factor in the fall of FSH and LH to very low levels by the 8th week of pregnancy.

ADRENAL GLAND

Total corticosteroids increase progressively to term. This could account, to some extent, for a pregnant woman's tendency to develop abdominal striae, glycosuria, and hypertension.

THYROID GLAND

The thyroid gland enlarges during pregnancy, occasionally to twice its normal size. This enlargement is mainly due to colloid deposition caused by a lower plasma level of iodine, consequent on the increased ability of the kidneys to excrete during pregnancy. Oestrogen stimulates an increased secretion of thyroxin-binding globulin. In consequence both T_3 and T_4 levels rise. The raised levels do not indicate hyperthyroidism as both the thyroid-stimulating hormone (TSH) and the free thyroxin levels are in the normal range. When tests are made to determine thyroid function these changes must be taken into account.

Genital tract changes

UTERUS

The effect of the hormonal stimulation is most marked upon the tissues of the genital tract, and the uterine muscle fibres grow to 15 times their prepregnant length during pregnancy, whilst uterine weight increases from 50g before pregnancy to 950g at term (*Fig. 5.1*). In the early weeks of pregnancy the growth is by hyperplasia, and more particularly by hypertrophy of the muscle fibres, with the result that the uterus becomes a thick-walled spherical organ. From the 20th week, growth almost ceases and the uterus expands by distension, the stretching of the muscle fibres being due to the mechanical effect of the growing

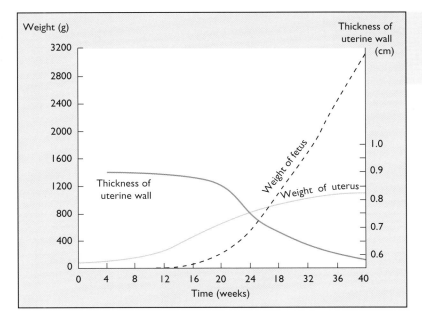

Fig. 5.1 Relation of the weight of the uterus and the thickness of the uterine wall to the weight of the fetus at varying times in normal pregnancy.

fetus. With distension the wall of the uterus becomes thinner and the shape cylindrical (*Fig. 5.2*). The uterine blood vessels also undergo hypertrophy and become increasingly coiled in the first half of pregnancy, but no further growth occurs after this, and the additional length required to match the continuing uterine distension is obtained by uncoiling the vessels.

The uterus is derived from the two Müllerian ducts and the myometrium is made up of a thin external, largely longitudinal, layer; a thin inner, largely circular layer; and a thick, intricately interlaced middle layer, which comprises two spiral systems of interdigitating muscles derived from the two Müllerian ducts. The proportion of muscle to connective tissue is greatest in the fundal area and diminishes as the lower segment of the uterus and cervix is approached, the lower half of the cervix having no more than 10% of muscle tissue.

The effect of the uterine distension is to stretch both interdigitating spiral systems, and to increase the angle of crossing of the fibres, in the thinner lower segment area where the fibres cross at an angle of about 160° and are less stretched. Incision of the myometrium in this zone is anatomically more suitable, and experience of lower segment caesarean section confirms that healing is better (*Fig. 5.3*).

The lower uterine segment is that part of the lower uterus and upper cervix lying between the line of attachment of the peritoneum of the uterovesical pouch superiorly and the histological internal os inferiorly. It is that part of the uterus where the proportion of muscle diminishes, this muscle being replaced increasingly by connective tissue (mainly collagen fibres), which forms 90% of the cervical tissues (*Fig. 5.4*). Because of this the lower uterine segment becomes stretched in late pregnancy as the thickly muscled fundus draws it up from the relatively fixed cervix.

Fig. 5.2 Enlargement of the uterus in normal pregnancy, drawn from radiographs.

Fig. 5.3 Representation of the obliquity of decussation and interweaving of myometrial fibres. The obtuse angle of decussation in the lower segment can be seen.

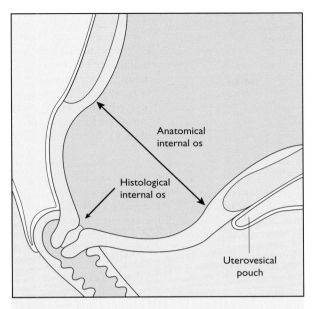

Fig. 5.4 *The lower uterine segment in late pregnancy (see also Fig. 7.8).*

CERVIX

The cervix becomes softer and swollen in pregnancy with the result that the columnar epithelium lining the cervical canal becomes exposed to the vaginal secretions. This change in the cervix is due to oestradiol, which increases the hygroscopic properties of the cervical connective tissue and loosens the acid mucopolysaccharides (glycosaminoglycans) of the collagen-binding ground substance.

Prostaglandins act on the collagen fibres, especially in the last weeks of pregnancy. At the same time, collagenase is released from leucocytes, which also helps in breaking down collagen. The cervix becomes softer and more easily dilatable, the so-called ripening of the cervix. In this way the cervix is more easily able to dilate in labour.

VAGINA

The vaginal mucosa becomes thicker, the vaginal muscle hypertrophies and there is an alteration in the composition of the surrounding connective tissue, with the result that the vagina dilates more easily to accommodate the fetus in parturition. The changes, initiated by oestrogen, occur early in pregnancy and there is an increased desquamation of the superficial vaginal mucosal cells with increased vaginal discharge in pregnancy. Should pathogens, whether bacterial, fungal (such as candida) or parasitic (such as trichomonads) enter the vagina they can more easily establish themselves and, consequently, vaginitis is more frequently found in pregnancy.

Cardiovascular system

The changes which occur during pregnancy to the blood volume, the plasma volume, and the red cell mass are shown in *Figures 5.5* and *5.6*. The plasma volume increases to fill the additional intravascular space created by the placenta and the blood vessels. The red cell mass increases to meet the increased demand for oxygen. Because the increase in the red cell mass is proportionately less than the increase in the plasma volume, the concentration of the erythrocytes in the blood falls with a reduction in the haemoglobin concentration. Although the haemoglobin concentration falls to about 120g/L at the 32nd week, the woman has a larger total haemoglobin than when not pregnant. Concurrently the number of white blood cells increases (to about 10,500 per ml) as does the blood platelet count.

CARDIOVASCULAR DYNAMICS

To deal with the increased blood volume and the additional demand for oxygen, the cardiac output increases by 30–50% in pregnancy (*Fig. 5.7*). Most of the increased cardiac output is due to an increased stroke volume, but the heart rate increases by about 15%. The increased cardiac output is balanced by a decrease in the peripheral resistance (*Fig. 5.8*). For these reasons the woman's blood pressure is altered only minimally in the first three-quarters of pregnancy, unless pregnancy-induced hypertension occurs. After the 30th week of pregnancy, there is a tendency for the blood pressure to rise.

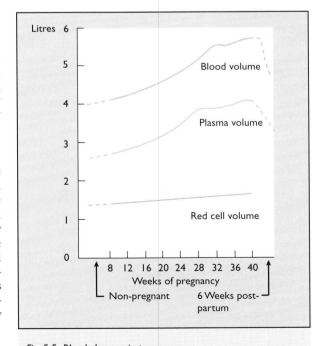

Fig. 5.5 *Blood changes in pregnancy.*

	Non-pregnant	Weeks of pregnancy		
		20	30	40
Plasma volume (ml)	2600	3150	3750	3850
Red cell mass (ml)	1400	1450	1550	1650
Total blood volume (ml)	4000	4600	5300	5500
Body haematocrit (%)	35.0	32.0	29.0	30.0
Venous haematocrit (%)	39.8	36.4	33.0	34.1

Fig. 5.6 Plasma volume, red cell volume, total blood volume and haematocrit in pregnancy

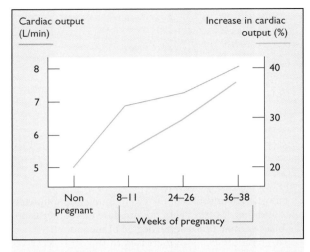

Fig. 5.7 Cardiac output in pregnancy.

In common with other blood vessels, the veins of the legs become distended. The leg veins are affected particularly in late pregnancy because of the obstruction to venous return caused by the higher pressure of the venous blood returning from the uterus and the mechanical pressure of the uterus on the vena cava. This may lead to varicosities in the leg veins (and occasionally the vulval veins) of susceptible women.

REGIONAL DISTRIBUTION OF THE BLOOD

The uterus receives the greatest proportion of the blood flow, which is vital to perfuse the placenta properly. Renal blood and plasma flow increase to 400ml per minute above non-pregnant levels by the 16th week of pregnancy and remain at this high level to term. Blood flow through the capillaries of the skin and mucous membranes increases, reaching a maximum of 500ml per minute by the 36th week. The increased skin blood flow is associated with peripheral vasodilatation. This is the reason why pregnant women 'feel the heat', sweat easily and often profusely and may complain of nasal congestion.

Respiratory system changes

Breathing remains diaphragmatic during pregnancy, but because of the restricted movement of the diaphragm after the 30th week, pregnant women breathe more deeply, increasing tidal volume and ventilation rate, thus permitting an increased mixing of gases and an increased oxygen consumption of 20%. It is thought that this effect is due to the increased secretion of progesterone. It may lead to overbreathing and a lower arterial PO_2. In late pregnancy the lower rib cage flares out to some extent and may not return to its prepregnancy state, causing some concern to figure-conscious women.

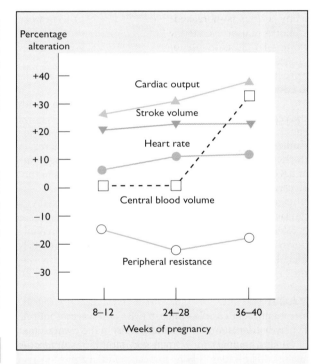

Fig. 5.8 Cardiovascular dynamics: percentage alterations over non-pregnant levels occurring in pregnancy.

Alimentary system changes

In the mouth, the gums may become 'spongy', probably induced by intracellular fluid retention, a possible progesterone effect. The lower oesophageal sphincter is relaxed, which may permit regurgitation of gastric contents and cause heartburn. Gastric secretion is reduced and food remains longer in the stomach. The intestinal musculature is relaxed, with lower motility, which permits a greater absorption of nutrients, but may lead to constipation.

Renal system changes

The smooth muscle of the renal pelvis and ureters relaxes, causing their dilatation. This increases the capacity of the renal pelvis and ureters from 12ml to 75ml and increases the chance of urinary stasis. The bladder musculature relaxes, which also encourages urinary stasis. In consequence, urinary tract infection is more common in pregnancy. The muscles of the internal urethral sphincter relax and this, together with the pressure of the uterus on the bladder, may cause some degree of incontinence.

The renal blood flow increases to the 16th week of pregnancy and then levels off. The glomerular filtration rate increases by 60% in early pregnancy and remains at the new level until the last 4 weeks of pregnancy when it falls. As tubular re-absorption is unaltered, the clearance of many solutes is increased. Up to 300mg of protein per 24 hours may be excreted, which is normal. The increased glomerular filtration rate together with natruretic effect of progesterone would cause an increased loss of sodium were it not for increased production of renal renin and, in consequence, angiotensin.

Immune system changes

Human chorionic gonadotrophin can reduce the immune response of pregnant women. In addition, serum levels of IgG, IgA and IgM decrease from the 10th week of pregnancy, reaching their lowest level at the 30th week and remaining at this level to term. These changes may account for the anecdotal increase in the risk of infection among pregnant women.

Weight gain in pregnancy

The better absorption of nutrients from the gut, the reduction of muscle tone and a reduction in thyroid activity produces a quiescence in the maternal metabolism. The body adapts to preserve and nourish the growing fetus.

During pregnancy a woman inevitably gains weight. A healthy person may expect to gain 12.5kg (range 9–15kg) in pregnancy, of which 9kg is gained in the last 20 weeks. The 'ideal' weight gain is only a guide and an allowance should be made for individual variations. However, a woman whose prepregnancy weight is in the normal range (body mass index, BMI, 19–24.9) or who is overweight (BMI 25–29.9) should avoid excessive weight gain (more than 15kg) as she may find it difficult to regain her prepregnancy weight after the birth. This is of concern to many women, who want to be reassured that they will regain their body shape and prepregnancy weight as soon as possible after the baby has been born.

After the birth there is a great variability in weight loss. Six weeks after the birth, an average woman weighs 3kg more than her prepregnancy weight. Six months after the birth, she will weigh about 1kg more than she weighed before she became pregnant.

The situation is different for obese and underweight women, both during pregnancy and after birth. An obese woman (BMI greater than 30) should be encouraged to limit her weight gain during pregnancy as she has an increased risk that pregnancy-induced hypertension may occur and that she will have a large baby. She should have a glucose tolerance test performed to exclude gestational diabetes mellitus and she should be advised to eat a prudent but not a very low calorie diet as such a diet does not confer any benefit on mother or fetus. An underweight woman (BMI less than 19) should avoid becoming pregnant until she has gained weight as she has a 20% of giving birth to a low-birth-weight baby.

ELEMENTS OF WEIGHT GAIN IN PREGNANCY

Weight gain in pregnancy is caused by several factors:
- The products of conception – the fetus, placenta and amniotic fluid
- The maternal factors – the uterus and breasts, the increased blood volume, the increased stores of fat, water retention.

Fetus, placenta and amniotic fluid

In the first 20 weeks of pregnancy, the fetal weight gain is slow; in the second 20 weeks, it increases more rapidly. The weight gain of the placenta shows the reverse of that of the fetus (Fig. 5.9). The amniotic fluid increases rapidly from the 10th week, being 300ml at 20 weeks, 600ml at 30 weeks, and peaking at 1000ml at 35 weeks. After this a small decline in the total quantity of amniotic fluid occurs.

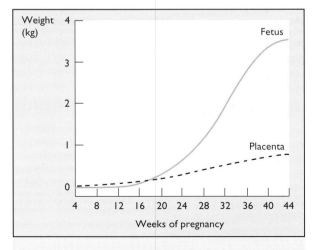

Fig. 5.9 Fetal and placental weight curves compared at various gestational periods.

Maternal factors

The weight of the *uterus* increases throughout pregnancy. It is more rapid in the first 20 weeks, when myohyperplasia is occurring, than in the second 20 weeks when most of the enlargement is due to stretching of the muscle fibres. The *breasts* increase in weight throughout pregnancy due to deposition of fat, increased retention of fluid, and growth of the glandular elements. The *blood volume* also increases throughout the pregnancy (see *Fig. 5.5*). The amount of fat deposited in adipose tissues depends on the amount of fat and carbohydrate in the diet. A gain of 2.5–3.0kg of fat is usual, of which 90% is deposited in the first 30 weeks of pregnancy. The fat contains 90–105MJ of energy, which can be released after birth for various activities, including breast feeding. In normal pregnancy, the *total body fluid* increases by 6–8L, of which 2–4L is extracellular. Most of the fluid is retained before the 30th week but a pregnant woman who has no clinical oedema, retains 2–3L of extracellular fluid in the last 10 weeks of pregnancy.

The elements of weight gain in pregnancy and their weight at 40 weeks are shown in *Figure 5.10*.

Fig. 5.10 The elements of weight gain (g) in pregnancy at 40 weeks	
Fetus	3300
Placenta	600
Uterus	900
Breasts (glandular tissue)	400
Blood	1200
Fat deposited	2500
Fluid (extracellular)	2600
Total	11000

ENERGY

The resting metabolic rate (RMR) in pregnancy is 10–15% higher than in non-pregnant women. The extra energy required in the 40 weeks of pregnancy for the increased RMR, the growth of the fetus and placenta, the increase in size of the uterus and breasts, and the extra fat is about 250MJ. This works out at about 0.9MJ a day – an amount provided by two slices of bread and 100ml of milk. A pregnant woman does not need to eat for two!

There are exceptions to this statement. Poor women in developing countries, particularly where starvation is not uncommon, benefit by having food supplements during pregnancy. These supplements aid modestly in increasing the birth weight of the baby, and giving her or him a greater chance of survival.

CHAPTER 6

Antenatal care

The aims of antenatal care are to ensure that:
- The mother reaches the end of the pregnancy as healthy as, or even healthier, than she was before she became pregnant.
- Any physical or psychological problems arising during the pregnancy are detected and treated.
- Any complication of pregnancy is either prevented or detected early and managed adequately.
- The mother gives birth to a healthy baby.
- The mother has the opportunity to discuss her anxieties and fears about the pregnancy.
- The mother is informed about any proposed procedures, the reason for the procedure and the probable outcome.
- The couple are prepared for the birth and for child rearing, including receiving information about diet, child care and family planning.

The provider of antenatal care may be a general practitioner or an obstetrician, working in conjunction with nurse–midwives. Shared antenatal care is becoming increasingly common and may take place in a doctor's rooms, in a hospital clinic or in a clinic conducted by a nurse–midwife. The opportunity should be available for an expectant mother to choose which facility she would prefer, but she should know that, if a complication arose, she would be transferred, if necessary, quickly and efficiently, to a facility staffed by experienced obstetricians.

Whichever facility a pregnant woman has chosen she should have the opportunity to talk to a health professional about matters which concern her during the pregnancy in an unhurried way and have her questions answered by an informed, communicative doctor or nurse–midwife.

Psychological preparation for motherhood

Some women appear confident that their pregnancy will proceed normally and that the birth of the baby will be easy. Most women, however, have concerns about the pregnancy and the process of childbirth. In the early weeks of pregnancy many women fear that the pregnancy may terminate as a miscarriage. Later in pregnancy many women fear that the baby will be malformed or retarded, or that childbirth will be dangerous and painful. A few women are concerned that, after the birth, they will not be able to regain their prepregnancy body shape. These fears may not be expressed unless the woman feels confident that she is able to ask her doctor about them and may expect to receive a reasoned answer. Fears about the difficulty and pain of childbirth can be reduced by simple explanations of the nature and course of labour.

Studies have shown that women who obtain social and psychological support during pregnancy are less likely than women who do not, to have negative feelings about their pregnancy and the forthcoming birth. They are more likely to feel that they are 'in control' during the pregnancy, to have a worry-free childbirth, to communicate more effectively with their doctor or nursing staff and to be more satisfied with the care they receive.

Many women are helped by antenatal classes run in conjunction with antenatal clinics, or privately. Other mothers are helped by reading books written for women (one of which is *Everywoman. A Gynaecological Guide for Life,* published by Penguin Books).

Antenatal depression

Between 5 and 10% of women develop depression at some time during their pregnancy, as judged by psychometric scales such as the Edinburgh Postnatal Depression Scale (EPDS). The vulnerable women tend to be primigravid, have poor social support, have either a partner who is unemployed or none at all, to be ambivalent about being pregnant or to be anxious about the health of their fetus. Vulnerable women require empathetic support from their attending health professionals and time to talk about their feelings when they are seen at an antenatal clinic or in a doctor's rooms. These women are also likely to develop postnatal depression (see page 98).

Diet in pregnancy

Many pregnant women are confused about what they should eat during pregnancy to make sure that the fetus is properly nourished. What should a pregnant woman eat? To a large extent this will depend on her cultural background, her eating behaviour and her income level. As a general principle, a woman should be advised to eat more fruit and vegetables, and less-fatty foods including confectionery and cakes. This is termed a prudent diet (*Fig. 6.1*). However, the woman should be able to choose and should follow a diet which is similar to that of her family.

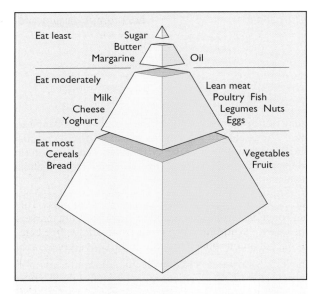

	Eat least	Sugar

Fig. 6.1 A prudent diet.

In terms of nutrients a woman should try to obtain, each day, the following amounts:

Kilojoules	9000kJ (2200kcal)
Protein	51g
Calcium	1g
Iron	30mg
Vitamin A	750µg
Vitamin D	10µg
Thiamin	1mg
Riboflavin	1.5mg
Niacin	1.5mg
Ascorbic acid	50mg
Folate	400µg

If this is translated into the foods a household buys, a pregnant woman should try to eat the following each day:

- Fish or meat 120g and an egg.
- Milk 500ml or cheese 30g.
- An orange, an apple or some other fruit.
- Green leafy vegetables at least three times a week.

When the woman has complied with the above, she can eat any other foods to satisfy her hunger as long as this is in agreement with the earlier suggestions for a prudent diet.

Most pregnant women who eat a prudent diet do not need vitamin supplements, with the exception of folate. It is now recommended that a woman who intends to become pregnant should take folate 0.5mg a day before conception and during the first quarter of pregnancy. The vitamin may be obtained from food or preferably a prescribed folic acid supplement (0.5mg). Women carrying a multiple pregnancy should continue taking folate throughout the pregnancy. Also, it should be noted that if a pregnant woman ingests excessive amounts of vitamin A (more than 8000IU a day) from dairy foods, oily fish and, particularly, liver the fetus may develop abnormalities. The current recommendation is that pregnant women should avoid eating liver.

Healthy women living in the industrialized countries, whose haemoglobin is within the normal range and who eat a good diet, do not need iron supplements mainly because between 30 and 60% of the iron in food is absorbed during pregnancy. However, some women in the developed countries, particularly if poor and single, and most women living in the developing countries, require iron supplementation. This is discussed in Chapter 16, Cardiovascular, respiratory and haematological disorders.

Often pregnant women are prescribed additional calcium. Most women in the developed countries obtain all the calcium they need from the diet suggested above, as 75% of the dietary calcium is absorbed when a woman is pregnant (compared with 58% in non-pregnant women).

Preconception advice

In recent years, clinics have been established to provide preconception advice (the cost benefits of such clinics have not been determined). At these clinics the family history is discussed, relating particularly to diabetes, hypertension and fetal defects. The immune status of the patient is explored, particularly relating to her ABO group and rhesus factor, and immunity to rubella, and to hepatitis B and C. If diabetes is identified the woman should make sure that the diabetes is under control before trying to become pregnant. This is discussed on page 135.

Other women who probably benefit from the advice given by such clinics are those who have given birth to a baby with spina bifida or anencephaly. There is evidence that if these women increase their intake of folate in the weeks before becoming pregnant and for the first 10 weeks of pregnancy the risk of a second affected baby is considerably reduced. Folate intake can be increased if the woman eats more green leafy vegetables, but these should be eaten raw or lightly cooked as folate dissolves in boiling water. Doctors may prefer to prescribe folate 5mg a day during the prepregnancy weeks.

Antenatal screening

A great deal of prenatal care is spent in detecting potentially dangerous conditions early; screening is one strategy used. In its simplest form blood pressure measurement is a screening strategy, as is discussed later. Currently, much interest is being shown in screening for congenital defects, such as Down's syndrome, neural tube defects and single gene defects, using DNA probes (Fig. 6.2).

Fig. 6.2 Possible indications for genetic diagnostic tests in first half of pregnancy

---

- Pregnancies in women over 35 years of age
- Pregnancies at increased risk for fetal neural tube defects (i.e. previously affected child)
- History of Down's syndrome or other chromosomal abnormality in the family
- Previous pregnancy resulting in the birth of a chromosomally abnormal child, or one with multiple malformations
- Known chromosomal abnormality in either parent
- History of sex-linked disease (eg thalassaemia, haemophilia, Duchenne muscular dystrophy)
- Couples at risk for detectable inborn errors of metabolism

SCREENING FOR GENETIC DEFECTS

Screening for Down's syndrome and certain other genetic defects (for example, cystic fibrosis, thalassaemia, haemophilia, Huntington's disease, some muscular dystrophies) can be carried out by chorionic villus sampling or amniocentesis. Before using these methods, an ultrasound examination of the fetus is made to exclude gross abnormalities.

Chronic villus sampling

A sample of chorionic tissue is removed from the placental edge between the 9th and 11th week of pregnancy, by introducing a needle transabdominally and advancing it to the edge of the placenta under ultrasonic guidance. About 20mg of chorionic tissue is sucked into a syringe. The karyotype of the sample is determined within 24 hours.

Amniocentesis

The procedure is carried out at about the 15th week of pregnancy. A needle is thrust through the abdominal wall and into the amniotic sac, guided by ultrasound to avoid the placenta and fetus, and a sample of amniotic fluid is removed. This is centrifuged and the fetal cells obtained are cultured for 3 weeks. They are then harvested and a karyotype is made.

Chronic villus sampling or amniocentesis?

The choice between chronic villus sampling (CVS) and amniocentesis is controversial. CVS is performed in the first quarter of pregnancy, and the karyotype is obtained within 24 hours, so the parental anxiety about the result is reduced. However, compared with amniocentesis, the karyotyping is slightly less accurate, and the risk of abortion following CVS is claimed to be slightly higher (1% above the background rate compared with 0.5% following amniocentesis). Concern has been expressed that CVS may be

followed in late pregnancy by oligohydramnios and limb defects. A multicentre study of over 140,000 patients has shown no increase in these defects when CVS is compared to amniocentesis. On the other hand the karyotype is only obtained 3 weeks after amniocentesis, which increases the psychological stress on the parents, and if the fetus is abnormal and termination of pregnancy is suggested, the process is more painful and psychologically disturbing.

Down's syndrome

At present, screening for Down's syndrome is only made in women over the age of 35 years, or who have had a previously affected baby. As this misses over half of all affected babies, a new strategy has been put in place. This is to obtain a serum sample and to measure serum markers for Down's syndrome. At present two markers, free beta-human chorionic gonadotrophin (β-hCG) and pregnancy associated protein A (PAPP-A), measured between the 8th and 14th week of pregnancy seem to be the most accurate markers. A low level of PAPP-A and a high level of free beta-hCG indicates a probable Down's syndrome-affected fetus. Used in conjunction with maternal age, in a multicentre trial, a detection rate of 63% (with a false positive rate of 5%) was obtained. If a positive finding is obtained CVS or amniocentesis is recommended. More information is awaited.

An alternative, or complementary marker, is also used in some obstetric units. This is to measure the nuchal neck thickness (as determined by the fluid behind the fetal neck) between the 10th and 14th week of pregnancy. If the nuchal thickness is greater than 3mm, the risk of Down's syndrome is increased to approximately 1 in 250. This risk is similar to that of a woman aged 35 years. There is some concern that if this strategy is adopted and all pregnant women are offered screening, although more babies with Down's syndrome will be detected, more women will require an amniocentesis, which may increase the miscarriage rate. In addition, more women will be caused anxiety whilst waiting for the results.

Screening for open neural tube defects

Open neural tube defects (NTDs) occur in 2–5 pregnancies per 1000. The Clinical Genetics Society in Britain has recommended that all pregnant women should be offered prenatal screening by measuring the alphafetoprotein (AFP) level at the 16th gestational week, but the cost effectiveness of this strategy has been questioned.

A blood sample is taken at about the 16th week of pregnancy. If the serum AFP level is more than 2.5 times the median for the week of pregnancy, the test is repeated. If it is raised in this sample an ultrasound examination is made to check the gestation period and exclude the presence of a multiple pregnancy. If this is excluded, an amniocentesis is made to measure the amniotic AFP. If the latter is raised (3 times the mean for the gestational week),

99.5% of the fetuses will have an NTD. The parents may choose to have the pregnancy terminated. It should be added that many units no longer use the AFP test, relying on ultrasound to detect a neural tube defect.

Counselling the patient

The screening procedures discussed can be traumatic to the parents for several reasons. First, the procedure itself is invasive; second, a delay occurs between taking the sample and obtaining the result; third, several of the procedures may have to be repeated before a diagnosis is obtained; and, last, false positives may occur.

The doctor has a responsibility to explain fully the reason for and the procedure of the investigation before it is made. If an abnormal result is obtained he must then explain the possible consequences and the choices open to the parents. To reduce the couple's anxiety the doctor must allow them time to absorb the information and he should answer their questions clearly, avoiding medical jargon. The doctor must inform, but not influence, the woman or her partner, who alone are responsible for making the decision whether to terminate or to continue the pregnancy.

MEDICAL IMAGING IN PREGNANCY

The development of ultrasound imaging, particularly using newer technologies, for example real-time ultrasound and colour Doppler imaging, has made a considerable impact on the care of the pregnant woman.

The role of ultrasound examination in obstetrics is shown in *Figure 6.3*. Examples of ultrasound imaging are shown in *Figures 6.4–6.14*. Ultrasound imaging has reduced the need for radiology, which, in obstetrics is limited to the determination of the pelvic dimensions in a few cases of breech presentation at term and to some cases of 'trial of labour'. In these cases a single lateral X-ray is taken.

The one controversial issue about ultrasound used in obstetrics is whether a woman should be screened routinely at about the 18th week of pregnancy. The supporters of routine imaging claim that the information gained, such as the age of the fetus and the presence, or absence, of some fetal malformations, is valuable. The parents can be reassured that the fetus is healthy and normal, and can obtain a photograph for their Baby Book! The opponents of routine imaging point out that it is costly and that between 10 and 30% of malformations (particularly cardiac malformations) may be misdiagnosed or missed. If this occurs and the parents are wrongly informed that the fetus is normal, it may cause great distress and may have unpleasant legal consequences.

Who should conduct antenatal care?

Antenatal care may be conducted by nurse–midwives, with two or three antenatal visits to an obstetrician or the

Weeks	
	Fig. 6.3 Some indications for ultrasound imaging in pregnancy
0–10	Do not use ultrasound to diagnose pregnancy, but scan if there is any doubt about gestational age, particularly if chorionic villus sampling is considered. **Threatened abortion:** scan at time of bleeding; repeat scan only if fetal heart sounds are undetectable **Recurrent abortion:** scan at 6–10 weeks **Ectopic gestation:** if suspected clinically, but not confirmed **Hyperemesis gravidarum:** if admission required, scan to exclude hydatidiform mole and multiple pregnancy
11–20	**Many obstetricians routinely scan women at 18–20 weeks' gestation** In addition scanning may be used to: **Estimate fetal maturity,** if suspected from a uterus smaller (by 4 weeks) or larger than dates **Detect multiple pregnancy,** if suspected clinically **Exclude a fetal malformation,** if a previous malformation reported
21–30	**Detection of multiple pregnancy** **Diagnosis of fetal death** **Antepartum haemorrhage** **Clinical polyhydramnios**
31–40	**Placental localization,** particularly if a low-lying placenta is detected at 18th week scan **Antepartum haemorrhage** **Moderate or severe pregnancy-induced hypertension** **Diabetes** **Severe renal disease** **Malpresentation** suspected at or after 36 weeks **Multiple pregnancy,** repeat scan at 34 weeks

Fig. 6.5 The echogram shows an empty amniotic sac at 11 weeks' gestation. The patient aborted 1 week later.

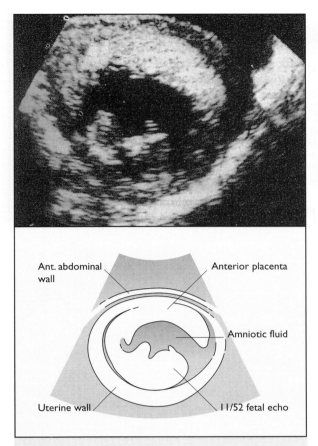

Fig. 6.4 Transverse scan showing normal fetus at 11 weeks' gestation.

Care of the pregnant woman

With this background information it is now possible to discuss the care of a pregnant woman. As mentioned in Chapter 1, Gyniatric history and examination, most women have a good idea that they are pregnant when they visit a medical practitioner to confirm the diagnosis. At this visit the doctor will inquire about the present pregnancy, the history of previous pregnancies, family history, previous illnesses or infections (including genital herpes and HIV-AIDS) and other matters and will examine the woman (including her breasts) as already described.

Two examinations require further discussion: blood pressure and weight, and whether the patient should be weighed at each antenatal visit.

BLOOD PRESSURE

A significant rise in blood pressure from the base line in early pregnancy, provides an early warning that the patient

woman's family doctor. In some centres a team of up to six midwives undertake antenatal care and one of the team attends the woman during childbirth. Alternatively the woman's antenatal care may be conducted throughout her pregnancy by an obstetrician or a trained family doctor.

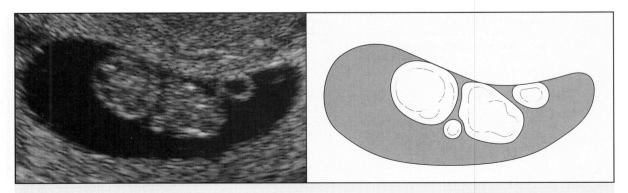

Fig. 6.6 Early intra-uterine pregnancy (9 weeks) (transverse scan).

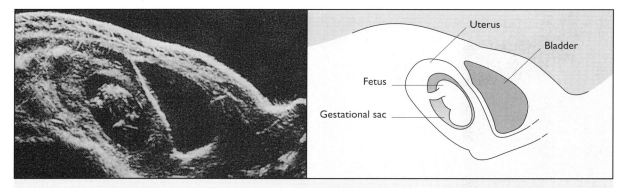

Fig. 6.7 Twelve-week fetus (sagittal scan).

Fig. 6.8 Fetal ascites.

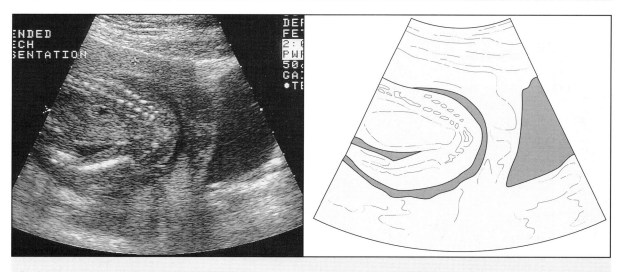

Fig. 6.9 Breech with extended legs at 22 weeks' gestation.

Fig. 6.10 Twins at 22 weeks' gestation. There is a slight discrepancy in the size. One is 21 weeks' gestation (left), the other 23 weeks' gestation (right).

Fig. 6.11 Hydrocephaly with distended cerebral ventricles and disturbances of the midline structures. The placenta is anterior (transverse scan).

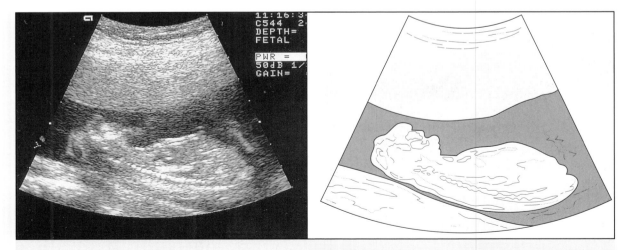

Fig. 6.12 Ultrasound scan showing an anencephalic fetus.

Fig. 6.13 Anencephalic fetus with large sacral meningomyelocele detected by ultrasound scan.

Fig. 6.14 Placenta praevia – Type two.

may develop pregnancy-induced hypertension (also known as pre-eclampsia or pre-eclamptic toxaemia). For this reason the woman's blood pressure should be measured at each antenatal visit.

In a normal pregnancy the blood pressure tends to remain at a constant level until the last quarter, when a rise of less than 10mmHg may occur. By convention a systolic pressure of more than 140mmHg and a diastolic pressure of more than 90mmHg are considered to indicate hypertension. However, a rise from the base line measurement of >30mmHg systolic pressure and more than 15mmHg diastolic pressure should be noted and a further reading made a few days later.

Problems in recording blood pressure, which may make the readings erroneous, occur in pregnant as well as in non-pregnant patients. These are associated with, for example,

the posture of the woman, the size of the cuff, the accuracy of the sphygmomanometer, the time of day and the emotional state of the patient ('White Coat' hypertension).

To reduce these variables, blood pressure recording equipment should be calibrated regularly, cuffs checked and the blood pressure taken with the patient seated or reclining with her arm at heart level. The brachial artery should be palpated and an appropriately sized cuff inflated until the pulsation disappears. Elevations of 2mmHg should be recorded, and if the rise is significantly above the baseline, a further estimation should be made after an interval.

The systolic pressure is easy to record. Although in Europe the change from a hard to a muffled sound, Korotkoff (K) 4, is used to identify the diastolic blood pressure, recent studies show that the disappearance of sounds (K5) is a more accurate marker of intra-arterial diastolic blood pressure. There is a greater concordance between observers when K5 is used to identify the diastolic pressure in pregnant women. If there is a significant difference between K4 and K5, both should be recorded.

WEIGHING THE PREGNANT PATIENT

It is customary to weigh a pregnant patient at each antenatal visit as it is believed that a small weight gain (or no gain) between visits is associated with restricted fetal growth, and that a weight gain of more than 1kg a week in the second half of pregnancy is an early marker for the possible development of pregnancy-induced hypertension. Careful studies show that the measurement of weight gain is of minimal value as a sign that the problems will develop and that therefore the medical indications for regular weighing can be abandoned. When the doctor chooses to continue to weigh the patient, a weight gain of less than 4kg may be expected before the 20th week of pregnancy; after that a gain of not more than 0.5kg a week should occur. Many pregnant women are concerned about their weight and wish to be weighed (or will weigh themselves). In such cases the doctor should offer to weigh the patient and offer sensible advice if the weight gain is 'abnormal'.

Women who are obese (body mass index more than 30) at the onset of pregnancy may require additional prenatal care, as they are more likely to develop gestational diabetes and pregnancy induced hypertension and may have a difficult labour.

LABORATORY TESTS

Several laboratory tests are made at the first antenatal visit, either by the health professional consulted or, if the woman is referred to a hospital antenatal clinic or to an obstetrician as a private patient, at the referral visit (*Fig. 6.15*).

Frequency of antenatal visits

There was, in 1929 in Britain, increasing concern that the maternal mortality rate had not fallen since 1880 (when it was 5 per 1000 live births). This led to the formation of a committee which recommended that a pregnant woman should visit an antenatal clinic every 4 weeks to the 28th week of pregnancy, then every 2 weeks to the 36th week, and thereafter weekly until delivered. Much discussion has arisen recently regarding whether this 70-year-old recommendation is appropriate today. One suggestion is that whilst a primigravida should be seen according to this schedule, a 'normal' multigravida need only been seen once in the first 10 weeks of pregnancy, then at the 22nd week and again at the 30th week before entering the later schedule of visits.

Whatever schedule is adopted, a pregnant woman should be asked at each antenatal visit if she has any problems she wishes to discuss and if she is feeling fetal movements. She

---

Fig. 6.15 Routine laboratory tests at the first or early antenatal consultation

At first antenatal visit

Blood:	Haemoglobin concentration (normal range 10.5–15.0g/L)
	Haematocrit (PVC) (normal >35)
	MCV* and MCH** (Especially if patient Southern European, Asian or African because of possible thalassaemia)
	ABO and Rhesus group. Rhesus antibodies
	All patients, irregular antibodies
	VDRL or similar test (to exclude syphilis)
	Hepatitis B surface antigen (HBsAG)
	Antirubella antibodies
	?HIV antibodies

Vaginal smear. If abnormal pathogens are detected, treatment should be given. This applies to bacterial vaginosis infection as it appears to be associated with an increased risk of preterm labour. Women do not commonly develop bacterial vaginosis after 16 weeks. For this reason metronidazole should be prescribed about this time.

Urine:	Urinalysis
	Mid-stream sample for bacteriuria culture

At subsequent antenatal visits

All women repeat the irregular antibody test at 36 weeks' gestation
Rhesus–negative women: rhesus antibody tests at 28 and 36 weeks
Haemoglobin: check between 32 and 36 weeks and/or measure serum ferritin

* MCV = mean cell volume
   There is some evidence that MCV may be the most useful measure of anaemia, as the MCV declines rapidly in iron deficiency.
** MCH = mean cell haemoglobin

should have her blood pressure measured, her urine tested for protein, and the height of her fundus estimated (see *Fig. 1.7, page 6*) or measured with a tape measure (*Fig. 6.16*) to evaluate the growth of the fetus. Some health professionals listen for fetal heart sounds after 'quickening' (fetal movements) has occurred. Quickening is usually noticed by the expectant mother between 16 and 24 weeks of pregnancy. Other health professionals apply a fetal heart sound machine so that they and the patient can listen to the fetal heart sounds.

In addition, after the 28th week the health professional customarily palpates the woman's abdomen to determine the growth, presentation and position of the fetus in the uterus. The technique used is discussed later in this chapter.

Preparation for breastfeeding

During pregnancy the health professional should ask the patient if she wishes to breastfeed her infant. If she intends to breastfeed, her wish should be positively reinforced. The benefits of breastfeeding should be discussed:

- Breast milk provides the ideal nutrition for infants and contributes to their healthy growth and development.
- For most women breastfeeding provides a sense of satisfaction and pleasure.
- Among poorer women, particularly in the developing countries, exclusive breastfeeding contributes to a woman's health by increasing the space between pregnancies.
- Breastfeeding reduces the chance that the baby will develop infections, particularly gastrointestinal infections, thereby lowering infant mortality.

Fig. 6.16 *Gestational age estimated from symphysis–fundal height.*

The health professional should examine the woman's breasts and note if her nipples are protractile, pseudo-protractile or inverted. Inverted nipples may be made protractile if, in the second half of pregnancy, the woman places her thumbs on the opposite sides of the base of her nipples and draws her thumbs apart in both the vertical and horizontal planes, to break supposed adhesions which are preventing the nipples from everting. Some doctors advise the woman to wear nipple shields, but the benefit of these is uncertain.

Nipple care should be discussed. The nipples should be washed daily with water to remove any crusts which have formed, and if the woman wishes she may apply anhydrous lanolin. Exposure of the nipples to the air also helps.

The health professional may provide the woman with a pamphlet about the breastfeeding groups which are available in her area.

Should the woman choose not to breastfeed, for whatever reason, the health professional should avoid making her feel guilty and should discuss the importance of preparing the breast-milk substitute according to the manufacturer's directions.

Growth of the fetus during pregnancy

As mentioned above, fetal growth can be determined roughly by the height of the fundus or the distance between the symphysis pubis to the top of the uterus. A more accurate assessment of the fetal growth and weight can be obtained by ultrasound imaging (*Fig. 6.17*), but this is only required in some pregnancies, for example, if the doctor suspects that the fetus is growth restricted. Until about the 28th week of pregnancy the position of fetal head (or buttocks) relative to the mother's pelvis is of little clinical importance. After that time it becomes increasingly important, and should be monitored by the doctor. For the purposes of communication descriptive terms are used:

- The *lie* of the fetus refers to the relationship of its long axis to the mother. By the 38th week the fetus may have a longitudinal lie (cephalic or breech) or an oblique or a transverse lie (*Fig. 6.18*).
- The *presentation* of the fetus relates to the fetal part which occupies the lower part of the uterus over the pelvic brim. If the fetal head presents it is termed a cephalic presentation; if the buttocks present it is a breech presentation; if a shoulder presents it is termed a shoulder presentation.
- The *presenting part of the fetus* is that portion of the fetus which is presenting against the cervix in the first stage of labour, or against the vagina in the second stage of labour. If the presentation is cephalic, the presenting part is usually the posterior part of the fetal head, the vertex or occiput, but it may be the face or the brow.

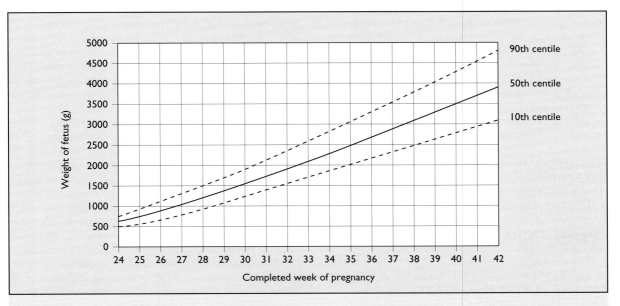

Fig. 6.17 Fetal weight at various weeks of gestation (from 24 weeks) among Scandinavian women as determined by ultrasound.

Fig. 6.18 The presentation of the fetus.

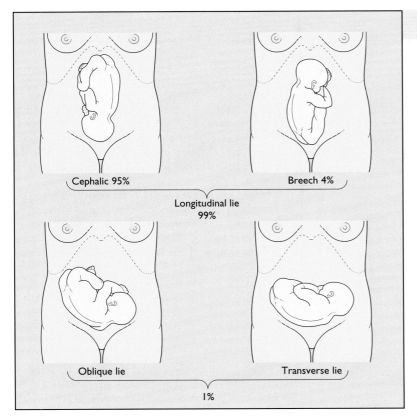

- The *attitude* of the fetus is defined as the relation of various fetal parts to other parts. Normally the fetus lies with all its joints flexed, but in some breech presentations the fetal legs are extended along its body.
- The *position of the presenting part* of the fetus is of little clinical significance until labour is established. It refers to the relationship of the presenting part to the bony pelvic walls, and will be discussed in Chapter 9, Course and management of childbirth.

TECHNIQUE OF ABDOMINAL EXAMINATION

The patient assumes a reclining position having emptied her bladder. The abdominal examination to the fetus is made by four 'manoeuvres', which are shown in *Figures 6.19–6.22*. The information is recorded in the patient's antenatal records.

ASSESSMENT OF THE SHAPE AND SIZE OF THE MATERNAL PELVIS

This procedure should be delayed until the 38th week of pregnancy because, firstly, it is, by then, more comfortable for the patient, and, secondly, the fetal presenting part may be expected to have descended into the pelvis

to some degree in most primigravidae. In multigravidae, the fetal presenting part may not descend into the pelvis until labour supervenes. Possible reasons for non-descent in primigravidae are shown in *Figure 6.23*. In most cases, pelvic assessment is only required in primigravidae, as the history of previous labours will give information about the pelvis.

The patient lies is a reclining position, with her legs flexed and her bladder empty. The doctor inserts two gloved fingers, lubricated with chlorhexidine cream, into the vagina. The condition of the vaginal walls and the cervix is noted. The degree of engagement of the fetal-presenting part is recorded (*Fig. 6.24*). If the fetal head presents and has not descended into the pelvis, a test can be made to determine if it will descend. This test estimates the relative size of fetal head and maternal pelvis (*Fig. 6.25*).

The architecture of the pelvis is explored by the fingers reaching diagonally upwards and backwards to determine if the sacral promontory can be reached. The curve of the sacrum is next palpated and the prominence of the ischial spines noted. The sacrospinous ligament is palpated and should accommodate two of the examiner's fingers. Finally the distance between the two sacral tuberosities is measured by the clenched fist.

Fig. 6.19 First manoeuvre – fundal palpation. The height of the fundus is estimated and the fundal area gently palpated in an attempt to identify which pole of the fetus (breech or head) is occupying the fundus.

Fig. 6.20 Second manoeuvre – lateral palpation. The examiner's hands gently slip down the sides of the uterus with quick palpation to try to identify on which side the firm back of the fetus or the soft belly and knobbly limbs can be detected.

Fig. 6.21 Pelvic manoeuvre. The examiner gently turns to face the patient's feet and slides his hands gently on the lower part of the uterus, pressing down on each side to determine the presenting part. If it is the fetal head it can be ballotted between the fingers.

Fig. 6.22 Pawlik's manoeuvre. This is not always necessary and must be performed gently. The presenting part is moved between the fingers and thumb of the examiner's hand, to determine whether it is the fetal head or breech and the degree of descent into the maternal pelvis.

Fig. 6.23 The causes of lack of engagement of the fetal head

• Lack of adequate formation of the lower uterine segment

• Malposition of the fetal head

• Cephalopelvic disproportion or contracted pelvis

• Tumours in the pelvis obstructing the entry of the fetal head

• Placenta praevia

• Incorrect estimation of the period of gestation

Fig. 6.24 Descent of the fetal head.

Completely above	Sinciput +++ occiput ++	Sinciput ++ occiput +	Sinciput + occiput just felt	Sinciput + occiput not felt	None of head palpable
5/5	4/5	3/5	2/5	1/5	0/5
'Floating' above the brim	'Fixing'	Not engaged	Just engaged	Engaged	Deeply engaged

level of pelvic brim

Fig. 6.25 Estimating the relative size of the fetal head and the maternal pelvis by Muller-Kerr 'head fitting' test.

Age and reproductive performance

TEENAGED PREGNANCY

More teenaged women are becoming sexually active at an earlier age than in previous decades. Studies in northern Europe and in North America have shown that by the age of 17 years, 50% of teenaged woman have had sexual intercourse and that by the age of 20 years, the proportion has risen to 70%. Only one woman in four uses contraceptives in the first 4–6 months of starting sexual intercourse. These two facts account for the increasing numbers of young women who become pregnant. In Australia and Britain, 5% of teenaged women, and in the USA 9% of teenaged women become pregnant each year. Of these women, 35–45% obtain an induced abortion, 5% miscarry, and the remainder continue the pregnancy and give birth.

Pregnant women under the age of 18 years have an increased risk of developing complications of pregnancy and childbirth. The woman is more likely to develop pregnancy-induced hypertension or anaemia, and to give birth to a low-birth-weight baby. The reasons appear to be:

- Low socioeconomic status.
- A nutritionally poor diet.
- Substance or drug abuse.
- A lack of antenatal care.

The problems can be avoided if the adolescent woman accepts the need for and receives antenatal care from helpful health professionals and social workers. If this occurs the proportion of adolescent pregnant women developing complications in pregnancy is no greater than among women aged 20–35 years.

PREGNANCY IN OLDER WOMEN

In the past decade the proportion of women choosing to delay their first pregnancy until they are in their 30s has increased in most developed countries. The women tend to belong to the upper socioeconomic group, to be well educated and to have a career. Births to women aged over 30 years now account for between 25 and 35% of all births, (and the proportion of all births to women over the age of 35 years is between 5 and 15%). Births to primigravidae aged 35 years or more account for about 3% of all births. These 'older primigravidae' have an increased risk of having essential hypertension and of developing pregnancy-induced hypertension, gestational diabetes and antepartum haemorrhage. They are also more likely to have a baby with Down's syndrome, but they have no increased risk of a preterm birth or of fetal growth restriction.

They have an increased chance of having a caesarean section or a vaginal operative delivery, but this may be due to concern by the obstetrician that the woman's fecundity is reduced and the desire to obtain a 'perfect baby', as much as to a medical or obstetric complication.

Provided pregnant women over the age of 35 years receive antenatal care, sound genetic diagnosis and counselling early in pregnancy, the outcome in terms of a live healthy mother and a live healthy child is excellent.

Preparing for childbirth

A woman who knows what to expect in childbirth, is better able to cooperate and to find the experience less painful. Antenatal classes are available in many hospitals and are provided by private obstetric physiotherapists for childbirth training. Childbirth training has broadened in recent years along with the expansion of the original technique of psychoprophylaxis first developed in Russia. Psychoprophylaxis is based on the belief that fear and anxiety about pain and danger in childbirth, learned before the woman becomes pregnant and during pregnancy, sink deeply into her memory and produce a 'conditioned reflex'. Because of this reflex, every time a woman thinks of childbirth a mental image of pain and danger is conjured up, with the result that she enters labour anxious and tense. The tension and fear may increase the pain and delay the birth of the baby. Psychoprophylaxis seeks to eliminate the 'conditioned reflex' and to replace the negative image of childbirth with a more positive one. This is achieved by education during pregnancy in the hope that knowledge and insight will change the woman's perceptions of labour.

Psychoprophylaxis also seeks to alter the brain's perception of pain and to convert it into a sensation of discomfort, which can be relieved by muscular activity. This is based on the concept of 'pain dissociation'. Pain becomes less intense if the woman keeps her mind busy by concentrating on something else. The suggested mental activity usually involves concentrating on a learned pattern of breathing, counting breaths, focusing on a particular point in the room or consciously commanding the body to release its tension. However, it is very difficult for most women to maintain control and remain in a calm state during the particularly painful stages of labour. The distraction techniques of psychoprophylaxis are therefore unrealistic and unsatisfactory for many women during childbirth.

As anthropologists, psychologists, physiotherapists and midwives have become increasingly active in the development of prepared childbirth, new strategies for pain management have been developed which offer more than the original psychoprophylaxis concept.

The social environment in which the baby will be born, and its effect on the woman, is now becoming an important consideration. Many women want their partner or some other 'support person' to be with them during childbirth. The presence of an informed loved one during labour gives the woman familiar and personal support to reduce the clinical environment of a delivery ward.

The discomfort and pain of childbirth is decreased if the attending nursing and medical staff treat the woman as an intelligent individual, who has needs and who can make choices, and who is perceived as a woman having a baby, rather than as a patient requiring medical attention. Some hospitals are trying to make the place of birth as non-clinical as possible by providing a supportive environment with floor mattresses, functional beds, soft fabrics and colours, and a shower. These innovations decrease a woman's anxiety and enable her to cope more efficiently with the process of childbirth.

Techniques of auditory and visual imagery provide an additional means of managing pain in labour. Instead of dissociating from her pain (as in psychoprophylaxis) the woman uses the sensations of labour to assist her in creating an image of what is happening inside her body. For example, she may visualize her cervix opening each time she has a contraction; the baby's head moving deeper into her pelvis; or the baby opening her vagina in the second stage of labour.

Another development has been the use of relaxation techniques. In psychoprophylaxis, relaxation is taught as a method of control. The woman uses quiet, controlled breathing to convince herself that she is not experiencing pain. More recently, relaxation has been used by the woman as a method of 'letting go' and so reducing the pain. She may move and rock to achieve relaxation; she may stamp her feet, or bang her fists to release stress and diffuse the pain. She may discover that for her, the most effective form of pain control is a combination of floor positions, rhythmic groaning and belly rocking.

The proponents of active involvement in childbirth believe that the woman, if possible, should be given a free choice in the position she wishes to adopt and the movements she wishes to make during labour and the birth of the baby. The woman may choose to lie on her side, to squat, or to position herself on her hands and knees. She may prefer to be supported in a nearly upright position, with her partner in front of or behind her. In this technique there is much less focus on breathing as an exercise or pattern, and more focus on breathing as a method which helps the woman 'go with the flow'.

A current approach used by many obstetric physiotherapists is to stress women's differences, rather than adopting a rigid technique. Attempts are made to find out the woman's most preferred mode of behaviour, and to encourage her to use these in childbirth. A woman who is 'tactile', for example, will probably respond well to massage, hot packs applied to her back and showers, and will tend to move about a good deal during labour. Other women prefer 'visualization', or eye-to-eye focusing, or will respond to key words such as 'relax', 'go soft', 'let go'. A third group of women are able to relieve the pain of labour more effectively by using auditory strategies. They respond to their support person 'pacing' them during a contraction and to giving themselves positive messages.

When a woman responds to the pain in a way she naturally prefers, her behaviour ceases to be due to a technique or a method. This reduces the anxiety that comes from having to perform a technique with which she is not comfortable, and which she fears she may not perform well.

The philosophy adopted by numbers of childbirth educators is to provide information and to give permission to the woman to be herself. Some women prefer neither to attend class nor to employ a private childbirth educator. For them, training videotapes are available which enable the woman and her partner to learn at home.

Signs that labour is about to start

The signs which indicate that labour is soon to start or has started are described on page 72. An expectant mother should have these signs described to her or have access to a book which describes them so that she can be comfortable knowing when she is probably in labour. A question asked by many women during an antenatal visit concerns whether they will be given drugs to relieve the pain of labour. They should be reassured that analgesics are readily available should they be requested. This matter is discussed on pages 86–89.

Many women are fearful that they will be left alone during the course of childbirth. Today, many women want their husband or partner or a 'significant other person' to be with them through the childbirth process, and most hospitals agree to this.

Antenatal information

Certain matters affecting the mother during pregnancy should be discussed at the early visits.

ALCOHOL

Heavy alcohol consumption in pregnancy (greater than 120g or 12 standard drinks a day) is associated with fetal growth restriction, developmental delay and neurological complications in the baby. There is some evidence that moderate alcohol consumption (between 100 and 120g a day) may be associated with an increased risk of spontaneous abortion, and a smaller fetal head circumference. A consumption of 20g a day or less does not appear to have any damaging effects on the fetus or mother. Nevertheless, a pregnant woman should be advised to limit her consumption of alcohol during pregnancy.

CLOTHING

In general, the patient should wear the clothes she prefers and which enhance her self-esteem. These clothes should be comfortable and non-constricting. Unless she is accustomed to wearing a girdle or has abdominal muscles stretched by previous pregnancies, a maternity support is not needed. As pregnancy advances the patient should be alerted to the fact that her centre of balance alters and that for comfort's sake, she should wear flat shoes.

DENTAL CARE

An early visit to the dentist is advised so that any dental care required can be carried out in the first half of pregnancy.

EMPLOYMENT

In the current economic conditions many pregnant women choose to or have to work. Provided she does not become too tired, that her enlarging abdomen does not interfere with the job and that industrial conditions in the office, factory or store are appropriate, work during pregnancy will harm neither the mother nor the fetus. In most developed countries paid maternity leave is granted for 6 weeks before the expected date of the childbirth.

EXERCISE

Exercise is to be encouraged if this is the usual habit of the mother, but need not be insisted upon if the patient is usually sedentary. She should take walks and other light exercise if she wishes. The woman should neither become a fanatic for exercise nor refrain from all physical activity. If she enjoys swimming, she may continue to swim. In general, she should not alter her regimen of exercise just because she is pregnant, unless the exercise regimen is very strenuous and may raise the woman's body temperature significantly.

IMMUNIZATION

If about to travel overseas, antityphoid or cholera inoculations may be given. All pregnant women who have not been immunized against poliomyelitis, or whose immunity has lapsed, should be immunized in early pregnancy.

SEX DURING PREGNANCY

Many doctors fail to discuss sex during pregnancy, and many women feel inhibited about asking. Because of this many couples are inadequately informed, and have considerable misconceptions.

Studies have shown that many women have reduced sexual desire and activity, especially in the early weeks of pregnancy and after the 30th week. The reason for this decline in libido is unclear. Some women find sexual intercourse uncomfortable; others fear that coitus and orgasm may damage the fetus or bring on premature labour. Others see themselves as unattractive, or find the physical awkwardness of coitus in late pregnancy inhibiting.

It is appropriate to talk with the couple. There is no evidence that coitus, cunnilingus or masturbation, whether leading to orgasm or not, have any damaging effect on the fetus, or induce labour prematurely. All forms of sexual enjoyment are permissible in pregnancy, with the proviso that, during cunnilingus, the man should be warned not to blow, forcing air into the woman's vagina, as this has led to air embolism in pregnancy.

Many pregnant women want additional closeness from their partner, and he should be supportive and gentle at all times. In late pregnancy, coitus with the man on top may be uncomfortable, but other coital positions are not, and non-coital sexual satisfaction may be preferred. Coitus can continue, if the couple wish, up to term without any damage to mother or baby. The principal medical contraindications to coitus are ruptured membranes and known placenta praevia.

SMOKING

Pregnant women should be advised not to smoke cigarettes or, if they are unable to break the habit, to restrict smoking to one cigarette after a main meal. This advice is given because female cigarette smokers (particularly women who smoke more than 20 cigarettes a day) have a slightly greater chance of aborting, and because their baby's weight, at all stages of gestation, is between 150 and 300g less than the weight of a baby of a non-smoker; additionally, the perinatal death rate may be slightly higher. One reason for the damaging effect of smoking in pregnancy is that smokers have a reduced intervillous blood flow and higher blood levels of carbon monoxide. Smoking is associated with a 1.2-fold increased risk of the baby having a cleft palate. These findings suggest that if the adverse effects of cigarette smoking are to be minimized, smoking should be avoided from the time of conception. However, smoking behaviour is affected by many psychosocial factors, and the woman may find smoking an appropriate method for her to reduce stress and tension, with the result that the success of a non-smoking campaign in pregnancy may be limited. This is important to know as fortunately there is no evidence that smoking during pregnancy has any effect on the long-term mental or motor development of the child.

TRAVELLING
Provided the journey can be made in a leisurely and comfortable way, there need be no restriction on travelling during pregnancy.

CHAPTER 7

Mechanical factors in childbirth

To be born, the fetus has to negotiate the birth canal propelled by contractions of the uterus. Factors which can delay or prevent this are:

- The shape and size of the bony and soft tissues of the woman's pelvis (the passages).
- The size of the fetus (the passenger).
- The quality and frequency of the uterine contractions (the powers).

The passages

BONY PELVIS

The bony pelvis is made up of four bones, the two innominate bones, the sacrum and the coccyx, united at three joints. When a woman stands erect, the pelvis is tilted forward. The pelvic inlet makes an angle of about 55° with the horizontal. The angle varies among individuals and between races; for example, black Africans have a lesser angle. An angle of more than 55° may make the descent of the fetal head into the pelvis difficult (*Fig. 7.1*).

The 'true' pelvis is bounded by the pubic crest, the iliopectineal line and the sacral promontory. An 'ideal obstetric' pelvis is described in *Figure 7.2* and the brim is shown in *Figure 7.3*. The true pelvis is cylindrical in shape, with a bluntly curved lower end and is slightly curved anteriorly. Anteriorly the pubic bones form its boundary,

measuring 4.5cm. Posteriorly, the curve of the sacrum forms its boundary, measuring 12cm. Laterally its walls narrow slightly distally (*Fig. 7.4*). The walls are penetrated by the obturator foramen anteriorly, and the sciatic foramen laterally which is divided into two parts by the sacrospinous and sacrotuberous ligaments.

	Fig. 7.2 The ideal obstetric pelvis
Brim	Round or oval transversely No undue projection of the sacral promontory Anterior–posterior diameter 12cm Transverse diameter 13cm The plane of the pelvic inlet not less than 55°
Cavity	Shallow with straight side-walls No great projection of the ischial spines Smooth sacral curve Sacrospinous ligament at least 3.5cm
Outlet	Pubic arch rounded Subpubic angle >80° Intertuberous diameter at least 10cm

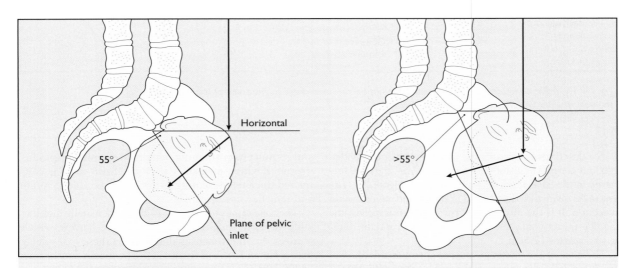

Fig. 7.1 Effect of the inclination of the pelvic brim on the engagement of the fetal head.

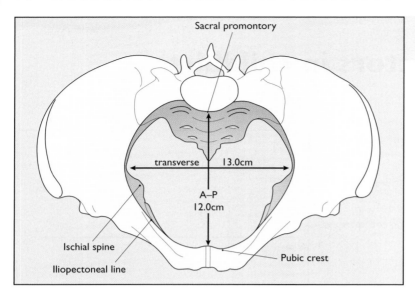

Fig. 7.3 The 'ideal obstetric' pelvis: pelvic inlet. A–P = anterior–posterior.

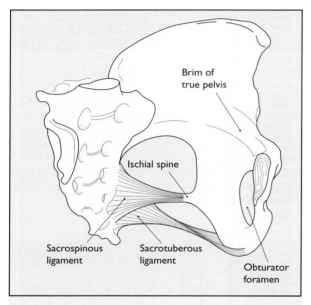

Fig. 7.4 The pelvic cavity. The right innominate bone has been removed in order to show the extent of the cavity.

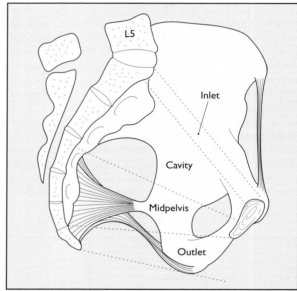

Fig. 7.5 The zones of the pelvis.

For descriptive purposes the true pelvis can be divided into four zones. These are shown in *Figure 7.5*. The measurements of the *zone of the inlet* are shown in *Figure 7.3*. The *zone of the cavity* is wedge-shaped in profile and almost round in section. It is the most roomy part of the true pelvis, the anterior–posterior diameter measuring 13.5cm and the transverse diameter 12.5cm.

The *zone of the midpelvis* passes through the apex of the pubic arch, the spines of the ischia, the sacrospinous ligament and the tip of the sacrum. It is the smallest zone and its most important diameter is the ischial–bispinous diameter, which measures 10.5cm. If this zone is contracted the fetal presenting part may not be able to rotate and may become arrested.

The *zone of the outlet* (Fig. 7.6) does not usually interfere with the birth unless the pubic rami are narrow, which reduces the intertuberous diameter. In these cases delay may occur and the soft tissues of the perineum may be torn and damaged.

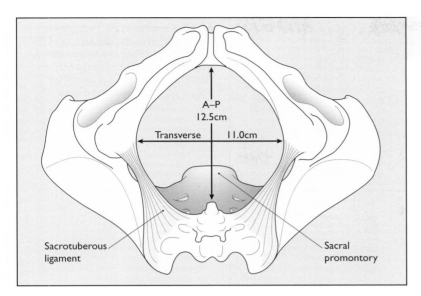

Fig. 7.6 The female pelvic outlet viewed from below. A–P = anterior–posterior.

Fig. 7.7 Inclination of the pelvic brim and the axis of the birth canal. The plane of the pelvic brim makes an angle of about 55° with the horizontal in the erect patient, and the plane of the outlet about 10° with the horizontal. The axis of the birth canal is angled, the alteration in direction occurring at the pelvic floor.

The *axis of the birth canal* corresponds to the direction the fetal-presenting part, usually the head, takes during its passage through the birth canal (*Fig. 7.7*).

Factors influencing pelvic shape and size

Minor alterations in pelvic shape have been found in many women receiving routine radiological pelvimetry, but only in a few instances has the abnormality been found to delay the birth. Smaller women tend to have a smaller bony pelvis but also tend to have smaller babies. More-severe alterations occur among populations where rickets or osteomalacia is found but are uncommon in the developed countries today.

SOFT TISSUES OF THE FEMALE PELVIS

These include the uterus, the muscular pelvic floor and the perineum.

Uterus

The uterus in pregnancy can be divided in three parts:
* The upper uterine segment.
* The lower uterine segment.
* The uterine cervix.

Upper uterine segment

This portion of the uterus consists of the fundus and that part of the uterus lying above the reflection of the vesico-uterine fold of peritoneum. During pregnancy, it undergoes the greatest degree of myometrial hyperplasia and hypertrophy. In labour, it provides the strong contractions which push the fetus along the birth canal.

Lower uterine segment

This portion of the uterus lies between the vesico-uterine fold of the peritoneum superiorly and the cervix inferiorly. During pregnancy, the upper part of the cervix is incorporated into the lower uterine segment, which stretches to accommodate the fetal-presenting part (*Fig. 7.8*). In late pregnancy, as the upper segment muscle contractions increase in frequency and strength, the lower uterine segment develops more rapidly and is stretched radially to permit the fetal-presenting part to descend (*Fig. 7.9*). In labour the entire cervix becomes incorporated into the stretched lower uterine segment.

Fig. 7.8 Formation of the lower uterine segment based on the observations of CP Wendell-Smith. Cone, the condensation of muscle at the junction of the body of the uterus and the cervix; AIO, anatomical internal os; HIO, histological internal os.

Fig. 7.9 (a) The lower uterine segment in late pregnancy. (b) The lower uterine segment in late labour. It is dilated circumferentially and has thinned but is shorter. (c) In obstructed labour the dilated and thinned lower uterine segment stretches and is in danger of rupture.

Cervix uteri

The cervix uteri is that part of the uterus which extends from the fibromuscular junction superiorly to the external cervical os inferiorly. The upper margin is not a fixed point as most of the myometrial fibres end as a cone of muscle which protrudes into the collagenous tissue which comprises 90% of the cervix. Some attenuated muscle fibres are present between the collagenous bundles and form 10% of the cervical tissue. The endometrium ceases at the level of the muscular cone and becomes a single layer of cubical endocervical cells which are folded into clefts. In late pregnancy the cervix becomes softer because of chemical changes in the collagen fibres, and shorter as it is incorporated into the lower uterine segment. It also undergoes

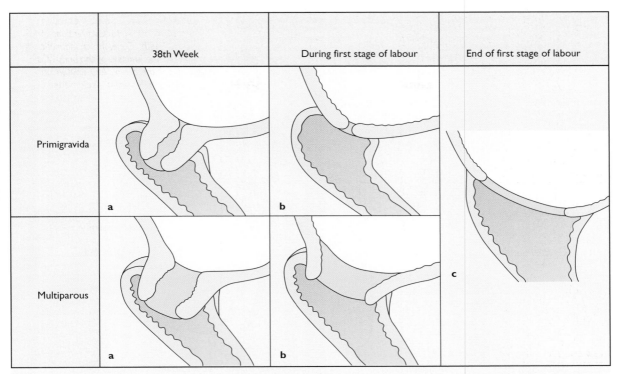

	38th Week	During first stage of labour	End of first stage of labour
Primigravida	a	b	c
Multiparous	a	b	

Fig. 7.10 Progressive effacement and dilatation of the cervix in late pregnancy and labour.
Primigravida. (a) Little or no effacement or dilatation has occurred. (b) Effacement has occurred but dilatation is not yet marked.
(c) The cervix is fully effaced and dilated.
Multiparous. (a) Dilatation has begun but no effacement has yet occurred. (b) Effacement and dilatation are occurring simultaneously.
(c) The cervix is fully effaced and dilated.

a variable degree of dilatation. Collectively, these changes are termed cervical 'ripening'. The changes may occur abruptly or gradually at any time after the 34th week of pregnancy, but usually occur nearer term, especially in primigravidae. At the 34th gestational week, the cervix is 2cm or more dilated in 20% of primigravidae and in 40% of multigravidae; and the proportion increases towards term (Fig. 7.10).

At the onset of labour, the cervix of a primigravida is ripe, and is either partly, or not, effaced (ie incorporated into the lower uterine segment).

Pelvic floor

The pelvic floor consists of the levator ani group of muscles, which arise on each side of the pelvis; (i) from the posterior surface of the pubis, (ii) from a condensation of fascia (the white line) which covers the obturator internus muscle, and (iii) from the pelvic aspect of the ischial spine (Fig. 7.11). The muscle has several designated parts – the pubococcygeus muscle, the levator ani muscle and the coccygeus muscle (Fig. 7.12). The fibres of these muscles slope downwards and forwards and interdigitate with muscle fibres of the opposite levator ani group to form a muscular sling through which the urethra, the vagina and the rectum pass. The muscles enclosed in fascia form the pelvic diaphragm (Fig. 7.13).

Perineum

The perineum (perineal body) is the tissue which lies distal to the pelvic diaphragm. It is pyramid-shaped and is bounded superiorly by the lower surface of the pelvic diaphragm; laterally by the bones and ligaments of the pelvic outlet; and below by the vulva and the anus. It can be subdivided into the urogenital triangle anteriorly and the anal triangle posteriorly by the transverse perineal muscles (Fig. 7.14). The perineum contains a number of superficial muscles, is very vascular and is filled with fatty tissue. Its importance in childbirth is that it is frequently damaged as the fetus is born.

Fig. 7.11 Lateral wall.

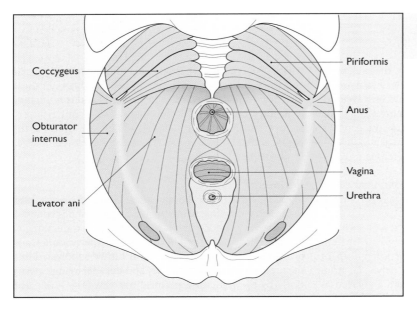

Fig. 7.12 The muscles which form the pelvic floor viewed from above.

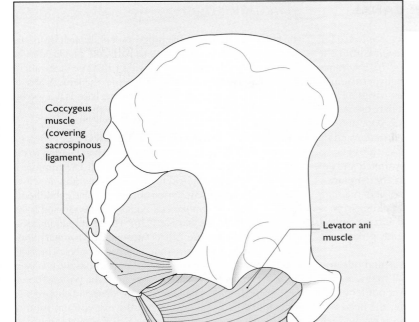

Coccygeus muscle (covering sacrospinous ligament)

Levator ani muscle

External sphincter ani

Vagina

Fig. 7.13 Pelvic diaphragm: lateral view.

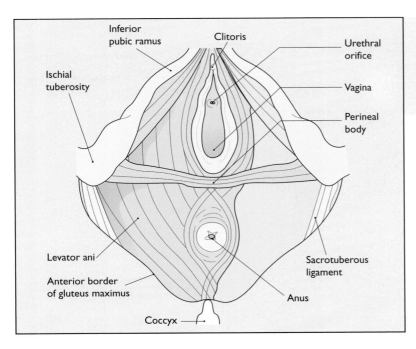

Inferior pubic ramus

Clitoris

Urethral orifice

Ischial tuberosity

Vagina

Perineal body

Levator ani

Anterior border of gluteus maximus

Sacrotuberous ligament

Anus

Coccyx

Fig. 7.14 The muscles of the female perineum. In the left half of the diagram the fat pad which fills the space has not been drawn, to show the lower surface of the levator ani which forms the roof of the space.

FORMATION OF THE BIRTH CANAL DURING LABOUR

When myometrial contraction and retraction has led to full dilatation of the cervix the fetal head descends into the vagina, which expands to encompass it (*Fig. 7.15*). Normally an apparent space, the vaginal muscle has hypertrophied and the epithelium become folded during pregnancy so that it can accommodate the fetus without damage. As the fetal head descends it encounters the pelvic floor and the leading point is directed forwards by the gutter formed by the levatores ani. The fetus must now pass through the urogenital diaphragm. The levator muscles stretch and are displaced downwards and backwards so that the anus receives the full force of the descending head and, dilating, gapes widely to expose the anterior rectal wall. Pressure is also exerted on the lower part of the vagina and the central portion of the perineum, and as the head is born the tissues may tear.

The descent of the fetus from the uterus and out into the world is straight to the level of the ischial spines; it then moves in an anterior curve around the lower border of the symphysis pubis. If the pubic arch is wide, the head will stem close behind the symphysis, and the perineum will not be so stretched. If the angle is narrow, the head is forced back, the direction of the curve is more obtuse and perineal damage is likely.

The passenger

The fetus may influence the progress of childbirth by its size and its presentation. Of all the fetal parts, the fetal head is the least compressible and pliant. However, because of the ability of the skull bones to override each other, the fetus is able to negotiate the birth canal provided that the fetus is not too big and the uterine contractions are sufficiently strong.

ANATOMY OF THE FETAL SKULL

The face of the term fetus is relatively small in relation to the cranium, which makes up most of the head. The cranium is made up of five bones held together by a membrane which permits their movement during birth and in early childhood. The bones are the two *parietal* bones, the two *frontal* bones and the *occipital* bone (see *Fig. 7.16*). The membranous areas between the bones are called sutures. The *coronal suture* separates the frontal bones from the parietal bones. The *sagittal suture* separates the two parietal bones, and the *lambdoid suture* separates the occipital bone from the parietal bones (*Fig. 7.17*). The *anterior fontanelle* is the diamond-shaped area of the junction of the sagittal and the two coronal sutures. The *posterior fontanelle* is the smaller Y-shaped area at the junction between the sagittal suture and the two lambdoid sutures. The configuration of the posterior fontanelle permits the occipital bone to be displaced under the two parietal bones during childbirth, thus reducing the volume of the fetal skull. This is called *moulding*. During moulding, the parietal bones may also slip under each other (*Fig. 7.18*).

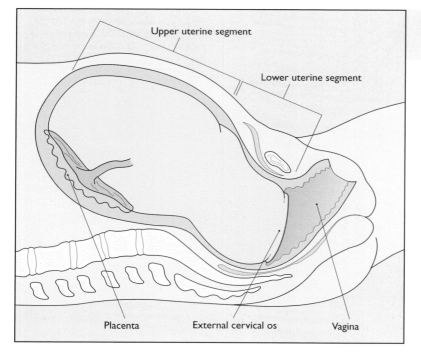

Fig. 7.15 Birth canal of a patient in the second stage of labour.

Upper uterine segment

Lower uterine segment

Placenta External cervical os Vagina

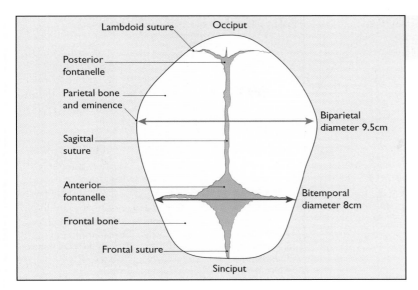

Fig. 7.16 Fetal skull from above – showing important obstetrical diameters.

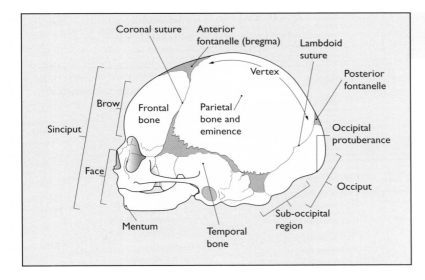

Fig. 7.17 Fetal skull from the side – showing landmarks.

Regions of the fetal skull have been designated to aid in the description of the presenting part felt at vaginal examination during labour. The *occiput* is the area lying behind the posterior fontanelle. The *vertex* is the area of the skull lying between the anterior and posterior fontanelle and between the parietal eminences. The *bregma* is the area around the anterior fontanelle. The *sinciput* is the area lying in front of the anterior fontanelle: this can be divided into two parts, the *brow*, which is the area between the anterior fontanelle and the root of the nose, and the *face*, which is the area below the root of the nose.

The region of the skull which presents in labour depends on the degree of flexion of the head. The diameters are shown in *Figure 7.19*, along with degrees of flexion or deflexion of the head on presentation to the maternal pelvis.

In labour, after the amniotic sac has ruptured releasing amniotic fluid, the dilating cervix may press firmly on the fetal scalp reducing both lymphatic and venous return from the fetal scalp. This may cause a tissue swelling beneath the skin called a *caput succedaneum* (Fig. 7.20). It is soft and boggy to the touch and disappears within a few days of birth.

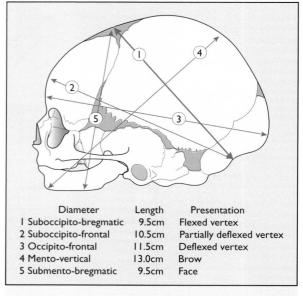

Diameter	Length	Presentation
1 Suboccipito-bregmatic	9.5cm	Flexed vertex
2 Suboccipito-frontal	10.5cm	Partially deflexed vertex
3 Occipito-frontal	11.5cm	Deflexed vertex
4 Mento-vertical	13.0cm	Brow
5 Submento-bregmatic	9.5cm	Face

Fig. 7.19 Diameters of the fetal skull.

Fig. 7.18 Moulding of the fetal skull. (a) Lateral view.
(b) Posterior view. The dotted line shows the shape before
moulding.

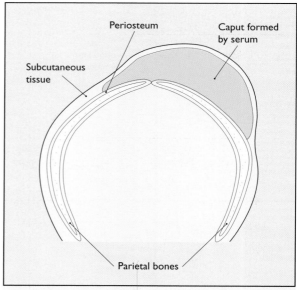

Fig. 7.20 Caput succedaneum.

The powers

The myometrium is formed from interdigitating muscle
fibres of the two Müllerian ducts. The middle parts of the
ducts adhere and the central septum is lost to form a single
hollow organ – the uterus. The myometrium has three
layers:

- An outer longitudinal thin layer.
- A thick middle spiral layer, the size of which diminishes
  towards the cervix and occupies only 10% of the
  cervical tissue.
- A thin circular inner layer. Each muscle fibre is made
  up of bunches of fibrils, which in turn are made up of
  spindle-shaped cells averaging 200mm in length and
  7mm in diameter. These cells are composed of smaller
  contractile fibres comprising interdigitating chains of
  actin and myosin, surrounded by a permeable membrane (Fig. 7.21).

CHARACTERISTICS OF MYOMETRIAL CONTRACTIONS

The uterus, although composed of many individual muscle
fibres, functions as a single hollow muscular organ. The
myometrium is never completely relaxed. It has a resting
tone of between 6 and 12mmHg. From early until late pregnancy the uterus contracts at intervals; the contractions

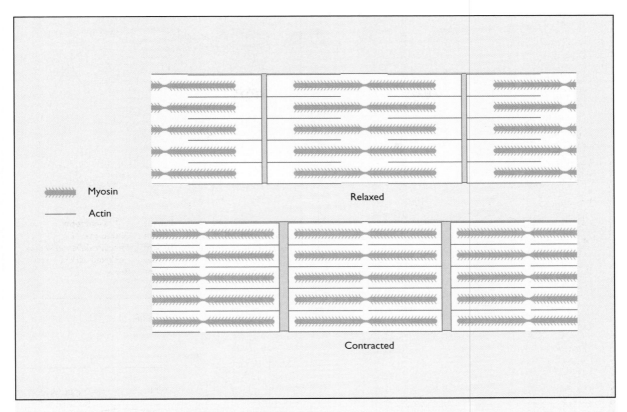

Fig. 7.21 Arrangement of myosin and actin in a muscle fibre.

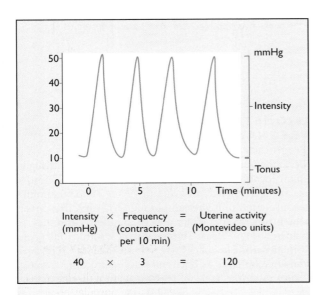

Fig. 7.22 Quantitative measurements of tracings of uterine contractions.

(Braxton Hicks contractions) are painless. Each contraction causes a rise in intra-uterine pressure of varying amplitude or intensity. This has two elements: a rapid rise to a peak and a slower return to the resting tone. For descriptive purposes the intensity of the contraction multiplied by the frequency of the contractions (per 10 minutes) provides a measure of uterine activity, which is expressed in Montevideo Units (Fig. 7.22). With the development of tocography, a different measure of uterine activity can be obtained. With a cardiotocograph linked to a computer, the area under the contraction can be measured and expressed in kilopascals per 15 minutes. These two methods of measuring uterine activity relate fairly closely to each other.

SPREAD OF UTERINE CONTRACTIONS

A uterine contraction starts from a pacemaker located at the junction of the Fallopian tube and the uterus on one side. The contractile wave passes inwards and downwards from the pacemaker at a rate of 2cm per second to involve the entire uterus in the contraction. In a normal labour the intensity and incremental phase of the contraction is greater in the upper uterine segment as the muscle is thicker and

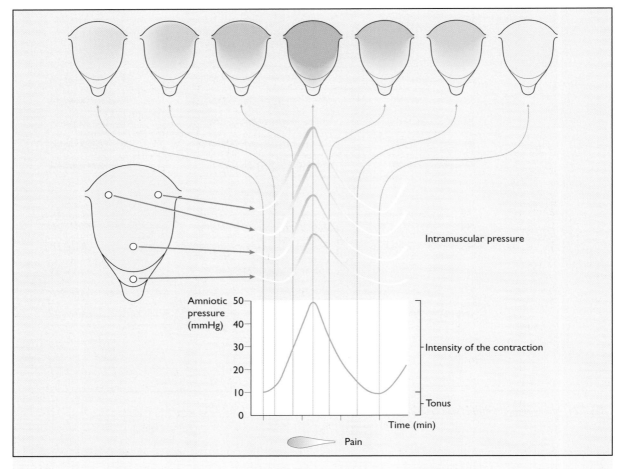

Fig. 7.23 *Normal wave of contraction passing over the uterus shown diagrammatically. The small uteri show how the wave starts and spreads, finally fading. The large uterus shows the four points at which the intramyometrial pressure was recorded with microballoons. The contraction phase is shown by the thick ascending line. Note how the peak of contraction occurs in all parts of the uterus simultaneously.*

there is a greater amount of actinomyosin to contract. This permits the contraction to be coordinated, the maximal intensity occurring in the upper part of the uterus, with a reducing intensity as the wave passes down towards the cervix; the peak of the contraction occurs simultaneously in all parts of the uterus. The phenomenon is known as the *triple descending gradient* (Fig. 7.23).

The intensity and frequency of the uterine contractions varies during labour, increasing as labour progresses. It has been found that uterine activity is greater if the woman walks about during early labour.

MYOMETRIAL ACTIVITY IN PREGNANCY AND LABOUR
Pregnancy
Up to the 30th week of pregnancy uterine activity is slight, small localized contractions of no more than 5mmHg occurring at intervals of 1 minute. Every 30 to 60 minutes a contraction of higher amplitude (10–15mmHg) arises which spreads to a wider area of the uterus and may be palpated (*Fig. 7.24a*). These palpable contractions occur with increasing frequency and intensity after the 30th week and are referred to as Braxton Hicks contractions (see *Fig. 7.24b*). After the 36th week of pregnancy, uterine activity increases progressively until at a point in time labour starts (see *Fig. 7.24c*).

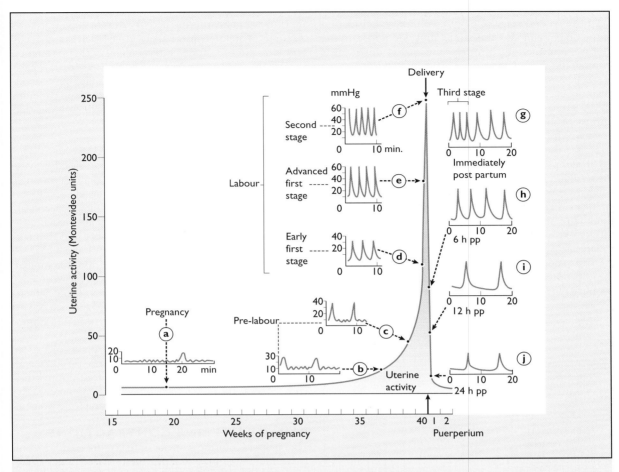

Fig. 7.24 Evolution of uterine activity in pregnancy and labour. For further explanation of a–j see text.

Onset of labour

This is difficult to determine with accuracy, and consequently difficult to define. At the most it can be said to be the time after which uterine contractions cause the progressive dilatation of the cervix beyond 2cm, and painful contractions usually occur at least every 10 minutes (see Fig. 7.24d).

Labour

In true normal labour the intensity and frequency of the contractions increase, but there is no rise in the resting tone. The *intensity* increases in late labour to 60mmHg and the *frequency* to 2–4 contractions every 10 minutes, or 150–200 Montevideo units. The *duration* of the contraction also increases from about 20 seconds in early labour to 40–90 seconds at the end of the first stage, and in the second stage (see *Fig. 7.24e*). Contractions are most effective when they are coordinated, with fundal dominance, have a maximum intensity of 40–60mmHg, last

60–90 seconds, recur with a 2- to 4-minute interval between the peaks of consecutive contractions, and the uterus has a resting tone of less than 12mmHg. More-frequent contractions of higher intensity diminish the oxygen exchange in the placental bed and may lead to fetal hypoxia and clinical signs of fetal distress. The efficiency of contractions is greater when the mother walks about or lies on her side during the first stage of labour, and this position also improves the placental blood supply.

The coordinated contractions of labour cause a permanent shortening of the muscle fibres, and since this is maximal in the upper part of the uterus, a distending tension is placed upon the less muscular lower part, and more particularly upon the scantily muscled cervix. The cervix therefore dilates circumferentially with each contraction, closing in at the end of the contraction; but, because of the retraction of the muscle in the upper uterus, a permanent but slight dilatation occurs with each contraction.

In the second stage of labour, voluntary contraction of the diaphragm and abdominal muscles, added to the uterine contraction, propels the baby downwards through the dilated vagina and overcomes the resistance of perineal muscles to its advance (see *Fig. 7.24f*). At the height of each bearing-down effort the total force exerted on the fetus is approximately 2kg/cm^2 and this is resolved into two components: one, a force propelling the head downwards, and the other, a dilating force, which stretches the birth canal against the resistance of the pelvic and perineal muscles. (If the membranes are intact the resultant propelling force is less, as the amniotic fluid balances it in part.) Since the pelvic floor muscles form an inclined groove, and since the head is ovoid, the additional pressure leads to the rotation of the occiput through 90° to lie anteriorly.

Uterine activity continues unaltered after expulsion of the fetus and leads to the expulsion of the placenta from the upper uterine segment, between 2 and 6 minutes after the birth of the baby. Once the placenta has left the upper uterine segment, uterine activity diminishes, but contractions of an intensity of about 60–80mmHg still occur regularly for 48 hours after delivery, the frequency decreasing as time passes (see *Fig. 7.24g–j*). These contractions, and those of the third stage, are usually painless, but painful contractions disturb some patients. Further painful contractions may occur with suckling, due to a reflex release of oxytocin.

INNERVATION OF THE UTERUS

The sensory nerve fibres from the uterus, together with sensory nerve fibres from the upper vagina, pass through the 'felted' plexus of nerve ganglia which lie adjacent to the lateral aspect of the cervix on each side (the juxtacervical, or Frankenhauser's plexus). The sensory fibres then pass to the hypogastric plexus, and the lumbar and thoracic chains to reach the spinal cord at T11, T12 and T13.

A few sympathetic nerve fibres derive from the lumbar sympathetic nerves. The function of these nerves seems to be limited to regulating vasodilatation. Uterine activity can continue without interruption in the absence of any nerve connection. Whether parasympathetic nerves supply the uterus has not been determined.

Motor nerves to the uterus leave the spinal cord at T6 and T7. They pass through the hypogastric plexuses and the juxtacervical plexus to reach and spread through the entire uterus. The uterus can contract without motor nerve stimulation as occurs in labour among paraplegic women.

PAIN OF UTERINE CONTRACTIONS

The pain of uterine contractions is, in part, due to ischaemia developing in a myometrial fibre. Since there are more fibres and the contractions are stronger in the upper uterine segment, pain is felt more strongly in the cutaneous distribution of cutaneous nerves T12 and L1. At the beginning of the contraction only slight pain is felt; it increases as the contraction grows stronger (*Fig. 7.25*).

Many women in labour complain of backache, which may be severe. It occurs during cervical dilatation when the lower uterine segment contracts more strongly than usual, or when the triple descending gradient fails to arise. In the second stage of labour the pain is due to uterine contractions and to the stretching of the vaginal, the pelvic and the perineal tissues. This pain is felt in the back, in the pelvis and down the thighs.

The perception of pain during labour is increased if the woman is apprehensive and has little knowledge of the process of childbirth. One of the reasons for childbirth training (see pages 50–51) is to reduce fear and improve the mother's understanding of childbirth.

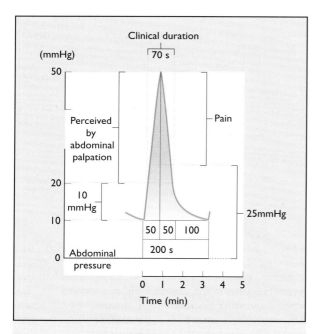

Fig. 7.25 Pain in labour. The initial part of the contraction is painless and not perceived by abdominal palpation. The duration of the contraction observed clinically (70 seconds) is shorter than the duration of myometrial activity (200 seconds).

CHAPTER 8

Physiological changes during childbirth

Labour or childbirth is the process whereby the fetus and placenta are expelled from the uterus by coordinated myometrial contractions. The reason why labour starts remains obscure in spite of much research and many theories. If the information was available, it might be possible to prevent premature labour with its increased perinatal mortality.

Currently the roles of oxytocin and prostaglandins in initiating labour are being explored. There is evidence that in late pregnancy increasing numbers of oxytocin receptors appear in the decidua and myometrial cells. Oxytocin binds to these receptors and induces the release of prostaglandins, particularly PGE_2. Oxytocin may also enhance the passage of calcium ions, which activate actin and myosin to produce contractions of the fibrils. It is also suggested that decidual prolactin is involved in modulating the effects of oxytocin. This remains a theory, and the statement made in 1965, that labour begins 'as the gradual accelerating convergence of a number of factors, structural, humoral, nervous, nutritional and circulatory which, at a specific time in each species, and adapted to morphological conditions present in each, are so associated that they lead to the evacuation of the uterus of its contents', still represents most of our knowledge on the subject.

Effect of childbirth on the mother

ENERGY EXPENDITURE

Labour is appropriately named for it is a period of considerable expenditure of energy, mainly on the contractions of the uterus, but to some extent on increased cardiac activity. The energy is provided initially from metabolism of glycogen from the glycogen–water pool in muscles. In current obstetric practice, women in labour are denied food, and thus the pool is rapidly depleted and energy is obtained by the oxidation of stored body fat. This may lead to the accumulation of ketones in the blood, predominantly D-3-hydroxybutyric acid and to a lesser extent lactic and pyruvic acids. In consequence, a mild metabolic acidosis develops. This is most marked in the expulsive stage of labour when a fall in the blood pH is usual, although the pH remains in the normal range of 7.3–7.4. It is compensated for by a mild respiratory alkalosis, resulting from hyperventilation, which is common during this time. The mild ketoacidosis is of little practical importance, provided that the woman enters labour in a good nutritional condition and the birth occurs in less than 12 hours.

This extra expenditure of energy leads to increased heat production, and sweating occurs with a loss of body fluid.

BODY TEMPERATURE

The body temperature rises slightly during childbirth, but remains lower than 37.8°C, unless the woman becomes ketoacidotic, at which point it may rise above this level.

CARDIOVASCULAR CHANGES

The cardiac output increases by 12% over the prelabour readings between contractions and by 30% during contractions. The increased cardiac output is effected by an increase in stroke volume and heart rate. The mean arterial pressure rises by about 10% and, in the expulsive stage of labour, the rise may be greater. These changes further increase cardiac work in response to a uterine contraction. The right atrial pressure rises and may reach 40–50mmHg in late labour, and the cardiopulmonary blood volume increases at the same time. Following the birth a further rise in cardiac output occurs. Since bradycardia is usual at this time, the rise is due to an increase in stroke volume. The effect lasts for 3–4 days.

For these reasons childbirth may pose a hazard to a woman who has uncompensated heart disease or who is severely anaemic.

GASTROINTESTINAL TRACT

In labour gastric emptying is delayed and partly digested food may remain in the stomach for more than 12 hours. Intestinal motility is also delayed.

TRAUMA TO THE TISSUES

Vaginal birth is always associated with some lacerations of the cervix, which usually cause no problems, the round cervical os becoming a slit. In some cases the damage is greater (see Chapter 24, Disorders in the puerperium). The vagina may suffer lacerations and the perineum is often torn, particularly among primigravidae; for these reasons an episiotomy may be deliberately made.

Because of damage to the pubococcygeal muscle by the pressure of the fetus in late labour, retention of urine may occur after delivery.

BLOOD LOSS DURING CHILDBIRTH

Clinical estimates of blood loss during childbirth show that a mean of 400ml is lost. This may be an underestimate. In a healthy woman this loss is of no clinical significance, as it is less than the increase in blood volume which occurs in pregnancy.

Effect of childbirth on the fetus

The entry of a child into the world is not gentle. Unlike other mammals, humans have developed a large head which has to traverse a relatively small bony birth canal, propelled by uterine contractions. During a contraction the uterus exerts a force on the fetus of $1kg/cm^2$ and during the expulsive stage the force doubles when voluntary expulsive efforts are added to the uterine contractions.

The effect of this force is mainly on the fetal head and so moulding of the fetal skull may occur. Normally the baby is unharmed, but if moulding is great because of cephalo-pelvic disproportion, an inexpert delivery of the baby by forceps or vacuum extraction may lead to intracranial oedema or damage.

During childbirth the fetus suffers some degree of hypoxia. If the fetus has obtained a good supply of glucose during pregnancy the hypoxia causes few problems. But if the fetus is growth restricted because of insufficient supplies of nutrients from the mother it may enter labour with diminished glycogen reserves and may be unable to compensate for the reduction of glucose and oxygen during an abnormal or prolonged labour. This means that it may have to use anaerobic methods of obtaining energy, with resulting fetal acidaemia, which may affect the fetal heart rate as it attempts to compensate for the relative hypoxia. The fetal heart rate is the result of a balance between the tachycardia produced by sympathetic nerve stimulation and the bradycardia produced by vagal nerve stimulation. Normally, the vagus is dominant and exerts a slowing effect on the fetal heart, which beats at a rate of 140 ± 20 times per minute. If fetal hypoxia occurs, the altered composition of the blood leads to a rise in sympathetic and vagal tones, which differ in effect. The sympathetic effect becomes dominant in mild hypoxia. Its onset is delayed, but if the hypoxia persists it leads to fetal tachycardia. This persists for 10–30 minutes after the cause of the hypoxia has ceased. Vagal stimulation occurs if hypoxia is moderate or severe in degree. Bradycardia occurs rapidly, lasts as long as the hypoxia and then resolves rapidly.

CHAPTER 9

Course and management of childbirth

Choices in childbirth

In most developed countries nearly all women give birth in hospital. In contrast, in the developing countries, particularly in the rural areas where 75% of the population live, most women have their babies at home. Health authorities attempt to select those women who would be more safely delivered in hospital and arrange for the transfer of other women to hospital should problems arise. To attend to emergencies occurring at home births, 'obstetric flying squads' are set up. The flying squad consists of an ambulance staffed by a doctor and nurse–midwife and is equipped to deal with haemorrhage, delay in birth and resuscitation of the newborn.

With the almost universal trend towards hospital birth in the developed countries, some groups of women are questioning if this is always appropriate, claiming that on admission to hospital a pregnant woman loses her autonomy, often is not told about proposed procedures, and may be treated impersonally by busy attending staff. In other words, childbirth has been medicalized. Some women want a return to home births, despite potential dangers; others seek birth in a hospital-based, but home birth oriented, birth centre; others accept the benefits of a hospital birth, but want some of the attitudes of the attending staff and some of the procedures changed.

Several international organizations have addressed these issues and have made recommendations, which are paraphrased as follows:

- A pregnant woman should have access to a family member during labour and childbirth, who will remain with her throughout the process if she wishes and if the doctor in charge agrees.
- A pregnant woman should participate in decisions regarding the birth experience, and the need for procedures (including episiotomy). The techniques involved should be explained to her.
- Routine pubic and perineal shaving and routine enema should be abandoned.
- Induction of labour by amniotomy or use of prostaglandins should be undertaken only on strictly medical grounds. Routine rupture of the amniotic sac early in labour is not justified.
- Analgesia and anaesthesia should be provided at the patient's request.
- During labour the pregnant woman should be able to walk about, lie, squat or sit to find the position most comfortable for her, unless medical reasons demand that she remain in bed. In this case she should be able to recline. The dorsal lithotomy position during delivery should only be adopted if a forceps delivery or other operative procedure is needed.
- The mother and the baby should have facilities for 'rooming-in'.
- Breastfeeding should be encouraged and the mother should have immediate access to her newborn baby, when this is practicable.

The criticisms advanced by women's groups have had an effect on obstetric practice and choices in childbirth are now provided in many places. These choices are:

- Prepared participatory childbirth.
- Conventional childbirth.
- Actively managed childbirth.
- Elective caesarean section.
- Home birth.

PREPARED PARTICIPATORY CHILDBIRTH

In this approach the parents undertake childbirth training, learning about the processes of childbirth and how to accept the pains of uterine contractions. This has been discussed on pages 50–51. Labour is managed by trained staff, and the principles mentioned earlier are observed by staff and patients. The birth takes place in a quiet environment and the baby is given to the mother at once so that she may offer suckling and celebrate the birth.

Women can have a prepared participatory childbirth in a normal hospital delivery room, but for some it is more satisfactory if there is a birthing centre.

Birthing centre

A birthing centre is usually attached to a hospital so that the patient can be transferred thereto or treated by an experienced obstetrician should complications arise. An individual suite in a birthing centre is furnished like a bedroom, containing a firm double bed, chairs and furnishings, with the necessary equipment for medical care and infant resuscitation discreetly hidden. The father of the child or a significant other person remains with the woman in labour, providing support. The woman may have hired her own nurse–midwife (accredited by the hospital) or is looked after by a hospital nurse–midwife or a doctor. After the birth the baby remains with its parents so that bonding and celebration may take place. Early discharge is usual and the mother is followed up at home by district nurse–midwives. Experience with established birthing centres shows that women choosing this form of childbirth require fewer inductions of labour, and less analgesia, and have a greater number of spontaneous deliveries, fewer episiotomies and fewer hypoxic babies than do women delivering in conventional delivery units.

They are carefully selected, of course. About 5% of women choosing a birthing centre require medical intervention, and most are transferred to the delivery floor.

CONVENTIONAL CHILDBIRTH

The woman gives birth in a delivery suite. She is generally content to leave the process of childbirth to be managed by the attending staff, and accepts their decisions about management. Although her partner is often present, he or a significant other person may not always be in attendance. She is cared for with skill and does not participate overmuch in the process of childbirth.

ACTIVELY MANAGED CHILDBIRTH

The development of the partogram and the appreciation that most women have delivered within 12 hours of admission to hospital has led to another approach; actively managed labour.

On admission to the delivery unit, the diagnosis of labour is either confirmed or rejected. If the woman is in labour, the time of admission is designated as the start of labour. A partogram is started and the progress of labour is marked on it (Fig. 9.1). Vaginal examinations are made every 2 hours and the cervical dilatation is recorded on the partogram. Action lines, printed on transparent plastic, are superimposed on the partogram (Fig. 9.2). In the active stage of labour the slowest acceptable rate of cervical dilatation is 1cm/h. If the cervical dilatation lies to the right of the appropriate action line, the membranes are ruptured and an incremental dilute oxytocin infusion is established in nulliparous women (and some multiparous women), provided that a single fetus presents as a vertex and there are no signs of fetal distress. If the first stage of labour lasts longer than 10 hours a caesarean section is performed.

Progress in the second stage of labour is judged by the descent of the fetal head and its rotation. One hour is allowed for the fetal head to reach the pelvic floor (the first phase) and a further hour for the birth to be completed (the second phase). If these targets are not met, either a caesarean section is performed (in phase 1) or a forceps delivery is attempted.

Proponents of actively managed labour claim that the incidence of a labour lasting more than 12 hours is less then 3%; the caesarean section rate is 7–12% and the forceps rate is 8%. Opponents point out that only three randomized studies have been carried out and that in these studies, there was no reduction in the caesarean section or forceps rate.

ELECTIVE CAESAREAN SECTION

A small number of women, particularly over the age of 35 years, inform their obstetrician during pregnancy that they wish to be delivered by caesarean section. The obstetrician should listen to the woman and discuss the effects of the procedure. If the woman confirms that she wishes to be delivered by caesarean section, the obstetrician should agree to her wish.

HOME BIRTH

A few women elect to be delivered at home arguing that as childbirth is a normal phenomenon, the home environment is more appropriate. Women choosing this type of delivery must receive good prenatal care; must be screened for any medical or obstetrical abnormality; must accept transferral to a hospital if an abnormality arises during pregnancy or childbirth; must have a named midwife; and must have a family doctor, trained in obstetrics, who is available should an emergency arise. Even then home birth is less safe than giving birth in a midwife-controlled birthing centre.

Onset of labour

In the weeks before labour starts, the painless uterine contractions which have been becoming increasingly frequent merge into a prodromal stage of labour which may last up to 4 weeks.

During this time the lower uterine segment expands to take the fetal head, which enters the upper pelvis. This relieves the pressure on the upper part of the abdomen ('lightening') but increases the pressure in the pelvis. Consequently constipation and urinary frequency become apparent, and some patients complain of increased pressure in the pelvis and an increased mucoid vaginal discharge.

FALSE LABOUR

As term approaches, many women complain of painful uterine contractions, which may seem to indicate the onset of labour. However, despite the contractions, progressive dilatation of the cervix fails to occur – this condition is termed *false labour*.

In it, the triple descending gradient of uterine activity fails to become established. A reverse gradient of uterine activity is present, the lower part of the uterus contracting nearly as strongly as the upper part. Because of this, cervical dilatation fails to occur and the pain of the uterine contractions is often felt as low backache.

Clinically, the painful contractions occur more often at night, but their frequency and intensity do not increase as time passes. A woman who complains of this pattern of uterine activity needs an explanation and, if the pains are distressing, requires treatment with analgesics, and perhaps a hypnotic so that she may enjoy a good night's sleep.

Often the pains of false labour recur on a number of days and, in some cases, the reverse gradient of activity changes and true labour starts.

ONSET OF TRUE LABOUR

True labour may start and progress rapidly, or the start may be slow, with contractions only occurring at long intervals, the so-called sluggish uterus, or, in a more modern idiom, prolongation of the quiet (latent) phase of labour.

If the woman is becoming distressed that labour is not progressing, a more effective pattern of uterine activity can be obtained by performing an amniotomy and by starting an intravenous infusion of oxytocin. This regimen should only

Fig. 9.1 A partogram.

be instituted if there is no cephalopelvic disproportion and if the cervix is partly or wholly effaced, 2cm dilated and soft.

The onset of labour is difficult to time with any degree of accuracy, and may be heralded by the following signs:

1. The false labour pains may become coordinate and regular, or painful contractions may alert the patient that labour has started.
2. A discharge of mucus mixed with some blood may occur. This is due to the effacement and dilatation of the cervix, allowing the 'plug' which previously filled it to be released. The blood comes from minute lacerations in the cervical mucosa. The passage of the mucus and blood is known as the 'show'.

The transition into labour is gradual, but labour may be said to have begun when the cervix is at least 2cm dilated and contractions become painful and regular with diminishing intervals between each contraction.

Because of the difficulty in establishing the time of onset of labour with any degree of accuracy, many obstetricians mark its onset from the time the woman is admitted to hospital. This has advantages if the graphic method of recording the progress of labour (the partogram) is adopted.

DURATION OF LABOUR

The duration of labour is not easy to determine precisely as its onset is often indefinite and subjective. In studies of informed women, whose labour started spontaneously, there was a wide variation in the duration of labour as can be seen in *Figure 9.3*.

Labour is usually shorter when the patient knows something of the physiology of normal labour, is in good health at the onset of labour, has confidence in her attendants and is mentally well adjusted.

Several factors influence the duration of labour. These include the age of the woman, her parity, her knowledge of the process of childbirth, and the size of the fetus and its position in the uterus. Labour seems to last longer among nulliparous women, particularly older primigravidae, and if the baby presents in the occipito-posterior position.

Delivery with 16 hours may be expected in 90% of nulliparous women (para 0) and the same proportion of multiparous women (para 1+) will deliver within 12 hours.

Progress and management of labour and birth

The management of labour begins when the woman seeks admission to hospital, which she does when she believes or knows that she is in labour. As labour is a time of anxiety and stress, the attitude of the member of staff who admits her is most important. The care of the woman during her labour and childbirth may be conducted by a midwife (see also page 71), or by midwives in partnership with an obstetrician or a general practitioner.

ADMISSION

On admission the woman may be offered a shower. During the time she takes it, her antenatal records are obtained and scrutinized for any past medical or obstetrical problems, to check the history of the current pregnancy and to make sure that the appropriate laboratory tests have been made. Pudendal shaving is no longer performed, but the hairs surrounding the vaginal entrance may be trimmed.

During these procedures the history of the present labour is obtained, the frequency and strength of the uterine contractions are noted, and information is obtained about a 'show' of blood or mucus and whether or not the membranes have broken.

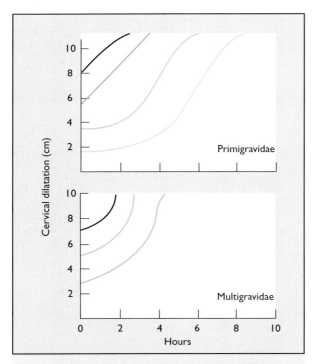

Fig. 9.2 Action lines for the partogram (Studd stencil). The lines show the slowest acceptable rate of cervical dilatation commencing with the degree of dilatation on admission to the delivery unit

Fig. 9.3 Duration (and range) of labour (in hours)		
	Nulliparae	**Multiparae**
1st Stage	8.25 (2–12)	5.5 (1–9)
2nd Stage	1 (0.25–1.5)	0.25 (0–0.75)
3rd Stage	0.25 (0–1)	0.25 (0–0.5)
	9.5 (2.25–14)	6 (1–10.25)

A general examination is made by a nurse–midwife or a doctor, the blood pressure, pulse and temperature being recorded. The abdomen is palpated to determine the presentation of the fetus and the position of the presenting part in relation to the pelvic brim (see *Fig. 6.24*, page 49).

A vaginal examination is made, with aseptic precautions, to determine the effacement and dilatation of the cervix and the position and station of the presenting part. The *station* of the presenting part is the level of the lowest fetal bony part (head or breech) in relation to an imaginary line joining the mother's ischial spines. It is measured in centimetres above or below the ischial spines (*Fig. 9.4*). If the amniotic sac (the membranes) has ruptured this is noted. It has recently been recommended, especially for developing nations, that during the vaginal examination done on admission, the midwife covers her sterile gloved examining finger with a solution of 0.25% chlorhexidine. This has been shown to reduce perinatal infection.

In many obstetric units a 20-minute cardiotocogram (CTG) is made on admission to establish that the fetus is not at obvious risk of becoming distressed during labour. The woman is transferred from the admission room to a bed in a delivery room (if she has not already been admitted to it) and a partogram is started, which shows the progress of labour at a glance.

FIRST STAGE OF LABOUR

The first stage of labour begins, as mentioned earlier, at an imprecise time. For convenience labour is estimated to start when the patient says that the pains are becoming regular, or on her admission to hospital when the signs of labour are evident. It ends with the full dilatation of the cervix.

At the beginning of the first stage of labour the fetal presenting part (usually it is the head, so this will be used in the rest of this chapter in place of the presenting part) has descended into the true pelvis to some extent. In a normally shaped pelvis the position of the occiput is in the transverse diameter of the pelvis in 75% of cases, in the oblique in 14% of cases, in the direct anterior position in 3% of cases and in a posterior diameter in 8% of cases (*Fig. 9.5*).

The first stage of labour can be divided into a latent (quiet) phase and an active phase. In the early part of the latent phase the uterine contractions are relatively painless, occur at intervals of 5–10 minutes and they do not usually distress the patient. As the latent phase progresses the contractions become stronger and more frequent but dilatation of the cervix is relatively slow. Towards the end of the phase the membranes may rupture spontaneously.

The active phase starts when the cervix is 3–4cm dilated. The cervix dilates more rapidly in the active phase and the process is considered to be normal if it dilates at a rate of 0.5–1.0cm/h. Towards the end of the active phase, when the cervix is 9cm dilated, many women complain of very painful contractions and may have a desire to push. As it is unwise to push at this stage, a vaginal examination should be made to establish whether the cervix is fully dilated.

The duration of the latent and active phases is shown in *Figure 9.6*. If they last for more than 12 hours in a nulliparous woman, or more than 9 hours in a multiparous woman, the cause should be investigated (see Chapter 22, Abnormal fetal presentations).

During the active part of the first stage of labour, the fetal head descends more deeply into the maternal pelvis and flexes (*Figs 9.7–9.9*).

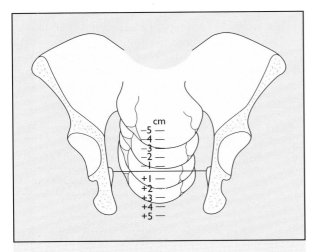

Fig.9.4 Station of the head.

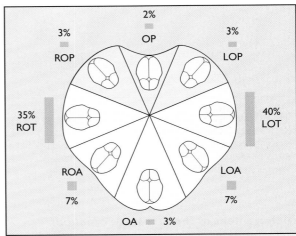

Fig. 9.5 The positions of the vertex at the onset of labour and their relative frequency; the shaded positions are associated with a more difficult labour and delivery. OP, occipito posterior; OT, occipito transverse; OA, occipito anterior.

Fig. 9.6 The phases of labour.

Fig. 9.7 Late pregnancy. The fetal head has engaged in the transverse diameter of the pelvic brim, and some flexion of the head on the chest has occurred. The cervix is soft but is not yet effaced and the amniotic membranes are intact.

Fig. 9.8 Early labour. There has been further flexion of the fetal head, and it has moved more deeply into the true pelvis, causing pressure on the bladder and rectum. The cervix has become effaced but has not yet begun to dilate and the membranes are intact.

Fig 9.9 Late first stage of labour. The cervix is now 7cm dilated and further flexion of the fetal head has occurred. The membranes are still intact.

Management of the first stage of labour

The patient should be made as comfortable as possible and should choose whether she prefers to remain in bed, walk about, sit on a chair and so on. If there is a common room on the delivery floor she may prefer to go there to be with other women. If the head has not descended into the pelvis, she should remain in bed, but should be propped up on pillows with a back rest so that the full weight of her uterus does not press on the descending aorta and inferior vena cava, impeding the flow of blood to the uterus and its return to the heart.

It is customary to withhold solid food during labour as the contents of the stomach remain therein, and if a general anaesthetic is required for a forceps or a caesarean delivery, the acid stomach contents may be regurgitated and inhaled causing Mendelson's syndrome. Today, few inhalational anaesthetics are given during childbirth and it is known that fasting does not reduce the acidity of the stomach contents. There seems no good reason why a woman at low risk of an operative procedure requiring general anaesthesia should not be permitted, if she wishes, to eat a low-residue, low-fat diet (such as tea, fruit juice, toast, lightly cooked eggs or biscuits). Food eaten during labour may reduce the chance of maternal ketoacidosis.

Obstetricians who believe that oral feeding should be withheld once labour has been established usually set up an intravenous infusion. It is now generally agreed that intravenous infusions are not required in the first 12 hours of labour, regardless of the presence of ketosis. The patient's lips can be kept moist and she may suck ice. If intravenous fluids are deemed necessary the amount should not exceed 1500ml in 12 hours, and normal saline (500ml) should alternate with Hartmann's solution (500ml). Glucose infusions providing more than 25g of glucose during labour should be avoided as they may cause fetal hyperinsulinaemia and neonatal hypoglycaemia.

Specific care in the first stage
The following steps should be followed:
- Support and comfort the patient and inform her about the progress of labour.
- Complete the partogram:
  1. Check pulse, temperature and blood pressure every 2 hours.
  2. Monitor the frequency, strength and intensity of the uterine contractions.
  3. Monitor the fetal heart rate once active labour has started, every 15 minutes in the first stage and every 5 minutes in the second stage of labour. The normal variation is 120–160bpm. If the rate remains below 100bpm between contractions and, particularly if meconium is passed, 'fetal distress' may be imminent and the situation should be assessed (see Chapter 21, The at-risk fetus). Although the fetal heart is usually monitored between contractions, a more informative way is to auscultate the heart immediately after a contraction. In some hospitals continuous fetal heart monitoring is practised using a transabdominal transducer.
  4. When labour has been established, perform a vaginal examination every 4 hours to determine the dilatation of the cervix and the descent of the fetal head (or breech).
  5. Discuss with the patient her need for analgesics or epidural anaesthesia (see pages 87–88).
- Determine the position of the head, in relation to the maternal pelvis, dividing the pelvis into 45° segments. Right refers to the right side of the woman, left to her left side. If the vertex presents, the occiput is the point of reference; if the breech presents, the sacrum is the point of reference; if the face presents, the chin is the point of reference. In *Figure 9.5* the positions and frequency of vertex presentations are shown.

SECOND STAGE OF LABOUR
The second stage of labour begins when the cervix is fully dilated, to complete the formation of the curved birth canal, and ends with the birth of the baby. The second stage of labour is the expulsive stage during which the fetus is forced through the birth canal. The uterine contractions become more frequent, recurring at 2–5 minute intervals and are stronger, lasting 60–90 seconds. The fetal head descends deeply into the pelvis, and, reaching the gutter-shaped pelvic floor, rotates anteriorly (internal rotation) so that the occiput lies behind the symphysis pubis (Fig. 9.10). Anterior rotation occurs in 98% of cases, though in 2% of cases the head rotates posteriorly with the result that the occiput lies in front of the sacrum.

The uterine contractions are now supplemented by voluntary muscle contractions. Simultaneously with the uterine contraction, the patient holds her breath, closes her glottis, braces her feet, and, taking a breath, holds it, grunts and contracts her diaphragm and her abdominal muscles, to force the fetus lower in her pelvis. The energy expended causes her pulse to rise, and she sweats. As the uterine contraction diminishes and ceases, she relaxes and often dozes.

As the fetal head is pushed deeper into the pelvis the patient may complain of intense pressure on her rectum or pains radiating down her legs, due to pressure on the sacral nerve plexus or obturator nerve. Some 15 minutes later the anus begins to open, exposing its anterior wall, and the head can be seen inside the vagina. With each contraction the fetal head becomes a little more visible, retreating a little between contractions but advancing slightly all the time (Fig. 9.11).

The head now presses on the posterior wall of the lower vagina and the perineum becomes thinner and stretched, its skin tense and shining. The woman complains of a 'bursting' feeling and a desire to push even without a uterine contraction. Soon a large part of the head can be seen between the stretched labia, and the parietal bosses become visible. The further sequence of the birth is shown in *Figures 9.12* and *9.13* and is now described. With an extra effort the baby's head is born, extending at the neck so that the forehead, the nose, the mouth and the chin appear in sequence. Mucus streams from the baby's mouth and nose. After a short pause, the head rotates into a transverse diameter (external rotation). This brings the shoulders into the anterior-posterior diameter of the lower pelvis. The shoulders are born next, the anterior shoulder stemming from behind the symphysis and the posterior shoulder rolling over the perineum, followed by the baby's trunk and legs. The baby gasps once or twice and cries vigorously. The uterus contracts to a size found at 20 weeks' gestation.

Management of the second stage of labour

In the second stage of labour the active cooperation of the expectant mother is needed, to add the voluntary muscle contractions of her diaphragm and abdominal muscles to the involuntary uterine contractions, which together increase the downward pressure on the fetus. As the contractions are very painful, the woman may need more analgesics, or if she has had an epidural anaesthetic it may need 'topping up'. Some women find relief by back massage or by moving into another position, including sitting up.

Throughout the second stage of labour a medical attendant (plus/minus the partner) should be present helping and encouraging the woman to bear down with each uterine contraction and to relax in between. As there is much energy expenditure, sweating usually occurs and the patient will feel more comfortable if she can have cool face cloths to wipe away the sweat.

During the second stage of labour most women prefer to recline on a bed at 45° to the horizontal, supported, if the woman wishes, by her partner. Some women choose to sit up, squat or kneel until the baby's head is visible at the vulva.

The actual birth of the baby is easier to manage if the woman is reclining on a bed, but there is no justification for putting her legs in stirrups.

The woman's contractions are recorded and the fetal heart is auscultated every 5 minutes. If the fetal heart falls below 100bpm, and the bradycardia persists for more than 2 minutes, action should be taken to determine the cause. This will include a vaginal examination to make sure that the umbilical cord has not prolapsed. The position of the patient should be changed as this may affect the fetal heart rate.

Traditionally, the second stage of labour is terminated by vacuum extraction or forceps if it has lasted 2 or more hours. If women have an epidural analgesic the second stage may be prolonged to 3 hours without any increased risk to the fetus, if the woman wishes to have a 'natural' birth and there are no significant fetal heart rate abnormalities.

Birth of the baby

HEAD

As the fetal head (for this is the usual presenting part) becomes visible between the labia, the woman should be prepared for the birth. With each contraction the patient pushes and the fetal head becomes more visible, retracting

Fig. 9.10 Early second stage. The cervix is fully dilated and the head is beginning to rotate at the level of the ischial spines. Rotation is through 90°, so that the occiput lies in the anterior segment of the pelvis and the sagittal suture of the fetal head in the anterior-posterior diameter of the pelvis. The membranes are intact and bulge in front of the head.

Fig. 9.11 Late second stage. The head is broaching the vulval ring 'crowning'. The membranes have ruptured, and the perineum is stretched over the head.

Fig. 9.12 Birth of the head. As the fetal head is pushed through the vulval ring it extends on the neck, and the perineum is swept over the face. The direction of movement of the head is now upwards. The uterus has retracted to fit closely over the fetal body. The shoulders are still in the transverse diameter of the midpelvis.

slightly between contractions. When the area of the visible head has increased to 5cm, and the perineum is thin and distended, the vulva should be swabbed with chlorhexidine (1:1000). The medical attendant who will deliver the baby now scrubs up and puts on gloves and gown. With each contraction, the fetal head is flexed by the index finger of one of the attendant's hands, whilst the perineum is 'protected' by a pad which covers the perineum and the distended anus and is held in the attendant's other hand. In some cases the perineum tears in spite of the protection; in others a deliberate incision (an episiotomy) is made to avoid the perineum tearing. This is discussed later.

The manoeuvres described permit the head to be born slowly, until the parietal bosses are visible (when the head is said to be 'crowned'). The mother now ceases to push with the contractions unless asked to do so by the medical attendant. Instead she is asked to pant during each painful contraction.

To be born the fetal head now has to extend, and this is aided by the attendant's left hand keeping the head flexed and the right hand holding the perineal pad pushing the chin upwards. The forehead, nose, mouth and chin emerge and the head is born, the perineum being pressed back behind the chin. The baby's eyes are swabbed with sterile water and the baby's head is rotated (or rotates itself) through 90°. The attendant now puts a finger inside the woman's vagina to feel if the umbilical cord is around the baby's neck. If it is, a loop of the cord is brought down.

Fig. 9.13 Birth of the head. A sequence showing the progressive distension of the perineum by the head, which extends on the neck as it is born. The perineum sweeps over the forehead, face and chin. Once the head is born it drops slightly and then restitution (external rotation) occurs.

SHOULDERS

As the baby's head rotates, mucus streams from its mouth and nose. With the next contraction, the rotated head is grasped gently between the attendant's two hands, which are placed over the side of the head, and the head is drawn posteriorly so that the anterior shoulder is released from behind the pubic bones (*Fig. 9.14*). Following the birth of the anterior shoulder, the baby is swept upwards in an arc to release the posterior shoulder, followed by the body and the legs (*Fig. 9.15*).

The mother should now be able to see and touch her baby. The baby is then laid between the mother's legs and, if necessary, its mouth and fauces are sucked clear using a suction apparatus or a soft tube and bulb. The baby is placed between the mother's legs so that it is below the level of the placenta and its circulation will receive an additional 60ml of blood as it drains from the placenta. One-third of this amount is received in the first 30 seconds after the birth and the remainder in the next 2–3 minutes. In normal cases (where the baby is not hypoxic) the attendant should not clamp, divide and tie the umbilical cord for about 2–3 minutes.

The Newborn baby

The neonate lies between its mother's legs, usually taking its first breath within seconds, and starting to cry and to move its arms and legs. It is checked for good respiratory effort and its colour and its alertness. Either an Apgar score is taken (*Fig. 9.16*) or the Basic Resuscitation Programme suggested in the UK is adopted (*Fig. 9.17*). Most babies establish respirations easily and quickly, but a few are born in a mild or severe hypoxic state. This problem is discussed further in Chapter 22, Abnormal fetal presentations. The baby is checked for gross malformations. It is then given to the mother for cuddling and suckling. This early mother–baby contact encourages (but is not essential for) bonding, and if the baby is put to the breast this helps to 'bring in' the milk.

Two other issues need discussion. These are the use of prophylactic eye drops to prevent gonococcal ophthalmic infection and the routine use of vitamin K.

PROPHYLACTIC EYE DROPS

There is no indication for the routine use of prophylactic eye drops or ointment as gonorrhoea is uncommon. In selected cases, tetracycline 1% eye ointment is the treatment of choice.

VITAMIN K

Most neonates develop vitamin K deficiency by the third day of life. This predisposes the baby to a bleeding diathesis (haemorrhagic disease of the newborn) caused by the depression of clotting factors II, VII, IX and X. The baby may bleed from the gastrointestinal tract, the umbilical cord or from skin punctures. A late onset variety of vitamin K deficiency may affect breastfed babies between 4 and 6 weeks after birth. It manifests as gastrointestinal bleeding or intracranial haemorrhage. To prevent these possible problems it is currently recommended that all

Fig. 9.14 Birth of the anterior shoulder. With the birth of the head the shoulders reach the pelvic floor and, directed by the levator 'gutter', rotate to lie in the antero-posterior diameter of the pelvic outlet. The head therefore rotates externally, or undergoes 'restitution' to its position at the onset of labour. The anterior shoulder (in this case the right one) is appearing from behind the symphysis. The birth of the shoulder is aided by downward and backward traction of the head by the accoucheur.

Fig. 9.15 The birth of the posterior shoulder. The accoucheur aids the birth by lifting the head gently upwards whilst maintaining traction. This prevents damage to the perineum.

newborn babies should be given phytomenadione (vitamin K₁) either 1.0mg intramuscularly at birth or 1.0mg orally at birth, at 3–4 days and at 6 weeks of age. The further care of the newborn infant is described in Chapter 10, The puerperium.

Third stage of labour

The third stage of labour extends from the birth of the baby to the expulsion of the placenta and membranes.

Separation of the placenta takes place through the spongy layer of the decidua basalis, as the result of uterine contractions being added to the retraction of the uterus which follows the birth of the child. The retraction of the uterus reduces the size of the placental bed to one-quarter of its size in pregnancy, with the result that the placenta buckles inwards, tearing the blood vessels of the inter-villous space, and causing a retroplacental haemorrhage, which further separates the placenta. The process starts as the baby is born and placental separation is usually complete within 5 minutes, but the placenta may be held in the uterus for longer because the membranes take longer to strip from the underlying decidua. Following the separation of the placenta, the lattice arrangements of the myometrial fibres effectively strangle the blood vessels supplying the placental bed, reducing further blood loss and encouraging the formation of fibrin plugs in their torn ends (Fig. 9.18).

MANAGEMENT OF THE THIRD STAGE OF LABOUR

There are two methods of managing the third stage of labour:
- Traditional management.
- Active management.

Traditional management

The placenta and membranes are allowed to separate without interference. The ulnar border of one hand is placed in the uterine fundus, and the signs of placental separation are awaited. These are:
- A gush of blood.
- The fundus rises in the abdomen and becomes spherical.
- That part of the umbilical cord which can be seen at the vulva, lengthens.
- If the fundus is lifted upwards the umbilical cord does not shorten.

Ten to twenty minutes pass before these signs appear. No attempt is made to hasten the separation, by 'fiddling' with the fundus, for example, unless haemorrhage demands action. Once the signs indicate that the placenta has been expelled from the uterus and is lying in the vagina, a uterine contraction is obtained by 'rubbing up' the uterus. The contracted uterus is pushed down towards the pelvis, so that it acts as a piston to expel the placenta and membranes from the vagina. The expelled placenta is grasped and twisted around with continuing traction to make the membranes into a twisted cord and so that they are expelled intact.

Active management

As the fetal head is being born, an intramuscular injection of Syntometrine 0.5ml or of Syntocinon 10IU is given. If the woman is hypertensive, Syntometrine is avoided as the ergometrine content may increase the hypertension. In this case an intravenous injection of Syntocinon 10IU is given with the birth of the anterior shoulder of the baby.

The delivery of the baby following the injection is conducted slowly over 60 seconds. The umbilical cord is

Sign	0	1	2
Colour	Blue; pale	Body pink; extremities blue	Completely pink
Respiratory effort	Absent	Weak cry; hypoventilation	Good; strong cry
Muscle tone	Limp	Some flexion of extremities	Active motion; extremities well flexed
Reflex irritability (response to stimulation of sole of foot)	No response	Grimace	Cry
Heart rate	Absent	Slow (below 100)	Fast (over 100)

Fig. 9.16 Apgar scoring method for evaluating the infant

Fig. 9.17 Basic resuscitation of the newborn.

Fig. 9.18 *The uterine muscle forms a 'living ligature' to occlude blood vessels.*

Fig. 9.19 *Controlled cord traction.*

divided and clamped 2 minutes after the birth. The slowness is because the oxytocic effect takes about 2 minutes to produce a strong uterine contraction. The attendant's left hand is placed on the uterus to detect the contraction. When it occurs, the hand is placed suprapubically and pushes the uterus upwards, whilst the right hand grasps the umbilical cord and pulls the placenta out of the vagina in a controlled manner (*Fig. 9.19*). The membranes are drawn out of the vagina intact by twisting them into a rope and pulling them out with a sponge forceps or the hand. In 1–2% of cases the placenta is retained, but no blood loss occurs. After a 10-minute delay another attempt is made to pull the placenta out by controlled cord traction. If this fails, manual removal of the placenta is necessary (see page 188). This is a disadvantage of the active management of the third stage of labour. The advantages of active management are that postpartum haemorrhage (a loss of more than 500ml of blood) is reduced from 4% to 2% of all deliveries and the third stage of labour is shortened.

INSPECTION OF THE PLACENTA AND MEMBRANES

The placenta and membranes are held up by the umbilical cord and the fetal surface is examined, attention being paid to the blood vessels to see if any run to the edge of the membranes, indicating a possible succenturiate lobe. The membranes are examined to make sure that no part remains in the uterus. The maternal surface of the placenta is examined next, any clots being washed away, so that the cotyledons can be inspected. The maternal surface is held in both hands and fitted together to make sure that no cotyledon has been left in the uterus. If any cotyledon is missing or if most of the membranes have been left in the uterus or vagina, a doctor should explore the vagina and the uterine cavity under sterile conditions.

Retained placenta

A retained placenta is one which has remained in the uterus for more than 1 hour. As a retained placenta may be associated with haemorrhage, action should be taken to remove it. The causes of a retained placenta are:

- Incarceration of a separated or partially separated placenta when, following the injection of an oxytocic drug, the closing cervix traps it.
- Uterine atony, which is accompanied by bleeding.
- A morbidly adherent placenta. In this relatively uncommon condition (1 in 1500 births), the trophoblast has invaded the decidua and myometrium to varying degrees (placenta accreta) or has penetrated to the serosal coat (placenta percreta).

MANAGEMENT

If postpartum bleeding is marked, attempts should be made at once to find if the placenta has separated as described earlier, and attempts should be made to deliver it. If these measures fail it should be removed manually (see page 188).

Should the placenta be retained for 1 hour with little bleeding the above procedures should be undertaken. A placenta accreta or percreta may resist attempts at manual removal and hysterectomy should be performed.

Inspection of the genital tract for damage

Following the expulsion of the placenta and membranes, bleeding usually ceases. If the perineum has been torn or an episiotomy made, the tear or incision is now repaired after inspecting the vagina for damage. If a difficult forceps delivery has been made, the cervix should be inspected to exclude a lateral tear.

Repair of an episiotomy or a perineal tear

EPISIOTOMY

Episiotomy, a deliberate incision in the stretched perineum and vagina, was first suggested about 200 years ago, to prevent a ragged perineal tear occurring which might extend to become a third or fourth degree tear. The idea was that episiotomy would prevent the development of such tears and would also prevent the later development of vaginal prolapse, although the evidence for this is dubious. However, the belief that the problems mentioned might occur has led to an episiotomy being performed in most primigravida labours, in some centres in the United States of America. A problem is that routine episiotomy has major disadvantages. The woman continues to have perineal pain and discomfort for longer than a woman who has not had the precedure. In addition sexual intercourse may be uncomfortable for up to 6 months after an episiotomy.

If the episiotomy has extended to produce a third or fourth degree tear, unless the anal sphincter is correctly sutured, the woman may develop anal or urinary incontinence.

If the doctor thinks that an episiotomy is required because the fetal head is overdistending the woman's perineum, he should explain what he proposes to the patient. If the woman agrees to the procedure, the doctor should infiltrate the perineum with a local anaesthetic, unless the woman has already had an epidural anaesthetic. The episiotomy incision may be midline or mediolateral (*Fig. 9.20*). The midline incision has the advantage that no large blood vessels are encountered and it is easier to repair. Its disadvantage is that it may extend into the rectum. If a large episiotomy is needed, for example when a difficult midforceps delivery is anticipated, a mediolateral episiotomy is preferred.

One method of repairing an episiotomy is shown in *Figure 9.21*. This repair is the least painful postoperatively, particularly when 2/0 polyglycolic suture material is used.

Another method is to use continuous suture to repair the vagina and interrupted sutures for the perineal muscles

and skin. The standard repair of an episiotomy is shown in *Figure 9.22*.

PERINEAL TEARS

Four degrees of perineal tears are recognized:
- *First degree* – damage to the fourchette and vaginal mucosa and the underlining muscles are exposed.
- *Second degree* – the posterior vaginal wall and the perineal muscles are torn but the anal sphincter is intact.
- *Third degree* – the anal sphincter is torn, but the rectal mucosa is intact.
- *Fourth degree* – the anal canal is opened, and the tear may spread to the rectum.

First degree tears are easy to repair; one or two sutures are all that is needed. Second and third degree tears need more care and their repair is shown in *Figure 9.22*. Third and fourth degree tears are uncommon, occurring in less than 1% of births. They usually follow a forceps delivery in a primgravida, the birth of a baby weighing more than 4kg, or the delivery of a fetus persistently maintaining an occipito-posterior position. Careful repair is essential but even then half of the women have persisting anal incontinence (usually only of flatus) for about 6 months due to poorly repaired sphincter damage, and 4% have faecal incontinence. Pelvic exercises may resolve the problem, but if this fails, surgery may be needed. Repair of fourth degree tears requires considerable skill, and it is essential to secure the apex of the tear otherwise a rectovaginal fistula may result. The anal sphincter retracts when torn and its exposed ends must be identified and rejoined by sutures (*Fig. 9.23*).

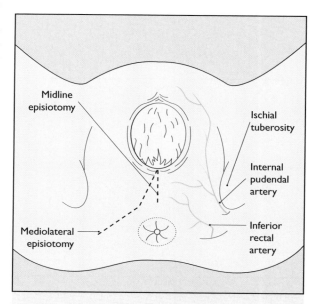

Fig. 9.20 *Types of episiotomy.*

POSTOPERATIVE CARE

The degree of postoperative pain and oedema depends on the method of delivery (forceps deliveries are followed by more oedema) and the quality of suturing. Most women need analgesics for a few days. A woman who has had the traditional interrupted sutures experiences more pain, but most patients can walk and have showers. Perineal swabbing is not usually necessary unless there is marked perineal oedema.

Episiotomies and perineal tears are not without longer-term discomfort. Twelve weeks after giving birth, 5% of women still experience some degree of pain and 15% have perineal discomfort. Sexual intercourse may be painful or uncomfortable for up to 20 weeks.

LACERATIONS OF THE LOWER GENITAL TRACT

After a difficult delivery the vagina and the clitoral area should be inspected for lacerations. Any large laceration should be sutured. Continued bleeding in spite of a firmly contracted uterus suggests an internal laceration. The vagina and cervix should be inspected with good illumination. If a

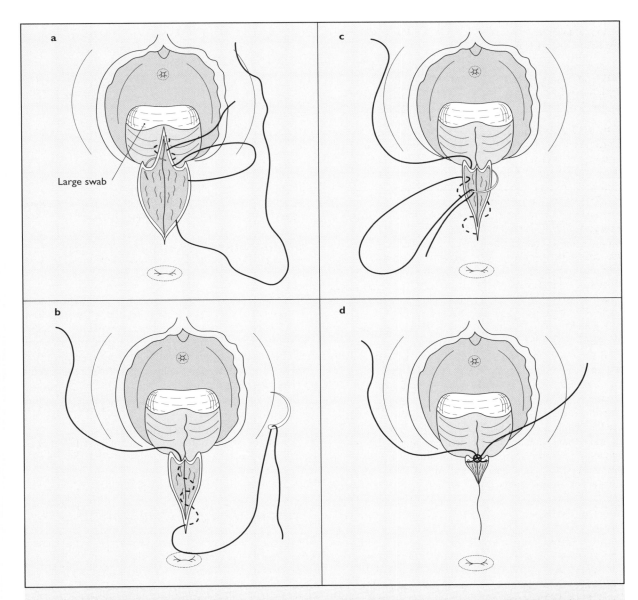

Fig. 9.21 (a) Suture of the vaginal wall. (b) The suture of the vaginal wall has been completed and the perineal muscles are being sutured. (c) The subcuticular suture of the perineal skin starting posteriorly and finishing deep to the hymen. (d) The two strands of catgut are tied, and cut short. The knot disappears beneath the vaginal mucosa.

Fig. 9.22 Standard method of repair of an episiotomy or perineal tear.

Fig. 9.23 Repair of a fourth degree tear.

lacerated cervix is found, the tear is sutured, care being taken to include the apex of the tear (Fig. 9.24).

Management of the immediate postdelivery period

The woman should remain in the delivery room for 1 hour. The medical attendants will check regularly that the uterus is contracted, that there is no excessive blood loss and that the vital signs are normal. During this time the baby will be checked thoroughly for abnormalities (see page 93), cleansed and returned to the mother to enable the parents to celebrate the birth.

Before the woman leaves the delivery room, the attendant must be sure that:

- The mother is in good general condition.
- The uterus is well contracted and contains no blood clots.
- The perineum has been properly repaired.
- The woman is not in pain from the repair.
- The woman does not have a full bladder.

Pain relief during childbirth

The pain of childbirth varies considerably between women. Because of this a woman has the right to know that analgesics and anaesthetics are available for her, and she can decide when she needs pain relief. If the medical attendants decide when a woman needs pain relief, the autonomy of the woman is reduced and the therapy is not always effective. In this context, surveys of women made some time after giving birth, in Britain, Norway and Australia,

Fig. 9.24 Repair of a cervical tear.

showed that between 15 and 20% were disappointed by a lack of effective pain relief during their labour.

The ideal obstetric method of pain relief should:
- Do no harm to the mother or her baby.
- Not prevent the patient cooperating, particularly in the second stage of labour.
- Not interfere with normal uterine activity.

Pain relief in labour

In early labour (the latent phase) when uterine contractions are not particularly painful, most women do not require pain relief. If the woman is very apprehensive a short-acting benzodiazepine drug may be given, but it is not requested by many women.

Most women seek pain relief once the active phase of the first stage begins. Several methods are available, including the use of drugs and nonpharmacological means.

NONPHARMACOLOGICAL METHODS

The *nonpharmacological* methods need to be taught during the pregnancy by a trained person, so that by the time labour begins the woman understands what she has to do. They include massage and touch, relaxation techniques, rhythmical movements, and hot and cold (e.g. showers or baths), transcutaneous electrical nerve stimulation (TENS). The effectiveness of these techniques is not clear, but some women find them very helpful in relieving pain.

Later in the active phase when the contractions become stronger, a woman may choose to continue with nonpharmacological methods, but must be made aware that if they do not provide adequate pain relief she may obtain treatment by a *pharmacological method*. She must not be made to feel that she has failed if she seeks *narcotics or epidural anaesthesia*.

PHARMACOLOGICAL METHODS

Of the narcotics, pethidine in a dose of 100–150mg intramuscularly at intervals is chosen by many women (the opioid is effective in about 15 minutes and the effect lasts for 2–3 hours). There is some concern that if pethidine is given within 2 hours of birth, the baby may have a delayed onset in breathing after birth. If this occurs it is easily and effectively treated by injecting an opioid antagonist, for example, naloxone into the umbilical vein, or intramuscularly.

An alternative method of giving pethidine, which is available in some hospitals, is patient controlled analgesia (PCA). Using PCA the woman controls the dose she is receiving (within limits). The method is attractive to some women, particularly after a caesarean section, but it is not widely used.

A recent (1996) well-designed study from Sweden shows that opioids do not relieve labour pain although they do reduce anxiety, discomfort and, in the case of pethidine, exhilaration in some women. This study is concerning as most health professionals and many patients are convinced of the value of opioids in pain relief. If, in advanced cancer, opioids provide pain relief, why do they not appear to do so in labour? Until the issue is settled many doctors will continue to prescribe pethidine to reduce labour pain, but others will increasingly recommend epidural analgesia.

NITROUS OXIDE AND OXYGEN

In most cases a 50:50 mixture of nitrous oxide and oxygen is given in an Entonox machine. The patient breathes the mixture during a contraction in the active phase of the first stage and during the second stage of labour. It can be used to supplement the pain relief provided by pethidine. To be effective it has to be used properly, and even if this is the case, rather less than 50% of women obtain satisfactory pain relief; 20% obtain some relief and 30% find the method ineffective.

EPIDURAL ANALGESIA

Epidural anaesthesia has become increasingly popular in recent years and would be chosen by more women if the service were more readily available. In Britain, for example, the Social Services Committee has recommended strongly that the Health Authorities should provide an anaesthetic service in all major obstetric units that is available within a few minutes of receiving a call. The Committee also recommends that only specifically trained doctors should give an epidural anaesthetic.

Epidural anaesthesia is the most effective way of relieving the pain of childbirth, and provides complete relief of contraction pain in 95% of labouring women. It also provides great flexibility in pain management. For example, should the delivery require forceps or vacuum extraction or be by caesarean section, epidural anaesthesia avoids possible adverse biochemical effects associated with a general anaesthetic, and can provide postoperative pain relief. The disadvantages of epidural anaesthesia are that a few women complain of dizziness or shivering and that it may increase the duration of the second stage and lead to an increase in operative vaginal delivery. A recent development is to use a low-dose epidural. This relieves the pain but permits the woman to walk about during labour without leg weakness or dizziness.

Serious side effects are uncommon. The most worrying are transient hypotension, which occurs in 20% of patients, and dural tap (in 1%), which is followed by severe headache in half of the women.

LOCAL ANALGESIA

Local analgesia is a choice in the relief of pain during childbirth for women who have not had an epidural anaesthetic and who require a forceps or vacuum extraction delivery; for the repair of an episiotomy or a perineal tear; and in some cases, for breech delivery. Two techniques are available. These are pudendal nerve block and perineal nerve infiltration. To understand the techniques, knowledge of the nerve supply of the vulva and lower vagina is needed.

Nerve supply of the vulva

The female vulva is innervated mainly by branches of the pudendal nerve. The pudendal nerve, derived from S.2, S.3 and S.4, leaves the pelvis medial to the sciatic nerve through the greater sciatic foramen. It then crosses the external surface of the ischial spine and re-enters the pelvis through the lesser sciatic notch and, passing along the lateral wall of the ischiorectal fossa, divides into branches which supply most of the perineum (Fig. 9.25). Further sensory branches to the skin of the perineum are derived from the ilio-inguinal nerve, the pudendal branch of the posterior femoral cutaneous nerve and the genital branch of the genitofemoral nerve (Fig. 9.26).

Technique of pudendal nerve block

A 10cm, 20-gauge needle and, if available, a needle director are required. Two fingers are introduced into the vagina to palpate the ischial spine, the guide containing the needle being introduced in the groove between the index and middle finger to impinge on the spine. The guide is then directed to lie just medial to, and below, the ischial spine and the needle is advanced 1cm beyond the guide (if no guide is available the needle is introduced between the fingers to the same site) and pushed through the sacrospinous ligament (Fig. 9.27); 10ml of 0.5% lignocaine is injected behind each ischial spine, and a further 10ml is used to make a perineal infiltration. Anaesthesia should be effective

within 5 minutes and it should be tested. The lower vagina and perineum become insensitive to pain. The use of pudendal nerve block is not without problems. For example, the needle may be difficult to introduce accurately in a relatively mobile patient, particularly when the fetal head is deeply engaged.

Technique of perineal nerve infiltration

Using a 7.5cm, 22-gauge needle, and 20ml of 0.5–1.0% lignocaine, the perineum is infiltrated in a fan-like manner, the base being the posterior fourchette at the midline. Three lines of infiltration are required, one medially as far as the anal sphincter and midway between the skin and the vaginal mucosa, and two others at 45° to block the nerves as they reach the perineum (see Fig. 9.27). The analgesia is effective in about 3 minutes and lasts between 45 and 90 minutes. It should be tested by pricking the skin with a sharp needle before any procedure is begun.

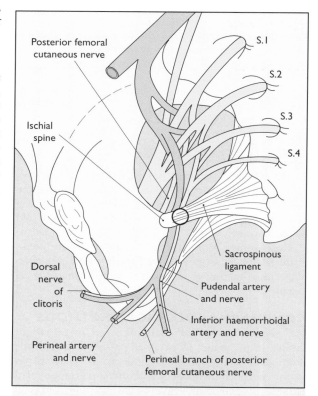

Fig. 9.25 The course of the pudendal nerve. The area in the circle which lies just medial to and below the tip of the ischial spine is the area into which the local anaesthetic is infiltrated.

Fig. 9.26 *Innervation of the perineum. On one side the nerves are shown, on the other, 'fanlike' local anaesthesia.*

Branch of ilio-inguinal nerve

Genital branch of genitofemoral nerve

Pudendal branch of post. femoral cutaneous nerve

'Fanlike' injections of local anaesthesia

Branches of pudendal nerve

Ischial tuberosity

Inferior haemorrhoidal nerve

Perforating cutaneous nerves

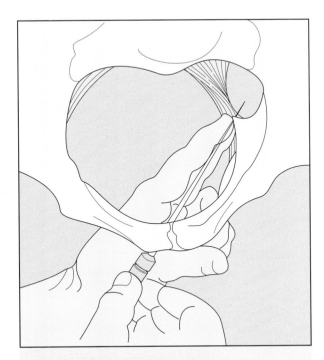

Fig. 9.27 *Transvaginal pudendal nerve block.*

CHAPTER 10

The puerperium

By convention the puerperium lasts for 6 weeks from the day of the birth of the child. During this time the physiological and morphological changes which occurred during pregnancy revert to the non-pregnant state. It is also a time when the woman takes on the responsibility of caring for a dependent, demanding infant. This may cause problems, particularly if she finds it difficult to adjust to being a mother.

Physiological and anatomical changes

The *endocrinological changes* which occurred during pregnancy rapidly revert. Within hours of the expulsion of the placenta the levels of the placental hormones, human placental lactogen (hPL) and chorionic gonadotrophin (hCG), fall rapidly. Within 2 days hPL is undetectable in serum and by the 10th day after birth, hCG can no longer be detected. The serum levels of oestrogen and progesterone fall rapidly in the first 3 puerperal days reaching non-pregnant levels by the 7th day after birth. They remain at this level if the woman chooses to breastfeed; if she does not, oestradiol begins to rise, indicating follicular growth. Among breastfeeding women human prolactin (hPr) levels rise following suckling.

The *cardiovascular system* reverts to the non-pregnant state during the first 2 puerperal weeks. In the first 24 hours the additional burden on the heart caused by the hypervolaemic state persists, after which time the blood and plasma volume return to the non-pregnant state. This occurs by the second puerperal week. In the first 10 days after birth the raised coagulation factors occurring during pregnancy persist but are balanced by a rise in fibrinolytic activity.

Morphological changes in the genital tract

Following the birth the *perineum* is either damaged or intact. The damage will have been repaired by the accoucheur, but oedema of the tissues may have occurred and will persist for some days. The *vaginal* wall is swollen, bluish and pouting. It rapidly regains its tonicity, although it is fragile for 1 or 2 weeks.

The uterus undergoes the most marked changes. At the end of the third stage of labour, the uterus is the size of a 20-week pregnancy and weighs about 1000g. It rapidly becomes smaller and by the end of the first puerperal week it weighs about 500g. Its involution can be demonstrated by the fact that its size is reduced on abdominal examination by one finger-breadth a day, to the extent that on the 12th day after the birth it cannot be palpated abdominally. Its involution continues after this time more slowly, but by the end of the 6th puerperal week it is only slightly larger than it was before the pregnancy.

Concurrently with the involution of the uterus, the *placental site* becomes smaller. It is rapidly covered after the birth with a fibrin mesh, and thrombosis occurs in the vessels supplying it. Beneath the placental site, macrophages, lymphocytes and polymorphs form a 'barrier' which also extends throughout the endometrial cavity. Within 10 days the placental site has shrunk to a diameter of 2.5cm, and a new growth of covering epithelium has occurred, which also covers the remainder of the uterine cavity. The superficial tissues of the uterine lining and placental site continue to be shed for 6 weeks, and form part of the lochia.

The *lochia* is the term used for the discharge from the genital tract which follows childbirth. For the first 3–4 days it consists of blood and remnants of trophoblastic tissue, mainly from the placental site. As the thrombosed vessels of the site become organized the character of the lochia changes. From the 3rd to the 12th day after the birth its colour is reddish-brown, but after this time, when most of the endometrial cavity has been covered with epithelium, it changes to a yellow colour. Occasionally some of the thrombi at the end of the vessels break, releasing blood, and the lochia becomes red once more for a few days.

Conduct of the puerperium

In contrast with 25 years ago, a recently delivered woman is no longer confined to bed. For instance, she may start walking about as soon as she wishes, go to the toilet when required and rest when she feels tired. Often an afternoon nap is all that she needs. Some women prefer to remain in bed for the first 24 hours after the birth, and women who have had an extensive repair of a torn perineum or a large episiotomy may choose to remain in bed for longer. Visitors are no longer restricted, but common sense must prevail and if the new mother is tired, they should be asked to leave.

A function of the medical attendants is to make sure that the tissues are healing properly, and that the uterus is involuting normally. But this function is less important than helping the woman to breastfeed if she chooses to do so, and providing information about the care of the infant when the mother goes home.

There is no longer a fixed time for remaining in hospital after the birth. A woman may choose to go home after 1 or 2 days or may prefer to remain in hospital for 5 days. An advantage of the longer stay is that lactation and breastfeeding are established during this time.

CARE OF THE PUERPERAL WOMAN

With early ambulation the care of the puerperal woman has become more simple. Regular checks are made of the temperature and pulse. The perineum is inspected each day to observe the degree of oedema (if any) and the sutures. Many women who have a damaged and repaired perineum experience considerable pain. The woman may need analgesics, and may find it more comfortable to sit on a rubber ring. This matter is discussed further on page 85.

The character and amount of the lochia is observed and recorded, and the height of the uterine fundus above the symphysis is checked daily.

Uterine contractions continue after childbirth. They are usually painless, but some women experience painful uterine contractions (afterpains) especially when breast-feeding. The woman may ask for analgesics.

URINARY TRACT PROBLEMS

Micturition may be difficult in the 24 hours after childbirth because of a reflex suppression of detrusor activity caused by the pressure on the bladder base during birth. As a diuresis occurs following the birth, the woman may be uncomfortable. If she is unable to pass urine, catheterization may be required. After catheterization, 60ml of chlorhexidine solution should be instilled into the bladder, to reduce the risk of urinary tract infection. This is more likely to occur in the puerperium rather than later because the pregnancy-induced dilatation of the renal pelvis and ureters and the relaxation of the bladder muscle take about 3 weeks to disappear.

About 10% of puerperal women experience urinary incontinence (usually stress incontinence). This incontinence persists for a few weeks and then ceases in all but a few women. Pelvic floor exercises (see page 307) may speed up the resolution of the problem more quickly.

BOWEL PROBLEMS

A few women become *constipated* in the puerperium. In most cases spontaneous relief is obtained; if not, stool softeners such as oral sterculia with frangula bark granules (Normacol) or bisacodyl rectal suppositories may be prescribed.

Women who have *haemorrhoids* during pregnancy often complain that they are more painful in the postpartum period. One woman in 20 develops haemorrhoids for the first time during the birth, but in most cases these settle in 2 or 3 weeks.

BACKACHE

Backache often occurs in the last quarter of pregnancy and persists after the birth, or it may occur for the first time in the puerperium. Backache affects about 25% of puerperal women, but over half of them had complained of backache before becoming pregnant. The pain can be considerable, particularly if the woman has no help in caring for her baby. It may persist for months but eventually settles.

Care of the neonate

Today in most hospitals, facilities exist for rooming-in, the baby lying in a cot close to the mother's bed, mother and baby being treated as a dyad. This has made the care of a healthy newborn infant much easier.

CHECKING FOR CONGENITAL ABNORMALITIES

A check for major abnormalities is made immediately after the birth and before the baby is given to the mother to celebrate the event. A full check is made during the baby's first day of life. The procedure is described in *Figure 10.1*.

CARE OF THE UMBILICAL CORD

The umbilical cord is inspected and the clamp removed, and the cord is tied and cut close to the umbilicus 24 hours after birth. The area is smeared with chlorhexidine cream, but no cord dressing or binder is used.

WEIGHT LOSS

A newborn infant may be expected to lose between 5 and 10% of its birthweight during the first 4 days of life. This causes no problems for a healthy mature baby. From the 4th day the infant will be obtaining sufficient breast milk (or breast-milk substitute) to start gaining weight. No fluids other than those obtained from the breast or bottle need be given. Extra fluids should be avoided in breast-fed babies as they interfere with the smooth establishment of lactation. The only reason for giving extra fluids is to counter the development of 'dehydration fever' in the baby.

DEHYDRATION FEVER

Because a neonate's temperature control is not very efficient, dehydration fever may affect a few infants in the first days of life in hot, humid weather. The infant develops a high fever, looks dehydrated, and has a dry mouth and a depressed anterior fontanelle. It is vigorous and thirsty, unlike an infected infant, which is languid and febrile. Dehydration fever rarely occurs in infants who room-in and breastfeed on demand. The treatment consists of replacing the fluid and salt lost by giving oral feeds of 200ml 1/5 normal saline per kg bodyweight per 24 hours.

THE STOOLS

In the first 2 days of life the infant's faeces are sticky and greenish-black in colour. As microorganisms invade the gut the colour of the faeces changes to yellow with the occasional passage of greenish faeces. Breastfed babies usually defaecate a soft stool which has little smell. Bottle-fed infants do not defaecate as regularly and the stool when expelled is firmer in consistency, dark yellow in colour and occasionally has an offensive smell.

JAUNDICE

Most babies develop transient jaundice which is benign and self-limiting. A few infants develop more marked jaundice. If this occurs within 24 hours of birth, persists, and the jaundice extends on to the infant's trunk or thighs, serum bilirubin measurements are made. A serum bilirubin reading of more than 250mmol/L is of concern as kernicterus may occur. Advice from a paediatrician should be obtained. Treatment consists of phototherapy or, in severe cases, exchange transfusion.

INFANT FEEDING

The establishment of maternal lactation and breastfeeding, or, if the mother chooses not to breastfeed, the establishment of feeding with breast-milk substitutes, is one of the most important tasks for those caring for the infant.

Lactation and breastfeeding

During pregnancy the breasts develop considerably. Fat is deposited around the glandular parts of the breasts. Oestrogen leads to an increase in the size and number of the ducts, and progesterone increases the number of alveoli; hPL also stimulates alveolar development and may be involved in the synthesis of casein, lactalbumin and lactoglobulin by the alveolar cells.

In spite of this activity, lactation is inhibited during pregnancy, although levels of human prolactin (hPr) rise throughout the pregnancy. The reason for this is that the high levels of oestrogen occupy binding sites on the alveoli which prevent them from responding to the lactogenic properties of hPr. In late pregnancy the breasts secrete a thickish, yellowish fluid, colostrum, which is rich in

---

Fig. 10.1 Examination of a newborn baby

Examine baby 1 hour after a feed when he/she is likely to be calm, quiet and have open eyes. Get mother to undress the baby.

1. Observe posture movements; check for skin abnormalities.

2. Palpate neck for goitre or sternomastoid tumour.

3. Look at eyes, see if he/she will follow side-to-side movement of examiner's face.

4. Measure occipito-frontal circumference; feel skull and fontanelles.

5. Get baby to open mouth; examine for cleft palate.

6. Examine the chest for signs of respiratory distress (note the respiratory rate should be <60).

7. Examine the pericardium for cardiac murmurs.

8. Palpate abdomen.

9. Examine external genitalia; feel for femoral pulses.

10. Check Moro and traction manoeuvres.
    Moro: When picked up, the baby extends and abducts arms and fingers and opens eyes; he/she then flexes and abducts arms.
    Traction: When lifted by grasping hands, the baby flexes arms and keeps head in the plane of trunk.

11. Pick up baby in prone position; check muscle tone, examine spine (scoliosis) and anus.

12. Examine hips.
    To examine the left hip, the doctor steadies the infant's pelvis between the thumb of the left hand on the symphysis pubis and the fingers behind the sacrum. The examiner grasps the child's left thigh in the right hand and attempts to move the femoral head gently forwards and then backwards out of the acetabulum. If the head of the femur is felt to move, with or without an audible 'clunk', dislocation, or dislocability is diagnosed. If there is any doubt after the examination, real-time ultrasound is used to detect a displaced hip. In about 10% of the cases the babies' hips produce a soft 'click' rather than a 'clunk', and there is no evidence of abnormal movement of the femoral head. These babies must be examined again before discharge from hospital. If 1 month later the click has changed into a clunk, and abnormal movement between the femoral head and the acetabulum is found, the ultrasound examination is repeated.

immune antibodies. The production of colostrum increases after the birth until it is replaced by breast milk production.

As mentioned earlier, the level of oestrogen falls rapidly in the 48 hours following childbirth. This permits circulating hPr to act on the alveolar cells to initiate and maintain lactation.

Lactation is encouraged by early and frequent suckling, as this reflexly causes the pituitary gland to secrete hPr (*Fig. 10.2*). On the other hand, negative emotions, including the fear of failing to breastfeed, may reduce the secretion of prolactin, by promoting the release of the prolactin-inhibiting factor (dopamine) from the hypothalamus.

By the 2nd or 3rd day after the birth, hPr has induced the alveolar cells to secrete milk, which is thin and bluish in colour. Initially the milk distends the alveoli and the small ducts, causing the breasts to become full, engorged and tender. Turgid veins can be seen beneath the skin, and the milk ducts can be felt as tender strings in the breast tissue. The engorgement is due to the absence of ejection of milk through the large ducts to the nipple.

MILK EJECTION REFLEX

The milk filling and distending the alveoli is unavailable to the infant until myoepithelial cells (*Fig. 10.3*) which surround the alveoli and smaller ducts contract in response to the milk ejection (or 'let-down') reflex. The reflex is initiated by suckling and is mediated via the hypothalamus and pituitary gland, which releases oxytocin into the bloodstream (*Fig. 10.4*).

The oxytocin causes contractions of the myoepithelial cells and milk is ejected from the alveoli and small ducts to flow to the large ducts and the subareolar reservoirs. Oxytocin may also inhibit the release of dopamine from the hypothalamus, further encouraging the secretion of milk.

Negative emotional and physical factors can reduce the let-down reflex with the result that for lactation to be established the mother must be confident that she can breastfeed. The medical attendants should encourage her to be confident.

A joint statement by WHO and UNICEF was published in 1989, which showed how the support needed for successful lactation could be obtained (*Fig. 10.5*).

NUTRITIONAL NEEDS IN LACTATION

The energy cost of lactation is 2095kJ per day. A woman who has been well nourished during pregnancy has fat stores of 125,700kJ, which can be used to supply the extra energy needs of lactation. The diet of a parturient woman provides over 10,050kJ per day and her energy needs for bodily functions and daily activity are about 8,400kJ a day, so that there is sufficient to meet the needs of lactation. But if she is anxious, she can be advised to eat an extra slice of bread with butter and cheese, which will provide the extra energy needed.

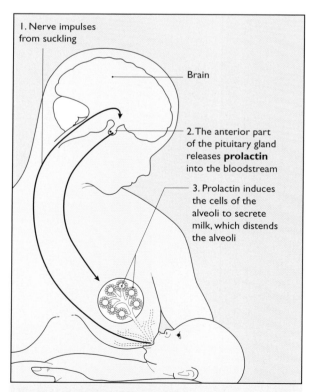

1. Nerve impulses from suckling

Brain

2. The anterior part of the pituitary gland releases **prolactin** into the bloodstream

3. Prolactin induces the cells of the alveoli to secrete milk, which distends the alveoli

Fig. 10.2 *The prolactin reflex.*

Fig. 10.3 *Myoepithelial cells surrounding a partially filled villus.*

1. Nerve impulses from suckling

Brain

2. The posterior part of the pituitary gland releases **oxytocin** into the bloodstream

3. Oxytocin causes tiny muscles around the alveoli to squeeze the milk to the nipple

Fig. 10.4 The milk ejection reflex.

Maintenance of lactation

The most effective way of maintaining lactation is regular suckling, so that both the prolactin and the milk ejection reflexes are initiated frequently, and abnormal distension of the alveoli by milk is prevented. If distension occurs, the alveoli are unable to secrete milk efficiently and at the same time suckling is avoided because of pain in the breasts. Consequently, the inhibition of the reflex which prevents the release of dopamine from the hypothalamus is lost and alveolar activity diminishes, with a further reduction of milk secretion.

ESTABLISHMENT OF BREASTFEEDING
The establishment of successful breastfeeding requires:
- That milk secretion occurs in the alveoli.
- That the milk ejection reflex is efficient.
- That the mother is motivated to breastfeed (she may need support to keep motivated).

As mentioned in *Figure 10.5*, breastfeeding is more readily established if:
- The baby is given to the mother to caress and suckle soon after birth.
- The baby rooms-in with the mother and the staff treat them as a dyad.
- The baby is allowed to suckle frequently from birth, for a short period each time, to help 'bring the milk in'.
- Once the milk is flowing the baby is fed on demand, including at night.

Fig. 10.5 Ten steps to successful breastfeeding

A joint WHO/UNICEF statement (1989).
Every facility providing maternity services and care for newborn infants should:

1. Have a written breastfeeding policy that is routinely communicated to all healthcare staff.

2. Train all healthcare staff in the skills necessary to implement this policy.

3. Inform all pregnant women about the benefits and management of breastfeeding.

4. Help mothers initiate breastfeeding within a half hour of birth.

5. Show mothers how to breastfeed and how to maintain lactation even if they are separated from their infants.

6. Give newborn infants no food or drink other than breast milk unless medically indicated.

7. Practise rooming-in. Allow mothers and infants to stay together 24 hours a day.

8. Encourage breastfeeding on demand.

9. Give no artificial teats or pacifiers (also called dummies and soothers) to breastfeeding infants.

10. Foster the establishment of breastfeeding support groups and refer mothers to them on discharge from hospital or clinic.

- No feeds of water or of glucose water are given to the infant by the nursing staff without the express agreement of the mother and her doctor.
- The nursing staff help the establishment of lactation by adopting a positive approach to the mother and are unhurried and supportive during the time she establishes breastfeeding.

TECHNIQUE OF BREASTFEEDING

The mother should be shown how to stroke the infant's mouth with her nipple, to induce the 'rooting' reflex in which the baby opens her or his mouth and searches for the nipple.

She then holds her breast with the nipple between her forefinger and middle finger, so that the nipple becomes more prominent and the infant is able to put its gums on the areola and not on the tender nipple (Fig. 10.6c). This technique enables the baby to breathe when suckling (Figs 10.7 and 10.8).

The mother is shown how to detach the infant's mouth from the nipple without causing her pain. This is done by putting her little finger into the corner of the baby's mouth to break the suction before detaching the baby from her nipple.

As mentioned earlier, very few babies managed in this way require additional fluids in the first 4 days of life. However, if the baby becomes clinically dehydrated, water may be given by a spoon or dropper after a feed. A feeding bottle should be avoided as it may stop the baby learning properly how to suck at the breast.

BREAST ENGORGEMENT

It takes a few days to adjust the supply of milk to the demand, mainly because the milk ejection reflex is not yet operating properly. During this time the breasts of some women become engorged as described earlier. Treatment depends on the severity of the engorgement. Many nurses claim that a successful remedy consists of hot and cold towels applied alternately to the breasts. They claim that the towels stimulate increased blood flow through the engorged areas of the breasts. Another method is to stimulate the milk ejection reflex using an electric breast pump (the Egnell pump). Severe and painful engorgement may be reduced by prescribing small doses of bromocriptine (a dopamine) for 24–48 hours.

If possible the mother should continue to breastfeed in spite of the engorgement of her breasts, to stimulate the milk ejection reflex.

BREAST PROBLEMS DURING LACTATION
Cracked nipples

Aggressive suckling by the baby may lead to cracked nipples, particularly if the nipple is not well within the infant's mouth (Fig. 10.6a and b). The nipple should be treated with chlorhexidine cream and a nipple shield used to protect the abraded area during feeding. If the cracking is severe, the baby should not be fed from the affected breast, which should be emptied manually or by using a breast pump.

Fig. 10.6 Ideal position of nipple in infant's mouth. In (a) and (b) the nipple is being chewed; in (c) the nipple is well within the baby's mouth.

Milk stasis

This may occur early in lactation and be associated with, or follow, breast engorgement. Milk stasis is due to pressure on the main duct of a lobule by the engorged alveoli and usually settles without treatment, but may lead to non-infectious inflammation of the breast. It is thought the pressure in some of the alveoli causes seepage of milk into the surrounding breast tissues, which results in the non-infectious breast inflammation. Treatment of both forms, if needed, is to try to help the mother feed her baby more often and to empty the breasts manually after each feed.

Acute mastitis

Most cases of acute mastitis in the mother are caused by organisms acquired from the infant's nasopharyngeal or umbilical areas, which harbour colonies of staphylococci or streptococci that develop within a few days of birth.

Acute mastitis occurs at the end of the first week following birth. The mother develops a fever and a tender, red, firm-to-hard area is felt in one of the breasts. Treatment consists of prescribing analgesics and antibiotics. As most infections are caused by staphylococci, currently flu-cloxacillin is preferred. If it is not too painful, the mother should continue suckling the baby. If pus develops in the infected area of the breast, causing a breast abscess, incision of the abscess and drainage for 24 hours may be required.

Proper attention to breastfeeding reduces the chance of acute mastitis developing. The breasts should be emptied after a feed, as incomplete emptying of the breasts leaves stagnant milk in the system, which may become infected.

Cracked nipples should be treated, as microorganisms may invade through the cracks. Rooming-in reduces the chance of cross-infection between babies and of mastitis in the mother.

SUPPRESSION OF LACTATION

Women who choose not to breastfeed or who stop breastfeeding may need to have lactation suppressed. Lactation will diminish and cease if the baby no longer suckles. At first the breasts become engorged, but, if supported by an appropriately sized bra, will become less engorged in a few days and lactation will cease. An alternative is for the woman to be prescribed a prolactin inhibitor (dopamine receptor agonist).

BREAST-MILK SUBSTITUTES

More than 95% of women can breastfeed if they want to, and although most women choose to breastfeed immediately after childbirth, by the 6th week of the puerperium, fewer than 60% of women are still breastfeeding.

Women who do not breastfeed choose one of the breast-milk substitutes (formula milks) available. They are based on cows' milk, modified as far as possible to have the same proportions of protein, fat, carbohydrates, minerals and vitamins as found in human milk. Provided that the formula milk is prepared according to the manufacturer's directions the baby will thrive, although she or he is not as well protected against infection as a breastfed infant. This is of importance in the developing countries and among poor women in all countries.

Fig. 10.7 The baby's lips are pursed awaiting attachment to the mother's breast.

Fig. 10.8 Good attachment of the baby.

Psychological problems in the puerperium

The birth of a baby places considerable 'stress' on the mother. She has the responsibility of caring for a demanding infant, she has to continue to care for her husband or partner, her nights are usually disturbed and she may not feel competent or confident about her ability as a mother. It is not surprising that it takes time for her to adjust to being a mother and that she may suffer psychological disturbances.

A large number of women become temporarily sad and emotional between the 3rd and 5th day after the birth (third day blues), and about 10% of women become more severely depressed. Postnatal depression is mentioned here and discussed more fully on page 190.

THIRD DAY BLUES

Why so many women develop third day blues is not known. Speculation about its aetiology includes hormonal imbalance (although none has been identified), reaction to the excitement of childbirth, and uncertainty by the mother about her ability to care for her dependent child. Another factor in Western culture may be the expectation that a mother immediately loves her baby, when in reality, mother love is a learned behaviour.

The condition leads to bursts of crying, to irritability and in some cases to general depression. Successful management of this malaise consists of one of the medical or nursing staff talking with the woman, explaining what is occurring, and if she wishes, restricting visitors. There is some evidence that third day blues are less likely to occur if maternal – infant bonding has occurred and if rooming-in is practised. Third day blues is a misnomer as the inability to adjust to parenthood, with feelings of inadequacy, tiredness, reduced sexuality, emotional lability and, in a small proportion of women, severe depression, may persist for weeks or months.

ADJUSTMENT TO PARENTHOOD AND PUERPERAL DEPRESSION

Few doctors understand that adjustment to parenthood is difficult for most women. Women have been brought up to believe that they should be good housekeepers, hard workers, excellent lovers and experienced mothers all at the same time. Yet on returning home after childbirth, the persistent demands of the newborn baby on the energy, the time and the emotions of a mother may cause considerable stress. This stress is aggravated by the nuclear family and the tendency for young people to live at some distance from their close relatives, who, in other cultures, are readily available to offer help and consolation. The stress becomes intensified as the mother realizes that she has the sole responsibility for a small, unpredictable infant who needs attention day and night. She may not have realized that the baby would cry so much, for so little apparent cause. Her sleep is constantly broken and fatigue is added to her feelings of maternal inadequacy. Her relationship with her partner also requires adjustment, and this can be emotionally disturbing, particularly if he does not do his share of parenting. As the baby occupies so much of her time, the mother finds that she cannot keep the house as clean as she would wish, and feels guilty that she is not the efficient person she believed she was.

The fatigue induced by the demands of the baby, the emotional readjustment in marital relations, the guilt experienced over an untidy house and lack of a helpful counsellor often induces depression. In about 10% of women the depression becomes so severe that medical help is sought, usually between the 2nd and 7th week of the puerperium. The presenting symptoms are mainly changes in mood: tearfulness, feelings of inadequacy and inability to cope predominate. These changes are labile, and tend to become worse towards evening, when associated psychosomatic complaints of fatigue, anorexia and nausea may occur. Doctors all too frequently offer sedation or psychotropic drugs, when explanation, reassurance and advice would be more useful.

It is also important to tell parents of community-based help organizations such as the La Lèche League in Britain and the USA, and the Nursing Mothers Association and Play Groups in Australia. These organizations provide 24-hour home counselling and home visiting when needed. Their activities in helping women adjust to parenthood can be of great value in reducing the incidence of puerperal depression.

Sexuality after birth

After childbirth the demands of the new baby occupy a good deal of a mother's time. Moreover, if the mother has had a perineal tear or an episiotomy repaired, her perineum and vagina may be tender for several weeks. It is not unexpected that her desire for sexual intercourse is reduced. Some women who breastfeed may have a reduced libido and develop vaginal dryness, both of which are reversed when the woman ceases breastfeeding. Sexual intercourse is not the only way of obtaining sexual pleasure and she may welcome touching, cuddling and stimulating her husband or partner to orgasm if he wishes. When she is ready the couple can resume sexual intercourse. Women may consult a doctor about their lack of sexual feeling after the birth and supportive advice is helpful.

Perinatal bereavement

About 12 babies in every 1000 are either stillborn or die in the first 28 days of life. They constitute perinatal deaths and many of these babies are born preterm, and are of low birth-weight, and about 25% have severe congenital malformations. Parents whose baby dies in the perinatal period have grief reactions similar to those which follow the loss of any loved person. At first the mother (and often the father) feel numb and shocked. After a few days the reaction changes to a desire to understand why the baby died, or to expressions of anger or guilt about events in pregnancy or during labour. Over the next 2 or 3 months many parents are likely to review the events surrounding the baby's death, often repeatedly. More than 50% of mothers suffer from depression and anxiety which may last for months, but in time, the couple adjust, the woman often embarking on a new pregnancy.

The severity and duration of the bereavement reaction may be reduced if the parents are given the opportunity to talk with the attending medical and nursing staff soon after the baby's death. The talk should take place in a quiet private area, not in an open ward. Most parents want to understand what has gone wrong; explained in clear, simple language. A few become angry, blaming the staff for the child's death. The doctor or nurse should listen to the parents with sympathy and understanding and explain as clearly as possible the events surrounding the death.

In addition, the staff member should give information to the parents about the grief reaction which may be expected and should provide reassurance that nothing the mother did, or failed to do, caused the death of the child.

Parents who wish to see their dead child (even if malformed) should be given the opportunity, so that they may mourn their loss. If they do not wish to see the child at that time, a photograph, a footprint and perhaps a lock of the child's hair should be kept with the mother's records, as later the parents may regret their decision not to have seen their child.

Before the parents see the baby they should be told how the infant will look. If deformities are present, they should be described (perhaps with the aid of a photograph). The baby is presented to the parents clothed and wrapped, and when they become accustomed to him or her, the baby is undressed by them. This procedure is often emotional, and support from a health professional may be invaluable. The parents should be told that they can spend as much time as they wish with the baby, and should be encouraged to name the child. Many parents wish to have a photograph of their dead baby. When the mother leaves hospital it is important to suggest that she makes contact with her family doctor (or health visitor), and she should be told about community-based help organizations in her area.

One woman in every five whose baby is stillborn, or who dies in the neonatal period, will suffer severe symptoms of bereavement (sleeplessness, depression and withdrawal). Women who have little or no support from husband, partner or family, who are cared for by insensitive health professionals and who lack a caring environment are more likely to be affected severely. These women, particularly, need help from sympathetic health professionals who listen, communicate and counsel.

There is some evidence that parents cope better, psychologically, with the next pregnancy if conception is delayed for a few months, but the decision has to be made by the couple, rather than imposed by a doctor. During the pregnancy, continuity of care is important, and supportive, communicating, sympathetic health professionals help to reduce possible mothering difficulties and puerperal problems.

Child abuse

Women who find difficulty in coping with their baby, or who have strange, disturbed behaviour whilst in hospital, are more likely to abuse their baby after discharge. The prevalence of child abuse before the age of 3 years is not known exactly, but it is probable that at least 6 per 1000 live-born children are abused. Mothers who have social problems, who have no supportive partner or relative, or who have marital problems are more likely to abuse their child. It is possible, by simple observation in the puerperium, to identify some vulnerable women, and this is part of postnatal care. Preventive intervention by family doctors, paediatricians and social workers has been shown to reduce the prevalence of child neglect and abuse.

Postnatal check

It is usual for the mother (and her baby) to be asked to return for a postnatal check 6–8 weeks after the birth. The purpose of this visit is for the woman to discuss her adjustment to parenthood, her need for information about child care, her sexual relationships and contraception. The doctor will refer to the records to recall if any complications arose in pregnancy or during childbirth which need follow-up. The doctor also examines the woman (and her baby if he or she is not being seen by a paediatrician).

The examination includes inspection of the perineum and vagina to ascertain that any damage has healed, to find out whether she has urinary or faecal incontinence and to determine the muscle tone. A vaginal speculum is used to visualize the cervix and a Pap smear is made if indicated. A bimanual examination is made to check that the uterus has involuted completely.

Most of the visit is spent in discussing the woman's problems, if she has any. Contraception is also an important area for discussion and advice (see Chapter 32, Conception control).

It should be noted, however, that if the woman has decided not to breastfeed, contraception should be discussed with her in the last quarter of pregnancy and started 21 days after the birth.

CHAPTER 11

Minor complications of pregnancy

The physiological and anatomical changes which occur during pregnancy may lead to complications which, although minor in medical terms, may cause considerable distress and discomfort to many pregnant women. They are listed below in alphabetical order.

Backache

Backache is common in late pregnancy and is felt over the sacroiliac joints. It is caused by relaxation of the ligaments and muscles supporting the joints, and is probably also induced by progesterone and, possibly, relaxin. It is usually worse at night and may prevent the woman from sleeping.

It is thought that if women avoid wearing high heels (whenever practicable) and have a good posture the incidence of backache decreases. However, this has not been shown in any well-designed study.

Cervical eversion and discharge

The high levels of oestrogen in pregnancy may increase the eversion of the endocervical columnar cells so that they appear as a red ring around the external cervical os. The cells may secrete mucus when exposed to the vagina – causing a non-infective vaginal discharge. The condition has erroneously been called a cervical erosion.

Constipation

The reduced gut motility aggravated in late pregnancy by the pressure of the enlarged uterus, makes constipation common in pregnancy. Treatment consists of increasing dietary fibre (for example by eating wholemeal instead of white bread) and attempting to defaecate after a meal. If the constipation is causing discomfort the woman may be prescribed oral sterculia with frangula bark granules (Normacol) or the contact laxative, bisacodyl.

Displacements of the uterus in pregnancy

PENDULOUS ABDOMEN

Women who have had several children and who have a wide separation of the recti abdominis muscles, may find in late pregnancy that the uterus becomes pathologically anteverted – the pendulous abdomen (Fig. 11.1). In late pregnancy this can cause considerable discomfort, and in labour may delay the birth because the fetal head does not enter the pelvis easily. Treatment consists of wearing a firm binder in pregnancy. In labour a binder should be applied and the woman should pull her uterus up.

PREGNANCY AFTER A VAGINAL REPAIR FOR PROLAPSE

This is considered on page 304.

RETROVERSION

In 10% of women the uterus is normally retroverted; moreover, retroversion of the uterus does not hinder conception, and so when examined vaginally in the early weeks of pregnancy some women will be found to have a retroverted uterus. In nearly all cases the uterus becomes anteverted spontaneously, usually between the 9th and 11th week of pregnancy. Very rarely the uterus remains retroverted until after the 14th gestational week and becomes incarcerated in the cul-de-sac. If this occurs the woman complains of frequency of micturition and dysuria. If the position of the uterus is not corrected, the symptoms increase in severity and eventually there is retention of urine and an enormously distended bladder. Finally, retention of urine with overflow occurs. Examination shows a smooth, soft cystic tumour arising in the pelvis and palpable abdominally in the midline. Treatment entails inserting a catheter and decompressing the bladder slowly. When this is done the uterus usually becomes anteverted but may need to be anteverted using the fingers by pushing up in the posterior fornix and manipulating the uterus to one side of the sacral promontory.

Fig. 11.1 Pendulous abdomen. The patient is age 36, gravida 4.

UTEROVAGINAL PROLAPSE

In multiparous women, particularly in the developing countries, uterovaginal prolapse may complicate pregnancy. In the early weeks of pregnancy the prolapse may become more prominent. As the uterus becomes an abdominal organ the pressure on the vagina is relieved, to some extent, and the prolapse becomes less obvious. Occasionally a swollen, infected cervix may protrude through the vulva. The prolapse causes few problems during labour and cervical dilatation is usually rapid.

Dyspnoea

By the 15th week of pregnancy 1 woman in 4 complains of dyspnoea on exertion. The proportion increases as pregnancy advances with the result that, by the fourth quarter of pregnancy, three-quarters of pregnant women are dyspnoeic. The condition is probably due to a lack of adaptation to progesterone-induced hyperventilation. There is no specific treatment and the patient should be reassured that the breathlessness will not harm her or her fetus.

Heartburn

Relaxation of the lower oesophageal sphincter permits the regurgitation of some of the stomach contents, causing irritation of the lower oesophagus. It is also possible that a similar relaxation of the pyloric sphincter permits a reflux of bile into the stomach, which may then be regurgitated into the lower oesophagus. The woman complains of heartburn, which increases as the pregnancy advances.

Treatment is difficult, but frequent small meals, avoidance of spicy food and cigarettes, and the use of antacids may relieve the discomfort. If antacids fail, floating antacids such as sodium alginate – sodium bicarbonate mixture (e.g. Gaviscon) – or metoclopramide may give relief. If the heartburn occurs predominantly at night, the use of extra pillows to prop up the expectant mother may help.

Haemorrhoids and varicose veins

Haemorrhoids and varicose veins of the legs, and occasionally the vulva, become increasingly common as pregnancy advances. Haemorrhoids often become larger or may appear for the first time during childbirth. They may persist for several months after the birth and cause pain.

Varicose veins increase in size in late pregnancy. Treatment entails the woman lying or sitting with her feet up as much as possible, and, if the veins are painful or disfiguring, wearing elastic stockings. The latter should be put on before the woman gets out of bed in the morning. Surgical treatment for either condition is generally contraindicated in pregnancy.

Insomnia

Many pregnant women find that their sleep pattern is altered. In early pregnancy they may sleep for longer than usual. In late pregnancy, because of the discomfort of the enlarged uterus, leg cramps and backache, sleep may be disturbed. The short-term use of hypnotics may help.

Leg cramps

The cause of leg cramps is not known. They tend to occur more frequently in the second half of pregnancy, usually at night. Various treatments, including calcium tablets have been tried, but have no value except as a placebo. Some women obtain relief if the foot of the bed is raised about 25cm.

Micturition

FREQUENCY OF MICTURITION

Increased frequency of micturition is common in early pregnancy, when it is due to a supranormal excretion of urine by the kidney, and in the last weeks when the pressure of the fetal head causes direct irritation of the trigone.

URINARY INCONTINENCE

Urinary incontinence affects over 50% of pregnant women to some extent and 15% of women complain that the leakage is bothersome. There is no specific treatment although pelvic floor exercises may help (see Fig. 40.3, page 307). Usually the leakage eases in the puerperium.

Nausea and vomiting

Nausea due to pregnancy affects over 75% of women and vomiting occurs in half of them. The symptoms usually begin at the 6th gestational week and cease by the 12th, although they may continue throughout the pregnancy. The symptoms are more common in women who have a history of unsuccessful pregnancies, or who are carrying a multiple pregnancy. One-quarter of women who have the symptoms will experience them again in a subsequent pregnancy.

The cause appears to be due either to the effect of the rising levels of oestrogen, or to the high levels of human chorionic gonadotrophin acting on the chemoreceptor trigger zone in the midbrain. Once the body has become habituated to the new hormonal environment, the nausea and vomiting cease in most women. In addition, psychological factors may act on the emetic centre in the cerebral cortex.

Nausea and vomiting may be graded as mild, moderate or severe.

MILD

Mild nausea (and occasional vomiting) affects 45% of pregnant women and is the most common form. The nausea usually occurs in the morning (*morning sickness*) but may be provoked by travel or emotional stress at any time of the day.

Treatment

The patient should be advised to eat frequent small meals during the day, to take fluid between (not with) meals, and to avoid fatty or spicy foods. If the vomiting is distressing she can be prescribed pyridoxine 50mg 6-hourly or metoclopramide (Maxolon) 10mg two to three times a day.

MODERATE

Moderate nausea and vomiting affects 5% of all pregnant women, and 10% of all women suffering from nausea. The symptoms may occur at any time of the day or night. The patient feels miserable and may become mildly dehydrated.

Treatment

The treatment suggested for the mild form of nausea applies to the moderate form, but most of the women choose to take a sedative. If the sedative used for the mild form does not relieve the symptoms, promethazine (25mg morning and evening) may be needed. The drug produces marked sleepiness, which reduces its value.

SEVERE

This form is uncommon, affecting 1 in 1000 pregnant women. The nausea is continuous and the vomiting frequent. This is the reason for its name – *hyperemesis gravidarum*. The woman rapidly becomes dehydrated and ketoacidotic.

Treatment

The patient should be admitted to hospital and treatment started urgently to avoid the possibility of liver damage. An intravenous line is established and dehydration and ketosis corrected by infusing 1L of 5% dextrose, followed by 1L of Hartmann's solution if electrolyte disturbance is detected. The infusion should provide 3–4L a day and is continued until hydration and electrolyte balance have been corrected. The fluid intake and output is recorded. The urine is checked twice daily for acetone, bile, sugar and specific gravity. Plasma electrolytes are measured daily. If vomiting persists, the patient should be given metoclopramide (10mg IM) as needed. During the time that the infusion is running, the patient can be given dry ice to suck, and oral feeding should be withheld. Once the vomiting has ceased the patient is treated in the same way as for the moderate form of nausea. She should remain in hospital for 2 days after the vomiting has ceased and until she has begun to gain weight.

Oedema

Oedema, particularly of the legs, is, in the absence of hypertension, a normal physiological adaptation to the pregnant state. The cause is water stored in the ground substance of connective tissue. In pregnancy the increased secretion of oestrogen alters the ground substance from a colloid-rich, water-poor matrix to a colloid-poor, water-rich matrix. In addition, in late pregnancy, increased mechanical obstruction to the venous return from the legs adds to leg oedema. Oedema around the ankles and lower legs is more common towards evening in hot, humid climates and in obese women. Treatment consists of the woman sitting or lying with her legs elevated. There is no place for diuretics.

Oedema, associated with a rise in blood pressure, requires further investigation, particularly when the hands or face become oedematous (see Chapter 15, Hypertensive diseases in pregnancy).

Palpitations, fainting and headaches

These symptoms are common in pregnancy and are caused by altered cardiovascular dynamics. The patient should be examined and reassured that she has no organic lesion. Auscultation of the heart may reveal a soft systolic murmur, which is due to the hypervolaemic circulation occurring during pregnancy. A murmur of this kind is not a sign of cardiac damage. Some women feel faint when lying on their back in late pregnancy because the pressure of the uterus reduces venous return to the heart (supine hypotension). Pregnant women should avoid lying flat on their backs. Headaches also appear to be due to the altered vascular dynamics.

Placidity and drowsiness

These symptoms are common in pregnancy and are due to the increase in circulating progesterone. There is no effective treatment available.

Pubic symphysis diastasis (pelvic osteoarthropathy)

In a few women abnormal relaxation of the ligaments surrounding the pubic joint permits the pubic bones to move on each other when the woman walks or exerts herself. This movement may put strain on the sacroiliac joints. Pubic symphysis diastasis may occur during pregnancy or start in the puerperium. The pain may persist for the remainder of the pregnancy or for several weeks after the birth, which makes care of the neonate difficult. The patient complains

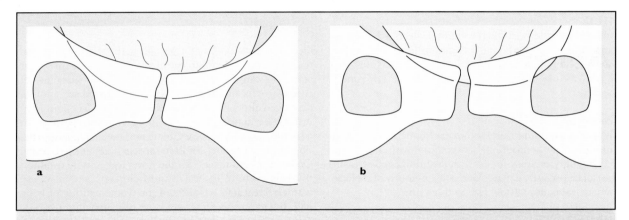

Fig. 11.2 Pelvic symphysis diastasis. The patient is 39 weeks pregnant. The sliding movement of the symphysis is shown when (a) the patient stands on her right leg; (b) the patient stands on her left leg.

of severe pubic pain, backache and sacral pain. Examination shows that the pubic joint is very tender when pressed. The diastasis can be confirmed by ultrasound or X-ray examination (Fig. 11.2). Treatment consists of bed rest on a firm mattress, with the patient nursed as far as is possible on one or other side. A firm binder may relieve some of the pain.

Sweating

Because of the vasodilatation and increased peripheral circulation, pregnant women 'feel the heat' and often sweat profusely, particularly in hot, humid climates. No treatment is available apart from frequent cool showers.

Vaginal discharges

In pregnancy the quantity of normal vaginal secretions increases and many women complain of a non-irritant vaginal discharge. Vaginal infections, particularly candidosis, are more frequent among pregnant women than among non-pregnant women. Vaginal discharges are discussed on page 259–261.

CHAPTER 12

Abortion

Abortion is defined as the expulsion of a fetus before it reaches viability. Because of different definitions of viability in different countries, the World Health Organisation (WHO) has recommended that a fetus is viable when the gestation period has reached 22 or more weeks, or when the fetus weighs 500g or more. As the term abortion does not differentiate between spontaneous and induced abortion, many obstetricians refer to the former as miscarriage. Most abortions occur naturally (or are induced) between the 6th and 10th week of pregnancy.

Data from several countries estimate that between 10 and 15% of clinically diagnosed pregnancies end as an abortion. Abortion is more frequent among women over the age of 30 years and increases further among women over the age of 35 years. It also increases in frequency with increasing gravidity: 6% of first or second pregnancies terminate as an abortion; with 3rd and subsequent pregnancies the rate increases to 16%.

Aetiology of spontaneous abortion

The causes of abortion are:
- Ovofetal.
- Maternal.

In the early weeks of pregnancy (0–10 weeks) ovofetal factors account for most abortions; in the later weeks (11–22 weeks) maternal factors become more common (Fig. 12.1).

OVOFETAL FACTORS

Ultrasonic examination of the fetus and subsequent histological examination show that in 70% of cases, the fertilized ovum has failed to develop properly or the fetus is malformed. In 40% of these cases chromosomal abnormalities are the underlying cause of the abortion and, in 20% of abortions, the trophoblast has failed to implant adequately.

MATERNAL FACTORS

Systemic maternal disease (e.g. systemic lupus erythematosis) and particularly maternal infections, account for 2% of abortions. A further 8% are associated with uterine abnormalities, such as congenital defects, uterine myomata, particularly submucous tumours, or cervical incompetence (see page 110). Psychosomatic causes have been suggested as leading to an abortion but the evidence is difficult to evaluate.

Mechanisms of abortion

The immediate cause of abortion is the partial or complete detachment of the embryo by minute haemorrhages in the decidua. As the placental function fails, uterine contractions begin, and the process of abortion is initiated. If this occurs before the 8th week, the defective embryo, covered with villi and some decidua, tends to be expelled en masse (the so-called blighted ovum), although some of the products of conception may be retained either in the cavity of the uterus or in the cervix. Uterine bleeding occurs during the expulsion process.

Between the 8th and 14th week the above mechanism may occur, or the membranes may rupture expelling the defective fetus but failing to expel the placenta, which may protrude through the external cervical os or remain attached to the uterine wall. This type of abortion may be attended by considerable haemorrhage.

Between the 14th and 22nd week the fetus is usually expelled followed, after an interval, by the placenta. Less commonly the placenta is retained. Usually bleeding is not severe, but pain may be considerable and resemble a miniature labour.

It is clear from this description that abortion is attended by uterine bleeding and pain, both of varying intensity. Although abortion is the cause of bleeding per vaginam in early pregnancy in over 95% of cases, less common causes such as ectopic gestation, cervical bleeding from the everted cervical epithelium or from an endocervical polyp, hydatidiform mole, and, rarely, cervical carcinoma must be excluded.

Fig. 12.1 Aetiological factors in 5000 abortions	
Factor	
Fetal or ovular	**Percentage**
Defective ovofetus	60
Defective implantation or activity of trophoblast	15
Maternal	
General disease	2
Uterine abnormalities	8
Psychosomatic	?15

Varieties of spontaneous abortion

For descriptive purposes the abortion is classified according to the findings when the woman is first examined, but one kind may change into another if the aborting process continues. If infection complicates the abortion, the term *septic abortion* is used. The various types of abortion are shown in *Figure 12.2* and each will be considered separately later.

Three other varieties of abortion are defined:

- *Recurrent abortion* is diagnosed if the woman has had three or more diagnosed abortions.
- *Induced (therapeutic) abortion* occurs when the pregnancy is terminated for medical reasons under rigid guidelines.
- *Illegal (criminal) abortion* is defined as termination of the pregnancy outside those guidelines.

THREATENED ABORTION

Threatened abortion is diagnosed when a pregnant woman develops uterine bleeding with or without painful uterine contractions; other causes of bleeding in early pregnancy should be excluded. A vaginal examination (or vaginal speculum examination) shows that the cervix is not dilated.

A real-time pelvic ultrasound examination will clarify the diagnosis. This may show:

- A normally sized amniotic sac and a fetus whose heart is beating.
- An empty amniotic sac.
- A missed or incomplete abortion.

Only if the first finding is obtained is the diagnosis confirmed. The ultrasound finding also provides the information that the pregnancy will continue (in 98% of cases), and the patient can be reassured. She should also be informed that in about 5% of cases the pregnancy will be curtailed and a preterm baby born.

The use of ultrasound examination has meant that the treatment of threatened abortion has changed in recent years. It is no longer normal practice to insist that the woman remains in bed until the bleeding has ceased. However, if the woman feels more comfortable there, she

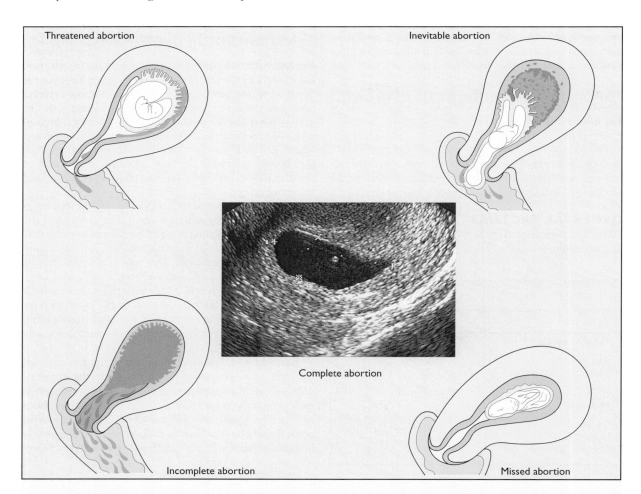

Fig. 12.2 *The types of abortion which may be seen. In complete abortion, the sac contains a small amount of debris.*

may do so. Drugs, hormones (e.g. progesterone) and sedatives have no effect except as a placebo, and should be avoided.

INEVITABLE, INCOMPLETE AND COMPLETE ABORTION

Abortion becomes *inevitable* if uterine bleeding is associated with strong uterine contractions which cause dilatation of the cervix. The woman complains of severe colicky uterine pains and a vaginal examination shows a dilated cervical os with part of the conception sac bulging through. Inevitable abortion may follow signs of threatened abortion or, more commonly, starts without warning.

Soon after the onset of symptoms of inevitable abortion, the abortion occurs either *completely*, when all the products of conception are expelled, or *incompletely* when either the pregnancy sac or the placenta remains, distending the cervical canal. In most cases the abortion is incomplete. Unless the doctor has been able to inspect all the material expelled from the uterus, or has had an ultrasound examination which shows an empty uterus (or one containing less than 10mm of tissues or blood clots), the abortion should be considered incomplete. This is treated by curettage; an alternative is to give misoprostol 400µg 4-hourly for three doses.

Treatment

A woman who is diagnosed as having an inevitable or an incomplete abortion and who is not in hospital should be transferred to one without delay. Before effecting the transfer, the examining doctor should give an analgesic to the patient (if required) and should make a vaginal examination. Any products of conception found protruding from the cervix should be removed by finger or sponge forceps, as leaving them may lead to vaso-vagal shock. If the woman is bleeding heavily an intramuscular injection of ergometrine 0.5mg should be given.

In hospital, intervention is required unless the abortion is proceeding quickly and with minimal blood loss. On admission of the patient a vaginal examination is made and any products of conception in the cervix are removed by finger or sponge forceps.

If there is any doubt about the completeness of the abortion, the patient should be taken to the operating theatre and the uterus evacuated using a sponge forceps (*Fig. 12.3*), followed by a careful suction curettage. Towards the end of the curettage, an injection of ergometrine 0.25mg is given intravenously.

Follow-up

Following a complete abortion, or one which has been completed surgically, bleeding usually ceases within 10 days. If placental remnants have been left in the uterus, the bleeding may persist beyond this time, varying in severity, and may be accompanied by uterine cramps. Examination will show a bulky uterus with a patulous os. Treatment is to perform an ultrasound and if this shows retained products of conception, recuretting the uterus carefully. The tissue removed should be sent for histopathology, as very rarely a choriocarcinoma is present.

Fig. 12.3 *The use of sponge forceps for clearing placental tissue from the uterus.*

A woman who is rhesus negative should be given a prophylactic injection of anti-D gammaglobulin, and a Kleihauer test should be performed to determine the amount of fetal blood cells in her circulation.

SEPTIC ABORTION

Although less common than formerly, because of better care in hospital and fewer 'backyard' abortions, infection may complicate some spontaneous and induced abortions. In 80% of cases the infection is mild and is localized to the decidua. The organisms involved are usually endogenous and are, most commonly, anaerobic streptococci, staphylococci or *E. coli*. In 15% of cases the infection is severe, involving the myometrium and may spread to involve the Fallopian tubes. If the infection spreads from the cervix it may involve the parametrium or the pelvic cellular tissues. In 5% of cases there is generalized peritonitis or vascular collapse, which is due to the release of endotoxins by *E. coli* or *Cl. welchii* and is termed endotoxic shock.

Clinical features

In infections limited to the decidua, production of a malodorous, pink vaginal discharge is usual and the patient may develop pyrexia. In more severe, spreading infections, pyrexia occurs, but its extent may not be related to the severity of the infection. Tachycardia usually develops: a pulse rate of more than 120 beats per minute indicates that spread has occurred beyond the uterus. Examination may show a tender lower abdomen; vaginal examination shows a boggy, tender uterus with evidence of extra-uterine spread.

Investigations

A high vaginal or cervical swab is made and, if the temperature is higher than 38.4°C, a blood culture should be taken. In severe infections, serum electrolytes and coagulation studies should be undertaken.

Treatment

Antibiotics are administered at once, the precise one chosen depending on local conditions, but in general a broad-acting antibiotic and one effective against anaerobes is selected. Twelve hours after starting antibiotics, or sooner if haemorrhaging is severe and the uterus is not empty, its contents are evacuated by careful curettage. If the infection is not controlled in spite of these measures hysterectomy may be indicated.

ENDOTOXIC SHOCK

As mentioned already this life-threatening condition follows 5% of septic abortions. Endotoxins released by *E. coli* and *Cl. welchii* are neutralized initially by phagocytes but if this protection fails, vasoconstriction of the postcapillary vessels occurs with resulting pooling of blood, a failure of venous blood to reach the heart and a reduced cardiac output. In addition, the Gram-negative endotoxins may act directly on the blood vessels and heart, releasing substances which profoundly affect the cardiovascular system.

Clinical signs include pyrexia, rigors, hypotension, tachycardia and hypoventilation. A patient with these signs is acutely ill and should be transferred to an intensive care unit with the least delay.

MISSED ABORTION

In a few cases of abortion, the dead embryo or fetus and placenta are not expelled spontaneously. If the embryo dies in the early weeks, it is likely to be anembryonic or blighted. In other cases a fetus forms but dies. Multiple haemorrhages may occur in the choriodecidual space, which bulge into the empty amniotic sac. This condition is called *carneous mole* (Fig. 12.4). It is thought that although the fetus has died, progesterone continues to be secreted by surviving placental tissue, which delays the expulsion of the products of conception.

If the fetus dies at a later stage of the pregnancy, but before the 22nd gestational week, and is not expelled, it is either absorbed or mummified. The liquor amnii is absorbed and the placenta degenerates. Fetal death after the 22nd week is discussed on page 112.

Clinical aspects

The patient usually has a history of threatened abortion, which settles down, but she complains of a dirty, brown discharge which persists. Examination, at intervals, shows that the uterus fails to grow (Fig. 12.5) and symptoms indicating early pregnancy disappear.

Fig. 12.4 *Carneous mole – a small fetus can also be seen in the centre.*

The diagnosis can not usually be made clinically for about 21 days, but can be established earlier by ultrasound examination.

Treatment

There is no medical need to treat missed abortion urgently as most cases end in a spontaneous abortion. Information and support must be given to the parents once they become aware that the fetus has died *in utero*, as this can be a very traumatic experience. The reason for delaying evacuation of the uterus if the uterine size is greater than 12–14 weeks gestational size must also be explained. Some women remain anxious after an explanation has been given and request that the abortion is completed. This is best effected using mifepristone and misoprostol or prostaglandins as described on page 111.

If a spontaneous abortion has not occurred within 28 days, the pregnancy should be terminated, as coagulation defects may result.

The termination procedure depends on the size of the uterus. If it is less than 12 weeks' gestational size, the uterus can be evacuated by sponge forceps and curette after cervical dilatation. If the uterus is more than 12 weeks' gestational size, the methyl ester of PGE_1 gemeprost (Cervagem) 1mg placed in the posterior vaginal fornix every 3 hours for a maximum of 5 doses in 24 hours is effective.

RECURRENT (HABITUAL) ABORTION

A few women (less than 1%) have the misfortune to miscarry successively. It has been estimated that after one abortion the risk of another is 20%; after two abortions it is 25% and, after three abortions, 30%. A woman who has three or more successive abortions is termed a recurrent aborter. As well as having a 30% chance of aborting again, if she avoids this outcome she is at greater risk than a non-aborter of delivering a preterm baby, but has at least a 75% chance of delivering a healthy infant at term.

The aetiological factors in recurrent abortion vary depending on the population studied, but two large series, of over 100 subjects in each, offer some idea of the aetiology (Fig. 12.6). In *Figure 12.6* the causes marked with a query are speculative.

Investigation and treatment of a recurrent aborter

A careful medical and obstetrical history may reveal systemic disease or suggest cervical incompetence. A vaginal examination may show uterine myomata or cervical incompetence, and the diagnosis can be clarified if a transvaginal ultrasound image is made. Ultrasound will also detect uterine malformations. *Submucous myomata* or *uterine septa* may be removed by abdominal surgery or under hysteroscopic vision. *Cervical incompetence* is discussed later.

If *endometrial infection* is considered a causative factor (as is the case with some specialists), endometrial tissue cultures may be made. However, it is doubtful if toxoplasmosis, cytomegalovirus, herpes virus, rubella or listeria are causes of recurrent abortion. Currently the role of bacterial vaginosis is being investigated.

Endocrine dysfunctions, for example, polycystic ovarian disease (see page 223) may be excluded by transvaginal ultrasound scanning. Other endocrine disorders, such as thyroid disease and diabetes, are no longer believed to be causes of recurrent abortion.

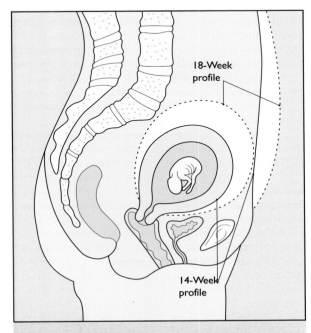

Fig. 12.5 Missed abortion. The duration of the pregnancy is 18 weeks but the uterus has failed to enlarge beyond the size of a 14-week gestation. Note that the abdomen is flat.

Fig. 12.6 Recurrent aborters		
	Percentage of abortions occurring	
Possible aetiology	**<12 weeks**	**>12 weeks**
Not known	62	35
Uterine malformations or abnormality	3	10
Cervical incompetence	3	30
Chromosome abnormality	<5	<4
?Endometrial infection	15	15
Endocrine dysfunction	3	3
Systemic disease	1	1
?Sperm factors	3	1
?Immune factors	?	1

Although it is usual to investigate both parents for *chromosome abnormalities*, such aberrations account for only 5% of recurrent abortions at the most, and no treatment is available.

Immunological causes for recurrent abortion have been investigated for the past 10 years. The theory is that if the two parents share several human leucocyte antigen (HLA) sites, the fetus may not be able to provide a sufficient stimulus to enable the mother to produce blocking antibodies to the allogenic fetus, with the result that the fetus is aborted. A clinical study which supports this theory found that if a woman who has had recurrent abortions changes her partner, her chance of aborting falls to that normally experienced by women in the community. The suggested treatment entails immunizing the woman between pregnancies with paternal leucocytes, pooled donor cells or trophoblast membrane preparations to enhance her immune system. Four of five clinical trials using this approach have failed to show any statistical benefit from immunotherapy.

A few women with an *autoimmune disease*, especially the antiphospholipid syndrome and systemic lupus erythematosus (SLE), have a strong blocking antibody reaction, which, it is believed, may lead to recurrent abortion. SLE must be excluded before immunotherapy is used as SLE may be aggravated. If SLE is identified by laboratory tests, treatment with low dose aspirin and low dose heparin improves the live birth rate from 10% to 70%.

General measures

Women who are recurrent aborters need considerable support and care. They should be advised to stop smoking, to avoid sexual intercourse and not to travel. The results from this regimen are as good as those following the use of multivitamins, hormones (including human chorionic gonadotrophin), metallic chemicals, thyroid extract and acupuncture, all of which are advocated from time to time.

Cervical incompetence

About 20% of women who have recurrent abortions in the second quarter of pregnancy will be found to have cervical incompetence. The diagnosis is based on:

- A history of recurrent abortions occurring after the 12th week of gestation, usually starting with painless leaking of amniotic fluid.
- The easy passage of a size 9 cervical dilator through the internal os of the cervix when the woman is not pregnant, and the absence of a 'snap' on its withdrawal.
- The gradual dilatation of the internal cervical os to more than 3cm during pregnancy as detected by ultrasound or repeated vaginal examinations.

If cervical incompetence is diagnosed, treatment entails placing a soft unabsorbable suture (such as Mersilk 4) around the cervix at the level of the internal cervical os (*Fig. 12.7*). The patient may return home the same night or stay in hospital for a day depending on the circumstances. There is no place postoperatively for the use of progesterone, uterine relaxants or narcotics.

Following cervical cerclage 10% of women abort, 10% give birth prematurely and the remainder give birth after the 36th week of pregnancy. Cervical cerclage should not be made if the membranes have ruptured. If abortion becomes inevitable following cerclage, the suture must be cut. In all other cases the sutre is left until about 7 days prior to term, at which time it is cut, and the woman may then be expected to give birth vaginally.

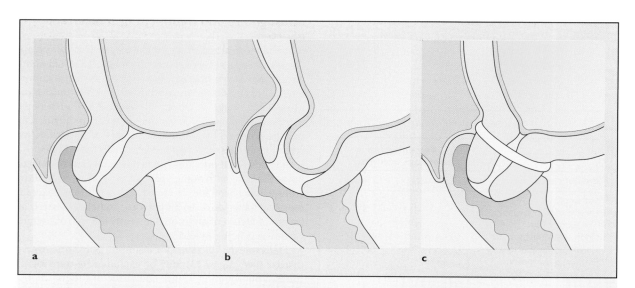

Fig. 12.7 Cervical incompetence. (a) Normal cervix at 16 weeks; (b) Incompetent cervix at 16 weeks; (c) Cerclage with an unabsorbable suture.

Psychological effects of spontaneous abortion

For most women a spontaneous abortion is a distressing occurrence: over 90% express a grief reaction which persists for a month in 20% of cases. During the period when the abortion threatens or is occurring, many women are distressed by not knowing what the outcome will be; others are distressed by being told to rest in bed without any further explanation.

Too little information is given by many doctors (both in general and hospital practice) after an abortion has occurred, about the reason for the abortion and the outcome of a future pregnancy. Women need counselling on these matters and need to have an opportunity to express their feelings. There are three main questions to which most women require answers:

• Why did the abortion occur?
• Is there anything that I did or did not do which caused the abortion?
• Is my next pregnancy likely to end in a miscarriage?

Some women are too embarrassed to ask these questions; even so the doctor should provide answers sensibly and sympathetically even if the questions are not asked. This will reduce the period of grief and distress that usually follows a spontaneous abortion.

Induced abortion

In many countries, induced (therapeutic) abortion is now legal. The exact conditions vary but the purposes of legalizing abortion are:

• To enable women, irrespective of social or economic status, after counselling to obtain an abortion performed by a trained health professional in hygienic surroundings.
• To reduce the frequency of illegal abortions performed in unhygienic surroundings, which are often associated with high morbidity and mortality.

The main reasons for the abortion are shown in *Figure 12.8*. In most developed countries where abortion is legal, over 95% are performed for social or psychiatric reasons. It should be stressed that women rarely seek an abortion without considerable thought, and are receptive to and welcome counselling during this difficult time. It is also evident that in many cases the pregnancy could have been prevented if effective contraceptive precautions had been taken.

TECHNIQUE OF INDUCED ABORTION

Abortion is safest when it is performed between the 6th and 12th gestational week. Only between 5 and 10% of terminations are made after the 12th week of pregnancy. Termination of the pregnancy may be surgical or medical.

The surgical approach is to evacuate the uterus using a suction curette, under local or general anaesthesia. Following curettage, uterine bleeding persists for about 6 days, often being light in the first 2 days after the termination. Most gynaecologists give the woman a course of doxycycline to prevent infection.

Medical methods of termination can be used if the pregnancy is less than 9 weeks' gestation. They include the administration of a single dose of the progesterone antagonist, mifepristone (200–600mg). The mifepristone tablet is followed 36–48 hours later by a prostaglandin E_1 vaginal pessary (gemeprost) 1mg every 6 hours for four doses. If the abortion has not started within 24 hours, gemeprost 1mg is given 3-hourly for up to four more doses. (An alternative is oral misoprostol 200μg repeated after 2 hours.) Bleeding usually starts during the interval between the mifepristone and the gemeprost vaginal pessary or oral misoprostol, and uterine contractions start within 4 hours of the administration of either drug. The pain may be severe and most women require narcotics. Nausea or vomiting affects one-third of patients. Bleeding persists for about 9 days, with a mean loss of 75ml (20–400ml). Over 98% of women abort using this regimen, but 10% require curettage for persistent heavy bleeding.

In countries where mifepristone is not available two commonly used drugs may be prescribed. Methotrexate 50mg per square metre of the body surface is given intramuscularly. This prevents folate from entering the fetal tissues with resultant death. Misoprostol 800μg is given intravaginally 5–7 days later and, following this, 75% of women abort within 24 hours. If the abortion does not occur, the misoprostol is repeated.

After the 12th gestational week the uterus may be evacuated using the following:

• Misoprostol 100–200μg given intravaginally every 12 hours for up to four doses.
• Prostaglandin $F_{2\alpha}$ (Dinoprost) vaginal pessaries.
• The mifepristone/gemeprost regimen mentioned earlier.

These regimens induce an abortion in 80–95% of patients and may replace dilatation of the cervix and uterine evacuation using sponge forceps and a curette, which can be a bloody and prolonged procedure.

Fig. 12.8 Indications for therapeutic abortion

Social

Psychiatric
Severe neuroses, psychoses

Medical
Severe cardiac disease; heart failure
Severe chronic renal disease; renal failure
Malignant disease, especially of breast or uterine cervix

Fetal
Viral infections
Haemolytic disease
Genetic defects
Congenital defects incompatible with normal life
(e.g. anencephaly, spina bifida)

Over 80% of women require narcotics for pain, and nausea or vomiting occurs in 30%. Following the abortion, one-third of women require evacuation of the uterus for retained products of conception.

SEQUELAE OF INDUCED ABORTION

An induced abortion performed before the 12th gestational week in a well-equipped and staffed clinic is followed by few complications. Less than 1% of women develop infection, and the mortality rate is less than 1 per 100,000 abortions. After the 12th gestational week the rate of complications rises to 3–5% and the mortality increases to 9–12 per 100,000. There is no reduction of the woman's fertility or any increase in the risk of spontaneous abortion, preterm birth or fetal loss in a subsequent pregnancy.

Psychological effects of induced abortion

An expert panel in the USA in 1990 reported that 'legal abortion of an unwanted pregnancy does not pose a psychological hazard for most women'. Most women feel grief and guilt after a termination but less than 10% show evidence of anxiety or depression persisting for more than a month. Most of the women adversely affected were ambivalent about having the abortion or were pressured by parents or partner into terminating the pregnancy. This finding emphasizes that a woman seeking an abortion should be counselled before the procedure takes place and should continue to receive support (if she chooses) during and after the operation.

Fetal intra-uterine death

The WHO has recommended that a fetus should be considered viable if the gestation period has reached 22 or more completed weeks or when the fetus weighs 500g or more. A fetus born after this time must be registered as a birth, either alive or stillborn. Not all countries have accepted the WHO recommendation. For example Britain categorizes a pregnancy ending before the 24th week of pregnancy as an abortion, and registration of a stillbirth is not required, although a live birth has to be registered.

Fetal intra-uterine death may follow pregnancy-induced hypertension, maternal diabetes mellitus and other complications of pregnancy. In most cases labour begins soon after the death and the baby is stillborn. In a few cases the dead fetus is retained in the uterus.

CLINICAL ASPECTS

The mother notices that fetal movements have ceased and Doppler examination fails to detect any fetal heart sounds. In addition to the psychological upset to the expectant mother when she realizes that her baby has died in the uterus and her concern that the dead fetus will decay and will infect her, medical problems are unlikely, at least in the first 3 weeks after the fetal death has been diagnosed. After this time, disseminated intravascular coagulation and hypofibrinogenaemia may arise with potentially serious consequences to the woman.

DIAGNOSIS

The history provides evidence that the fetus has died. This is confirmed by Doppler examination. In addition, an ultrasound examination may show overlapping of the bones of the fetal skull (Spalding's sign).

MANAGEMENT

The parents should be offered bereavement counselling and support. They should be made aware that the dead fetus will not cause any harm to the woman in the first 3 weeks after death and that, in most cases, labour will start before this time. The management of the labour should be discussed with the patient and she should be assured that she will be given analgesics to reduce or eliminate the pain of childbirth. In the event that she wishes to view and hold her fetus she should be made aware that it will be macerated.

The woman may choose to await spontaneous labour or to have labour induced. If spontaneous labour has not started by 3 weeks after the diagnosis, or if she chooses immediate treatment, labour is induced by prostaglandin E_2 vaginal pessaries or gel as described on page 193. Alternatives are to prescribe mifepristone 600mg a day for 3 days, misoprostol 100–200μg 12-hourly for four doses or the prostaglandin analogue, sulprostone, 1μg/min IV until the fetus is expelled. It is claimed that there are fewer gastrointestinal side effects if sulprostone is used. Using any of the methods, 50% of women will expel the fetus in 12 hours and 90% in 24 hours.

If the woman chooses to await the spontaneous onset of labour, frequent blood checks should be made by observing the clotting time of the blood or by estimating fibrinogen levels.

CHAPTER 13

Extra-uterine pregnancy – ectopic gestation

Most extra-uterine pregnancies occur in the Fallopian tubes (ectopic gestation) but, rarely, the fertilized ovum may implant on to the ovarian surface or the uterine cervix. Extremely rarely, the fertilized ovum implants on to the omentum (abdominal pregnancy).

The incidence of ectopic gestation is rising in the developed countries and is currently running at a rate of 1 in 80–150 pregnancies. The reason for the increase is not clear but the rise seen may be associated with increased sexual activity and an increased incidence of pelvic inflammatory disease or with earlier diagnosis using ultrasound.

Aetiology

The aetiology of ectopic gestation is not known. Implantation of the fertilized ovum can only take place when the zona pellucida has partially or completely disappeared. Premature implantation could occur if the passage of the fertilized ovum along the Fallopian tube is delayed because of tubal damage following infection. Premature implantation may occur in:

- The fimbriated end of the Fallopian tube (in 17% of cases).
- The ampulla (in 55% of cases).
- The isthmus (in 25% of cases).
- The interstitial portion of the tube (in 2% of cases) (Fig. 13.1).

Outcome for the pregnancy

In most cases the pregnancy terminates, in one of several ways (see below), between the 6th and 10th week.

TUBAL ABORTION

This occurs in 65% of cases and is the usual outcome in fimbrial and ampullary implantation (Fig. 13.2). Repeated small haemorrhages from the invaded area of the tubal wall detach the ovum, which dies and:

- Is absorbed completely.
- Is aborted completely through the tubal ostium into the peritoneal cavity.
- Is aborted incompletely, with the result that the clot-covered conceptus distends the ostium.
- Forms a tubal blood mole.

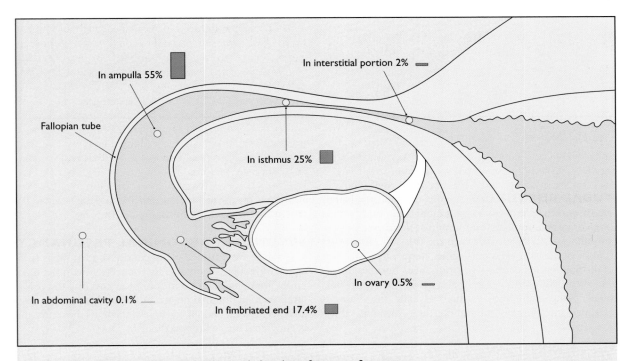

Fig. 13.1 Sites of ectopic gestation implantation, with the relative frequency of occurrence.

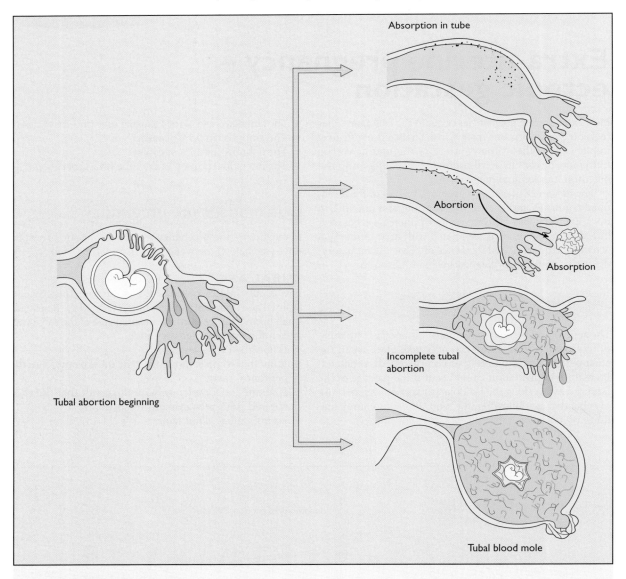

Fig. 13.2 Sequelae of tubal abortion.

TUBAL RUPTURE

This occurs in 35% of cases and is more common when the implantation is in the isthmus. Whilst the rupture of the ampulla usually occurs between the 6th and 10th week, rupture of the isthmus occurs earlier, frequently at the time of the first missed period. The trophoblast burrows deeply and eventually erodes the serosal coat of the tube, the final break being sudden or gradual. Usually the ovum is extruded through the rent and bleeding continues. If the rupture is on the mesenteric side of the tube, a broad ligament haematoma will form (*Fig. 13.3*).

SECONDARY ABDOMINAL PREGNANCY

Very rarely the extruded ovum continues to grow, as sufficient trophoblast maintains its connection with the tubal epithelium, and later the trophoblast covering the ovisac attaches to abdominal organs. A few of these pregnancies advance to term and, in a very few, the fetus dies early and is converted into a lithopaedion.

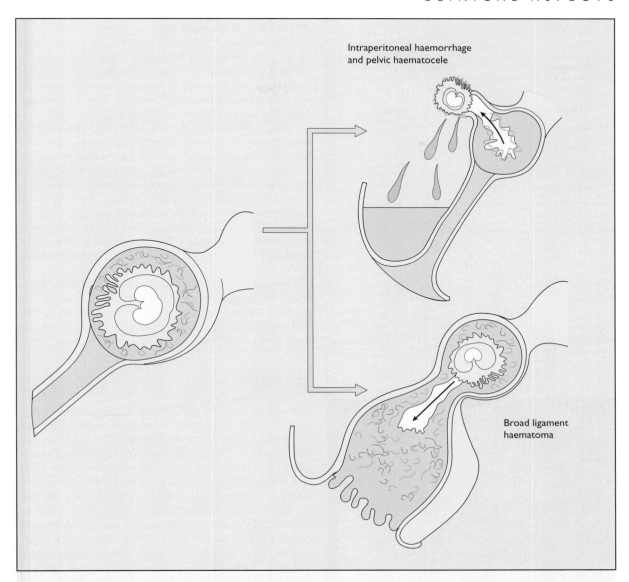

Intraperitoneal haemorrhage
and pelvic haematocele

Broad ligament
haematoma

Fig. 13.3 Sequelae of tubal rupture.

Clinical aspects

The possibility of an ectopic gestation should always be considered in a woman of childbearing age especially if there is a past history of acute salpingitis. The history is of greater importance than the physical signs, as these can be equivocal. Usually there is a short period of *amenorrhoea*, although in 20% of cases this may not be present. The *pain* is lower abdominal in site, but not distinguishable from that of abortion. However, in ruptured ectopic gestation *fainting* usually occurs, although this may only be momentary. *Vaginal bleeding* follows the pain, and may be mistaken for bleeding due to a delayed menstrual period or an abortion.

The bleeding is a slightly brownish colour and continuous, and clots are rarely present (*Fig. 13.4*).

Two clinical patterns occur, and are due to the extent of the damage to the tubal wall by the invading trophoblast. The first is subacute; the second acute.

SUBACUTE

After a short period of amenorrhoea, the patient experiences some lower abdominal discomfort, which may be so mild that she considers it normal for pregnancy. Occasionally there is an attack of sharp pain and faintness, due to an episode of intraperitoneal bleeding, and, if these symptoms are marked, and particularly if the episode is

Fig. 13.4 Symptoms and signs in ectopic gestation

Symptom/sign	Ectopic gestation (%)
Abdominal pain	90
Amenorrhoea	80
Adnexal tenderness	80
Abdominal tenderness	80
Vaginal bleeding	70
Adnexal mass	50

Fig. 13.5 Ectopic pregnancy.

ACUTE – DRAMATIC

Sudden collapse of the patient with little or no warning is more common when the implantation is isthmal, but is not the most frequent type of the acute clinical pattern. It is more usual for the acute rupture to supervene upon the subacute, but the mild symptoms of the latter may have been thought to be normal occurrences in pregnancy and ignored.

As the tube ruptures, the patient is seized with a sudden acute lower abdominal pain, sufficiently severe to cause fainting. The associated internal haemorrhage leads to collapse, pallor, a weak, rapid pulse and a falling blood pressure. Usually the condition improves after a short time, as the haemorrhage diminishes or ceases, but abdominal discomfort persists, and pain is felt in the epigastrium or is referred to the shoulder. A further episode of haemorrhage and collapse is likely, and continued bleeding can be suspected from increasing pallor and a falling haemoglobin level.

On examination the patient is shocked, and the lower abdomen is tender with some fullness and muscle guarding. Vaginal examination, which should only be carried out in hospital, shows extreme tenderness on movement of the cervix from side to side.

Diagnosis

Although in acute cases the presence of internal bleeding is obvious and the diagnosis not in doubt, in subacute cases the diagnosis can be extraordinarily difficult. Laboratory tests may help, but in most instances they are not particularly informative. A radio-immuno-assay for serum levels of β–human chorionic gonadotrophin (βhCG), should be made. A negative result (less than 1ng/ml) indicates that the woman is not pregnant, and ectopic gestation can be excluded. If the βhCG test is positive, a pelvic ultrasound examination should be made, preferably using a transvaginal probe. If this shows an empty uterus (Fig. 13.5), and particularly if it shows a sac and fetus in the Fallopian tube, the diagnosis is certain and a laparoscopy or a laparotomy should be made. On the other hand, if ultrasound shows an intra-uterine pregnancy, a concurrent ectopic pregnancy is extremely unlikely. If the diagnosis remains in doubt a laparoscopy will clear the matter up.

If ultrasound is not available, or is equivocal, the presumptive diagnosis should be confirmed by laparoscopy.

The diagnosis of suspected ectopic gestation is summarized in Figure 13.6.

Treatment

If the patient is seen in her home and ectopic gestation is suspected, she should be transferred to hospital without making a vaginal examination. If she is in shock, an

followed by slight vaginal bleeding, examination may reveal tenderness in the lower abdomen; vaginal examination may show a tender fornix or a vague mass, but the signs may be insufficient to make a diagnosis. If the patient is observed, further episodes of pain are likely, and the blood loss per vaginam persists until acute collapse supervenes (indicating tubal rupture or incomplete tubal abortion) or the symptoms cease (indicating complete abortion with or without a pelvic haematocele).

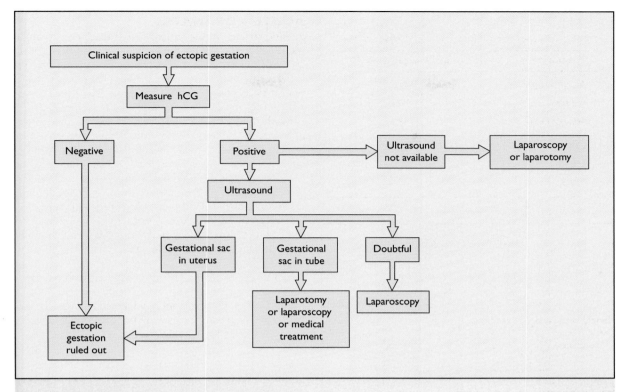

Fig. 13.6 Algorithm for diagnosis of suspected ectopic gestation.

intravenous line should be set up and transfer quickly arranged. Morphine may be given if the woman is in pain.

As mentioned, if there is any doubt about the diagnosis a pelvic ultrasound examination should be made to establish if the pregnancy is intra- or extra-uterine.

Once the ectopic gestation has been diagnosed, the treatment is surgical. Several approaches are possible. The gynaecologist may:
- Perform a laparotomy and either excise the Fallopian tube containing the ectopic gestation, or incise the tube over the ectopic gestation and 'milk' it out.
- Insert a laparoscope to inspect the Fallopian tube and, if possible, under laparoscopic vision incise along the superior border and suck the ectopic gestation out of the tube.
- If the tube has not ruptured, the gestation sac is small on ultrasound and the hCG level is not high, the gynaecologist may inject methotrexate into the ectopic gestation so that the viable trophoblast and embryo are absorbed, or give an intramuscular injection of methotrexate 50mg/m^2.

Following conservative surgery or if methotrexate is used, the woman should have serum hCG measurements made weekly until negative. If the woman complains of continuing symptoms, a second-look laparoscopy may be necessary.

Prognosis

Fewer than 60% of women who have had an ectopic gestation become pregnant again. Three-quarters of the women voluntarily avoid pregnancy, and one-quarter are involuntarily infertile. In a subsequent pregnancy the risk of a second ectopic gestation is 10% compared with a risk of less than 1% in other women. Because of this a woman who has had an ectopic gestation should be monitored carefully in the early weeks of her next pregnancy, a transvaginal ultrasound examination being made at 6–8 weeks' gestation, to establish that the pregnancy is intra-uterine.

CHAPTER 14

Antepartum haemorrhage

Antepartum haemorrhage is defined as significant bleeding from the birth canal occurring after the 20th week of pregnancy. The causes and proportions of cases of antepartum haemorrhage are shown in *Figure 14.1*. In fewer than 0.05% of cases the bleeding is due to a cervical lesion, such as a cervical polyp, or rarely, a cervical carcinoma. As a vaginal examination is usually made early in pregnancy, the local cervical conditions which may cause bleeding in the second half of pregnancy are usually diagnosed before the 20th week.

Fig. 14.1 The incidence of the causes of antepartum haemorrhage

	Incidence (%)
Placenta praevia	0.5
Accidental haemorrhage	
Unknown origin	3.0
Moderate grade	0.8
Severe grade	0.2
Cervical bleeding	0.05

Placenta praevia

In this condition the placenta is implanted, either partially or wholly, in the lower uterine segment and lies below (praevia) the fetal-presenting part. The extent of implantation may be minor, in which case vaginal birth is possible, or major, when it is not (*Fig. 14.2*).

Placenta praevia occurs in 0.5% of all pregnancies, and accounts for 20% of all cases of antepartum haemorrhage. It is three times as common in multiparous women as in primiparous, and no other aetiological factor has been detected.

The bleeding occurs when the lower uterine segment is increasing in length, and shearing forces between the trophoblast and the maternal blood sinuses occur. The first episode of bleeding occurs after the 36th gestational week in 60% of cases, between the 32nd and 36th week in 30% and before the 32nd week in 10%.

SYMPTOMS AND DIAGNOSIS

The bleeding is painless, causeless and recurrent. The presenting part is usually high and often not central to the pelvic brim. The diagnosis is made should an ultrasound image show that the placenta is praevia (*Fig. 14.3*).

If a routine ultrasound examination is made late in the second quarter of pregnancy, the report may show that there is a low-lying placenta. This does not mean that the placenta will be praevia later in pregnancy and a further ultrasound examination should be made at about the 30th week.

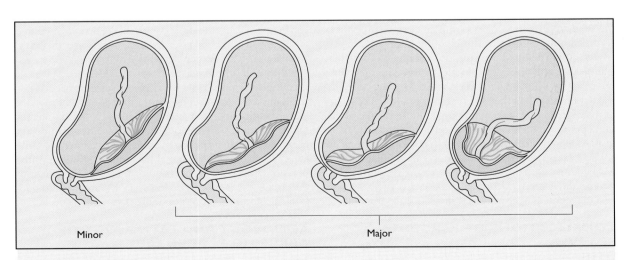

Minor   Major

Fig. 14.2 Degrees of placenta praevia.

Fig. 14.3 Placenta praevia – type two.

MANAGEMENT OF THE PLACENTA PRAEVIA

The first episode of significant bleeding usually occurs in the patient's home, and usually is not heavy. The patient should be admitted to hospital and no vaginal examination made, as this may start torrential bleeding. In hospital the patient's vital signs are checked, the amount of blood loss assessed and blood cross-matched. Heavy blood loss may require transfusion. The abdomen is palpated gently to determine the gestational age of the fetus, and its presentation and position. An ultrasound examination is made soon after admission, to confirm the diagnosis. Further management depends on the severity of the bleeding and the gestational age of the fetus.

In cases of severe bleeding, urgent treatment to deliver the baby (and the placenta) is required irrespective of the gestational age of the fetus. If the bleeding is less severe, expectant treatment is appropriate if the fetal gestational age is less than 36 weeks. As the bleeding tends to recur, the woman should remain in hospital and at the least, serum should be held in the blood bank in case urgent transfusion is required. An episode of severe bleeding may lead to urgent delivery but, in most cases, the pregnancy can continue until the 36th week, when the choice of delivery depends on whether the placenta praevia is of minor or major degree. Women who have a minor degree of placenta praevia may choose to await birth at term or may wish to have labour induced, provided that the conditions are suitable (see page 193). Placenta praevia of major degree is treated by caesarean section at a time determined by doctor and patient, although usually it is performed by 37–38 weeks, as a severe bleed may occur at any time.

COMPLICATIONS OF PLACENTA PRAEVIA

Episodes of heavy bleeding may occur at any time, during which the fetus may die from hypoxia. Following the birth, postpartum haemorrhage may occur because the trophoblast has invaded the poorly supported veins of the lower uterine segment. In most cases the haemorrhage ceases after administration of oxytocics, but occasionally the bleeding cannot be staunched and caesarean hysterectomy is required.

The perinatal mortality is less than 50 per 1000. The maternal mortality is low, provided the case is managed by an experienced obstetrician and no vaginal examination is performed before admission to hospital.

Accidental haemorrhage

The term 'accidental haemorrhage' derives from an observation made in 1775 that, in placenta praevia, haemorrhage is inevitable, whilst in the other group of antepartum haemorrhage it is due to some 'accidental' circumstance. About 4% of pregnant women develop accidental haemorrhage, which can be subdivided into three groups. In the first, the bleeding is slight, and when the placenta is examined after the birth, no retroplacental bleeding can be observed. This group is classified as *antepartum haemorrhage of unknown aetiology*. It accounts for 75% of cases of accidental haemorrhage.

In the second and third groups, there is evidence of retroplacental bleeding. The amount of blood lost to the circulation may be moderate or severe. These two groups are classified as *abruptio placentae*. Abruptio placentae accounts for 25% of cases of accidental haemorrhage. In four-fifths of cases of abruptio placentae the amount of blood lost to the circulation is moderate (less than 1500ml) and in one-fifth the blood loss is severe (more than 1500ml).

AETIOLOGY AND PATHOLOGY OF ABRUPTIO PLACENTAE

The aetiology is obscure, the only relevant associations being multiparity and cigarette smoking. Hypertensive diseases in pregnancy are associated with abruptio placentae in about 15% of cases, but it is not clear whether the hypertension is an aetiological factor.

The cause of the retroplacental bleeding is damage to the walls of the maternal venous sinuses supplying the placental bed. The bleeding spreads and causes detachment of the placenta to varying degrees. The blood then trickles down between the uterine decidua and the amniotic sac to appear in the vagina and vulva (revealed haemorrhage) or is retained behind the placenta (concealed haemorrhage). In a few cases of severe bleeding, the blood is forced by intra-uterine pressure between the myometrial fibres towards the serosal layer of the uterus. If the amount of blood is large, the uterus has the appearance of a bruised, oedematous organ, described as *apoplexie uteroplacentaire* or *couvelaire uterus*. This is a rare occurrence in today's obstetric practice.

In severe cases of abruptio placentae, shock may result from the distraction and separation of the myometrial fibres. Another complication is the release into the circulation of thromboplastins from the damaged vessels, which cause widespread intravascular coagulation. The microthrombi are dissolved by fibrinogens, mainly plasmin, with the release of fibrin-degradation products and the possible development of consumptive coagulopathy. In severe cases, some microthrombi escape lysis and are deposited in the endothelium of the vessels supplying the glomeruli of the kidneys. This may lead to tubular necrosis and oliguria or anuria.

SIGNS, SYMPTOMS AND TREATMENT OF ANTEPARTUM HAEMORRHAGE

The symptomatology is related to the degree of bleeding and the extent of placental detachment (*Fig. 14.4*).

Slight haemorrhage

The amount of blood lost is less than 500ml and there is no disturbance of the maternal or fetal condition. An ultrasound examination shows that the placenta is not lying in the lower uterine segment and no retroplacental clots can be seen. If the patient has been admitted to hospital she may go home once the bleeding ceases or, if the pregnancy has advanced to 37 weeks, she may choose to have labour induced by amniotomy, provided that the condition of the cervix warrants this.

Abruptio placentae: moderate placental detachment and haemorrhage

Usually at least one-quarter of the placenta has become detached and more than 1000ml of blood has been lost to the circulation. The woman complains of abdominal pain and the uterus is tender because blood has infiltrated between the muscle fibres of the uterus. The patient may be shocked, with a high pulse rate, but paradoxically in 5% of cases the pulse rate is within the normal range until delivery, at which time it rises precipitously. The fetus is hypoxic and may show abnormal heart rate patterns on a cardiotocogram.

Abruptio placentae: severe placental detachment and haemorrhage

In cases of severe placental detachment, at least 1500ml of blood has been lost to the circulation. The woman is usually in shock; her uterus is firm to hard and very tender. The fetus is almost always dead. As pregnancy-induced hypertension is only associated with about one-third of cases, the blood pressure may be in the normal range in spite of the shock. Most coagulopathies occur in this group.

Fig. 14.4 Comparison of the clinical picture in the various grades of accidental haemorrhage

| | Severity of bleeding | | |
	Mild	Moderate	Severe
Pulse	No change	Raised	Raised
Blood pressure	No change	Lowered	Lowered
Shock	None	Often	Always
Oliguria	Rare	Occasionally	Common
Hypofibrinogenaemia	Rare	Occasionally	Common
Uterus	Normal	Tender	Tender and tense
Fetus	Alive	Usually dead	Dead
Blood loss (litres)	<1	1–3	3–6

MANAGEMENT OF ABRUPTIO PLACENTAE

The management consists of restoring the blood lost, prevention of coagulopathy and monitoring urinary output:

- At least 1500ml of blood should be transfused in cases of moderate detachment, and 2500ml in cases classified as severe detachment. The first 500ml of blood is transfused rapidly. Rapid blood transfusion prevents renal 'shut down' and anuria. The central venous pressure is monitored and the remainder of the transfusion adjusted accordingly. The blood loss and the height of the fundus are monitored.

- Venous blood is examined 2-hourly for evidence of coagulopathy and, if present, this is treated. Adequate rapid transfusion and amniotomy or caesarean section usually prevent it from occurring.

- Urine output is measured 2-hourly. Oliguria may occur but diuresis follows the birth provided that sufficient blood has been transfused.

- If the fetus is alive the decision has to be made whether to perform a caesarean section or the artificial rupture of the amniotic membranes (ARM). If the latter procedure is chosen the circulating blood volume must be restored before performing an ARM. The fetal heart is monitored and, if the fetus develops distress, a caesarean section is performed.

MATERNAL AND FETAL LOSS

Maternal mortality depends on the speed and adequacy of treatment. Today, few women should die from abruptio placentae. Fetal mortality depends on the degree of placental separation.

CHAPTER 15

Hypertensive diseases in pregnancy

Between 5 and 8% of pregnancies are complicated by hypertensive diseases. These are pregnancy-induced hypertension, essential hypertension, and hypertension due to chronic renal disease. All of the hypertensive states may lead to eclampsia (fits).

Pregnancy-induced hypertension

Pregnancy-induced hypertension (PIH) was previously called toxaemia of pregnancy or pre-eclampsia. PIH accounts for 80% of all cases of hypertension in pregnancy and affects between 3 and 8% of patients, mainly primigravidae, in the second half of pregnancy.

CLASSIFICATION
There is no generally accepted classification of PIH. In each case the patient's blood pressure is measured at the level of the heart, with the woman propped up or lying on her side, after a rest of 10 minutes if she is an outpatient.

Potential PIH
The patient's blood pressure, measured as described, has risen by more than 30 points systolic or more than 15 points diastolic over her basal diastolic blood pressure. This should be taken as a warning that the woman may develop PIH, and she should be seen more frequently by a health professional.

Mild PIH (also known as gestational hypertension)
The patient's diastolic blood pressure is 90–99mmHg, and the elevation is detected on at least two occasions separated by 6 hours. The urine does not show significant protein (less than 300mg/L). Mild PIH poses little risk to the woman or to the fetus.

Moderate PIH
The patient's blood pressure lies in the range 140–170/100–110mmHg, confirmed on two occasions after resting. If significant urinary protein is found (more than 300mg/L) the category is changed to severe PIH.

A problem in determining whether the quantity of urinary protein is significant is that the 'dip stick' method is a poor predictor. A study, made in the USA, showed that the positive predictive value of protein 3+ or greater was only 36%. The authors recommend that urinary protein loss is measured in a 24-sample of urine before gestational proteinuric hypertension is classified.

Severe PIH (also known as pre-eclampsia or gestational proteinuric hypertension)
The patient's blood pressure exceeds 170/110mmHg or marked proteinuria is present. Severe PIH affects about 1% of primigravidae.

Imminent eclampsia
In addition to the signs of severe PIH, the patient complains of severe headache, blurring of vision or epigastric pain, and her reflexes are exaggerated.

Oedema
Oedema may occur in all grades of PIH, but it is of little diagnostic significance unless it is generalized, as oedema occurs as frequently in women who have no antenatal disorder.

PATHOGENESIS OF PIH
The aetiology of PIH is not known but there is increasing evidence that the disorder is due to an immunological disturbance in which the production of blocking antibody is reduced (see page 26). This may prevent the invasion of maternal spiral arteries by trophoblasts to any significant extent, leading to impairment of placental function. As pregnancy advances, placental hypoxic changes induce proliferation of cytotrophoblasts and thickening of the trophoblastic basement membrane, which may affect the metabolic function of the placenta. Normally the endothelial cells secrete a vasodilator substance. (This may be nitric oxide but the evidence is not strong.) Damaged cells, as in PIH, secrete less vasodilator. In consequence, endothelial cells of the placenta secrete less vasodilator prostacyclin and the platelets more thromboxane, leading to generalized vasoconstriction and decreased aldosterone secretion. The results of these changes are maternal hypertension, a 50% reduction in placental perfusion, and a reduced maternal plasma volume. If the vasospasm persists, trophoblastic epithelial cell injury may occur, and trophoblast fragments are then carried to the lungs where they are destroyed, releasing thromboplastins. In turn, thromboplastins cause intravascular coagulation and deposition of fibrin in the glomeruli of the kidneys (glomerular endotheliosis), which reduces the glomerular filtration rate and indirectly increases vasoconstriction. In advanced, severe cases fibrin deposits occur in vessels of the central nervous system, leading to convulsions.

PREVENTION OF PIH
Knowledge of the pathophysiology of PIH, although rudimentary, has suggested ways of preventing the disorder.

None has been successful. It was hoped that aspirin, which reduces platelet production of pro-aggregatory vasoconstrictor thromboxane A$_2$, would reduce the risk of recurrent PIH. However meta-analysis of trials showed it to be ineffective, except, perhaps, in women who have a raised diastolic blood pressure before 28 weeks of pregnancy. Another trial using calcium also showed no benefit.

MANAGEMENT OF PIH

The management of PIH is shown in *Figure 15.1*. The table shows that there is no consensus about treatment, and few double-blind studies have been made.

The aim of treatment is to permit the continued growth of the fetus until it is sufficiently mature to survive outside the uterus, or until the risk of intra-uterine death is estimated to be greater than that of extra-uterine death. The duration of treatment depends on:
- The severity of PIH.
- The duration of the pregnancy.
- The patient's response to treatment.

There is no cure for PIH except to terminate the pregnancy and deliver the fetus and placenta. The treatment is merely to buy time so that the fetus becomes more mature in the uterus.

Fig. 15.1 Summary of the management of pregnancy-induced hypertension

Classification	Nursing responsibilities	Obstetricians' treatment
Potential PIH	Report significant rise in blood pressure, or excessive weight gain, to obstetrician.	Usually no treatment required. See patient in 7 days.
Mild PIH	Report rise in blood pressure or excessive weight gain to obstetrician.	Possible admission to hospital, depending on socio-economic conditions. If not admitted, see patient in 3 days.
Moderate PIH	In hospital: Four-hourly recording of the blood pressure. Twice-daily urine testing for protein. Regular observation of the patient's condition, including fluid intake and output. Bed rest, but toilet privileges allowed.	Admit to hospital. Sedation (if indicated). Labetalol (starting) 100mg twice daily or atenolol (starting) 100mg in evening or oxprenolol (starting) 20mg three times daily or methyldopa (starting) 250mg three times daily. Nifedipine 10mg sublingually repeated as needed.
Severe PIH	Two-hourly blood pressure recording for 6 hours, then 4-hourly. Urine testing for protein and acetone twice daily. Fluid intake and output recorded. Careful observation of the patient for the signs of imminent eclampsia. Complete bed rest for 24 hours, thereafter possible toilet privileges.	Admit to hospital. Depending on the severity of the illness give: a) Magnesium sulphate (see page 126). This is the preferred medication b) Hydralazine intravenously Intravenous frusemide 20 mg or stable plasma protein substitute (SPPS), if persistent oliguria. ?Caesarean section.
Imminent eclampsia	The patient requires careful systematic observation as eclampsia is a possible outcome. The blood pressure requires frequent estimation, at intervals determined by the obstetrician. Fluid intake and urinary output must be measured meticulously, and the urine tested quantitatively for protein.	Magnesium sulphate (see page 126). This is the preferred medication. Hydralazine intravenously. Caesarean section.

PIH diagnosed before week 32 of pregnancy

Before the 32nd week of pregnancy the objective is to keep the fetus *in utero* until the 35th week or longer. Fetal well-being is monitored by daily fetal movement counts, or 3-weekly cardiotocograph examinations (see page 161). Two sinister signs are slow fetal growth detected by serial ultrasound examinations and abnormal Doppler umbilical blood flow measurements.

Platelet counts are made at intervals in cases of severe PIH. In most cases a reduced platelet count returns to normal after the birth, but a few patients who have severe PIH complain of upper abdominal pain, nausea or vomiting. If the platelet count is less than 100,000 the woman may have the HELLP syndrome (haemolysis, elevated liver enzymes, low platelets). Treatment consists of correcting the thrombocytopaenia and delivering the fetus.

If the PIH worsens the pregnancy must be terminated, usually by caesarean section.

PIH diagnosed between the 32nd and 35th week of pregnancy

PIH diagnosed between the 32nd and the 35th week is managed in the same way as before the 32nd week, but should delivery of the fetus be indicated the choice is caesarean section or induction of labour.

PIH diagnosed after the 35th week of pregnancy

PIH diagnosed after the 35th week of pregnancy should be controlled rapidly and labour induced, or a caesarean section performed, depending on the condition of the fetus and the state of the cervix (see page 193).

Women with PIH should not become postdates as the risk of intra-uterine death increases after term.

Care after birth

The woman needs to have 4-hourly blood pressure readings taken for 7 days after birth, and, if the blood pressure remains high, antihypertensive agents should be continued. Proteinuria often persists for longer and is of little consequence. One-third of the women will have non-proteinuric hypertension in a subsequent pregnancy, but the rate of recurrence of severe PIH is less than 5%.

If severe PIH presents before 34 weeks gestation a careful search for an underlying medical disorder such as renal disease, should be made.

Eclampsia

The purpose of the treatment of hypertensive disorders in pregnancy is to prevent eclampsia. The word arises from the Greek 'like a flash of lightning', and this is how the disease may occur.

Eclampsia is characterized by convulsions and coma, which usually occur in patients who have severe PIH or imminent eclampsia, and in patients in whom gestational proteinuria has been superimposed on chronic hypertension. In 10–30% of women there are no warning signs, the fits occurring 'like a flash of lightning'. With better antenatal care and early recognition and treatment of PIH and chronic hypertension, the incidence of eclampsia has fallen. In developed countries eclampsia occurs in 1:2000 pregnant women, but in the developing countries the incidence is higher.

PATHOPHYSIOLOGY

The changes which occur in severe PIH are more marked in eclampsia: vasospasm is intense, with tissue hypoxia; the glomerular filtration rate is further reduced and urinary output falls; intracellular water retention impedes cellular metabolism and cerebral oedema may occur; blood viscosity increases, platelet levels fall and coagulation defects arise.

CLINICAL PICTURE

The convulsion is preceded by a disorientation stage during which the woman becomes restless, twitches and develops spasmodic respiration. Within a minute she passes into the tonic stage of the convulsion: her back arches, her hands clench, she grimaces, her breathing ceases and she becomes cyanosed. In this stage she may bite her tongue. She then passes into the clonic stage of the convulsion, when her body jerks uncontrollably, frothy saliva may fill her mouth and her breathing becomes stentorous. Finally, she becomes comatose (*Fig. 15.2*). The coma may persist for an hour or longer, or recurrent convulsions may occur.

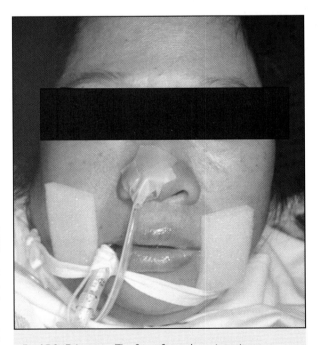

Fig. 15.2 Eclampsia. The face of an eclamptic patient.

The convulsions occur in late pregnancy in 40% of cases, intrapartum in 30% and a few hours after the birth in 30%.

MANAGEMENT OF ECLAMPSIA

The aims of treatment are:
- To control the fits by relieving the generalized vascular spasm and decreasing the sensitivity of the brain to stimuli.
- To reduce the blood pressure to prevent cerebral haemorrhage.
- To deliver the fetus.

Nursing care

The quality of the nursing care of an eclamptic patient is crucial. The patient is nursed on her side, with her head and shoulders raised, and a catheter is inserted into her bladder. The attending nurses must:
- Detect any changes presaging a second convulsion.
- Prevent the woman injuring herself during a convulsion.
- Provide continuous oxygen.
- Keep the mouth and fauces clear of any saliva by suction.
- Monitor vital signs and urinary output.

MEDICAL AND DRUG TREATMENT

Drug treatment – magnesium sulphate

Magnesium reduces the risk of recurrent seizures by relieving vasospasm and inducing cerebral vascular dilatation. It increases the release of prostacyclin, improving uterine blood flow, inhibits platelet activation and protects endothelial cells from injury.

Magnesium sulphate may be given intravenously or by deep intramuscular injection (*Fig. 15.3*). The intravenous route is preferred as the intramuscular injections are painful and are followed, in 5% of cases, by deep abscess formation.

The regimen is as follows:

Loading dose when the eclamptic patient is first seen: $MgSO_4$ 4g IV over 5–15 minutes, followed by $MgSO_4$ 1g/h (as an infusion of $MgSO_4$ 5g in 500ml of normal saline).

Continuing treatment: rate of infusion to provide 1g/h until 24 hours have passed since the last seizure, or the woman has given birth.

As useful as magnesium sulphate is in controlling the fits some problems may arise from magnesium toxicity. These and their management are:

Respiratory arrest: intubate, ventilate, and stop the $MgSO_4$ infusion. Give 1g calcium gluconate IV (the antidote to magnesium toxicity).

Respiratory depression: give oxygen by mask, calcium gluconate 1g IV and maintain a clear airway.

Absent patellar reflexes: if respiration is normal, stop the $MgSO_4$ infusion until reflexes return. If respiration is depressed, treat for this condition.

Poor urinary output (less than 100ml in 4 hours): if there are no other signs of magnesium toxicity, reduce the rate of the IV infusion to 0.5g/h and monitor fluid balance.

Antibiotics should be prescribed

If cardiac failure occurs, frusemide 20mg may be given intravenously, but because of the hypovolaemia it should be used with care.

Medical treatment

Once good control of the blood pressure and the convulsions has been gained, the pregnancy should be terminated. Depending on the period of the gestation, the health (alive or dead) of the fetus and its presentation, and on the condition of the cervix, delivery may be effected by caesarean section or labour may be induced using prostaglandins or by amniotomy. In most cases of eclampsia, induction of labour is followed rapidly by the birth of the infant. As post-partum haemorrhage may occur, prophylactic intravenous syntocinon should be given on the birth of the infant. The patient should continue to be monitored at least for the first 4 days of the puerperium.

PROGNOSIS IN PIH AND ECLAMPSIA

Today few women in the developed countries should die from severe PIH or from eclampsia. The situation in the developing countries is not so good: the maternal mortality after eclampsia varies between 3 and 20%, depending on the speed of starting treatment. Most deaths are from cerebral haemorrhage or cardiac failure.

Chronic (essential) hypertension

Most women with chronic hypertension have been diagnosed before the pregnancy; a few women are found to be hypertensive at the first antenatal visit. In the absence of a secondary cause for hypertension (for example renal artery stenosis or phaeochromocytoma), a raised blood pressure (greater than 140/90mmHg) which persists and is present before pregnancy or detected before the 20th gestational week, is diagnostic of essential hypertension. It is important to remember that the small physiological fall in blood pressure in the first half of pregnancy may be exaggerated in women who have chronic hypertension, and some cases may be missed.

Fig. 15.3 Magnesium sulphate treatment for eclampsia

Loading dose

$MgSO_4$ 4g intravenously over 5 to 15 minutes

Maintenance dose

$MgSO_4$ 1g per hour in solution of 5g in 500ml normal saline

Essential hypertension complicates 1–3% of pregnancies, and is more frequent among women over the age of 35.

PATHOPHYSIOLOGY

The generalized vasospasm of essential hypertension is counterbalanced by an increased stroke volume and heart rate, which maintains an adequate blood flow to most organs, with the exception of the uterus. Although uterine blood flow is increased in normal pregnancy, the increase is less in women who have essential hypertension and the higher the blood pressure the less the increase. This may reduce fetal growth and increase perinatal loss.

Pregnancy affects the course of essential hypertension. In 60% of affected women, a rise in blood pressure occurs, and, in 30%, significant proteinuria (more than 300mg/L) is detected. The changes usually occur after the 30th week of pregnancy. Essential hypertension with superimposed proteinuria is indistinguishable from severe PIH.

TREATMENT

The aims of treatment are:

- To obtain and to maintain as good a blood supply to the uterus as possible.
- To control the level of the blood pressure and prevent the superimposition of proteinuria.
- To terminate the pregnancy if the patient's condition deteriorates markedly, or if the fetus fails to grow adequately in the last quarter of pregnancy.

Maintenance of uterine blood supply

Usually the woman is instructed to rest more to improve the uterine blood supply.

Control of the hypertension

Most patients will be taking an antihypertensive drug and consultation should be made with a physician to confirm that the drug is required and that it is safe to be given during pregnancy. Diuretics should be avoided as these agents reduce plasma volume and uteroplacental blood flow. Most experience has been obtained using methyldopa, but it appears that beta-blockers such as atenolol, labetolol and calcium-channel blocker inhibitors are safe. Angiotensin-converting enzyme (ACE) inhibitors should be avoided.

Avoidance of problems

The woman should be seen more frequently during the antenatal period, the frequency depending on the severity of the hypertension. Her lifestyle should be checked, and if she is obese, a reduction diet should be prescribed. Her salt intake should be regulated.

If the fetus shows signs of growth restriction, biophysical tests for fetal well-being should be started (Chapter 21, The at-risk fetus), and if conditions deteriorate induction of labour should be discussed with the patient. It is safer for the fetus to be born earlier rather than later, and the patient should not become postdate as the perinatal loss increases.

Renal disease in pregnancy

Less than 0.2% of pregnant women, and less than 5% of women with hypertension in pregnancy, have renal disease. In most cases the diagnosis is known before pregnancy, but routine examination of a midstream urine specimen (which is made to detect symptomless bacteriuria) may occasionally detect an affected woman. Most affected women have no impairment of renal function, which is tracked by periodic serum creatinine measurements. If the level rises to more than 0.18mmol/L and there is evidence of poor fetal growth, either renal dialysis or induction of labour should be performed after consultation with a renal physician.

CHAPTER 16

Cardiovascular, respiratory and haematological disorders

Cardiovascular complications in pregnancy

It will be recalled that pregnancy places an increased strain on the heart because of the increased rate and stroke volume. The burden on the heart reaches its maximum at about the 28th week of pregnancy and continues into the puerperium. If a pregnant woman has heart disease, the increased strain may affect her well-being.

At present in the developed countries, between 0.2 and 0.5% of pregnant women have heart disease. In 30% of the cases, a woman has mitral valve disease; in 20%, ventricular septal defect; in 15%, atrial septal defect; in 15%, aortic stenosis; and in the remainder, other defects.

DIAGNOSIS

In most cases the diagnosis has been established before the pregnancy, but the doctor should auscultate the woman's heart at the first antenatal visit. Any suspicious signs, particularly a diastolic or loud systolic murmur, should lead to a referral to a cardiologist.

MANAGEMENT IN PREGNANCY

The initial assessment of the pregnant woman should be made in conjunction with a cardiologist, after which the medical management of the pregnancy can be carried out by the attending doctor, the patient being reviewed by the cardiologist at intervals. The aims of management are:

- To avoid those factors which predispose the woman to heart failure.
- Should failure occur, to treat it vigorously.

Factors which predispose to heart failure include anaemia, infections (particularly urinary tract infections) and the development of hypertension. If any of these are found, treatment should be started.

The woman's cooperation, and that of her family, should be obtained. Her daily activities should be evaluated and changes suggested if this is appropriate.

The patient should be seen at intervals of no more than 2 weeks up to the 28th week of pregnancy and, thereafter, weekly by a doctor (if it causes less stress on the woman, it could be her GP in collaboration with the obstetrician and the cardiologist). At each visit cardiac function is assessed by inquiring about breathlessness on exertion, or if she has a cough or orthopnoea. Her lungs are auscultated to detect rales.

Many cardiologists place pregnant women in categories suggested by the New York Heart Association and the management is planned on this. Initially most pregnant women are in class 1 or 2, but during pregnancy some degree of cardiac decompensation may occur.

Class 1

The patient has no symptoms, although signs of cardiac damage are present. She can undertake all physical activities. In this class, no additional treatment is needed.

Class 2

The woman is comfortable at rest, but ordinary physical exertion usually causes fatigue, palpitations and, occasionally, dyspnoea. Most patients in this class do not require treatment but if the woman's social conditions are unfavourable or if signs of a deterioration in cardiac reserve occur, she should be admitted to hospital.

Class 3

Less than ordinary physical exertion causes dyspnoea and fatigue, although the patient is comfortable when resting. Most women in this class should be admitted to hospital for rest, but home conditions and responsibilities have to be assessed and help provided if needed.

Class 4

Women in this class are seriously ill. The patient is breathless even when resting. Hospital admission is mandatory.

Heart failure

Should the woman develop heart failure the principles of treatment are no different from those of non-pregnant women. Digoxin is given to control the heart rate and increase the time for blood flow into the left ventricle. Diuretics (such as frusemide) are given when pulmonary oedema is present. There is no consensus if women who are not in cardiac failure should be given prophylactic digoxin, but most experts agree that if the woman is at risk of atrial fibrillation or has mitral heart disease and an enlarged left atrium, digoxin is indicated.

MANAGEMENT DURING CHILDBIRTH

Most women who have heart disease have an easy, spontaneous labour and there is no indication for inducing labour on account of the cardiac condition. During labour the patient should be nursed either on her side or well propped up, as compression of the aorta in the supine position may cause marked hypotension. The woman's fluid balance and her pulse rate should be checked at intervals. If her pulse rate is more than 110bpm between contractions and she has not been receiving digoxin, she should be 'digitalized'.

The place of prophylactic antibiotics is not clear, but many cardiologists recommend that they are given from the onset of labour and for the first 5 puerperal days.

Delay in the second stage of labour should be rectified by the use of forceps or vacuum extractor, but there is no place for a prophylactic instrumental delivery. The third stage is conducted in the same way as in non-cardiac patients, and active management using syntometrine is safe, unless the woman is in heart failure.

THE PUERPERIUM
The burden on the heart continues into the puerperium. For the first 24–48 hours the patient must receive constant observation for signs of decompensation. The woman should be nursed propped up and remain in bed for the first 2 days of the puerperium, and in hospital for 7 days.

PROGNOSIS FOR MOTHER AND BABY AND FOR FUTURE PREGNANCIES
With good antenatal care the risk to the mother or fetus is not increased during the current pregnancy. Only women in classes 3 and 4 should be dissuaded from having a further pregnancy until the condition of the heart has been assessed and further treatment, including surgery, discussed.

Thromboembolism in pregnancy

Thromboembolic disease affects between 50 and 60 pregnant or postpartum women per 100,000. Recent studies have shown that as many cases occur in pregnancy as in the puerperium. Women who have had the disease in a previous pregnancy have a recurrence rate of 10% and should be monitored (see also postpartum thromboembolism - page 189).

Treatment in pregnancy consists of prescribing heparin, initially intravenously (40,000U per day by continuous infusion in normal saline) to obtain a concentration of 0.6–1.0U/ml. Once full heparinization has been obtained for 3–7 days, the infusion may be replaced by calcium heparin given subcutaneously.

Respiratory conditions

ASTHMA
The effect of pregnancy on asthma is variable, but most asthmatic women experience fewer attacks. Asthma has no effect on the course of pregnancy, labour or the birth weight of the infant. Treatment is in no way different from that of a non-pregnant asthmatic woman.

PULMONARY TUBERCULOSIS
Although the prevalence of pulmonary tuberculosis is low in most developed countries, it appears to be increasing with increased movement of populations.

A patient diagnosed as having active tuberculosis in the first half of pregnancy should be treated with isoniazid and ethambutol. After the 20th week of pregnancy, rifampicin may be used.

The management of labour does not differ from that for a non-infected woman. If the mother's sputum shows acid-fast bacilli, the baby should be separated from her, vaccinated with bacille Calmette-Guérin (BCG) and remain separate for about 6 weeks. If the mother's sputum has no acid-fast bacilli, the baby should be vaccinated with BCG but may remain with her and be breastfed if the mother wishes to breastfeed.

Anaemia in pregnancy

In the developing countries, anaemia poses a considerable danger to pregnant women. In the developed countries, anaemia in pregnancy is less common, but some women, particularly of the lower socio-economic groups, become anaemic in pregnancy.

A healthy adult woman has a total body iron content of 3500–4500mg. Of this, 75% is held in the erythrocytes as haemoglobin; 20% is held in body stores, mainly the bone marrow and reticulo-endothelial system as a ferritin complex; and the remaining 5% is held in muscles and enzyme systems, mainly as myohaemoglobin.

The life of an erythrocyte is 100–120 days; each day erythrocytes die and release iron, and new erythrocytes are formed which use this released iron. However, each day a loss of 1mg of iron occurs through the death of epithelial cells. In women, iron is also lost each month in menstrual discharge. This averages about 1mg a day. Thus a non-pregnant woman needs 2mg of iron a day to maintain her iron balance. The average 'mixed' diet of a woman in the developed countries provides 12–15mg of iron of which 14–20% is absorbed. For most women this provides sufficient iron to maintain iron balance. In the developing countries, where the diet consists mostly of complex carbohydrates and vegetables, more dietary iron is needed daily as the cereals contain phytates which prevent iron absorption. In addition, many women living in these countries are infested with hookworm, which may cause a considerable loss of blood in the stools. These reasons (and malabsorption of iron in some women) provide the explanation of the higher prevalence of anaemia in pregnant women in the non-industrialized countries.

Pregnancy imposes an increased demand for iron, to meet the needs of the woman's larger red cell mass and additional muscle formation, particularly that of the uterus. This amounts to 425mg spread out over the 40 weeks of pregnancy. Also, the fetus requires about 300mg of iron, mostly in the last quarter of pregnancy, and the placenta, 25mg. Thus, pregnancy places a demand for 750mg of iron, less the 130mg saved from the cessation of menstruation. The demand is not constant throughout the pregnancy, but increases as pregnancy advances (*Fig. 16.1*). The increased demand for iron is, to some extent, compensated for by an increased absorption of iron from food. At 30 weeks' gestation, 30% of ingested iron is absorbed and, by 36 weeks 66% of the ingested iron is absorbed, a 9-fold increase over the absorption of iron at 16 weeks' gestation.

DIAGNOSIS

Most cases of anaemia in pregnancy are due to iron deficiency, but in areas where people from southeast Asia, southern Europe and Africa live, or in those areas they have migrated to, thalassaemia and sickle cell anaemia occur. In a few cases of severe anaemia (Hb less than 65g/L), megaloblastic anaemia may be present.

For these reasons all pregnant women should have a sample of blood tested for the presence of anaemia at the first antenatal visit. The test may be repeated at the 30th and 36th week of pregnancy. The number of tests varies, depending on local circumstances (*Fig. 16.2*), but a haemoglobin or a haematocrit estimation is always made.

If clinical anaemia is detected (Hb less than 105g/L), the mean cell volume (MCV) and serum ferritin should be measured, as a reduced Hb may merely indicate that the patient has a large blood volume.

TREATMENT

Treatment depends on the severity of the iron deficiency and the length of time available between diagnosis and the expected date of the birth. If the anaemia is detected before the 36th week of pregnancy and the haemoglobin level is greater than 65g/L, oral iron may be given. The dose should not exceed 200mg of elemental iron a day because of gastrointestinal upset, and the more severe the anaemia the greater the amount absorbed. Treatment should be started with one-third of the dose required and gradually built up. The iron tablets should be taken 8-hourly so that absorption may occur throughout the 24 hours. A daily increase of about 1.5g/L may be expected, and if this response has not occurred over a 2-week period, the case should be reviewed and megaloblastic anaemia suspected. If the woman is unable to take oral iron, if the time to delivery is short, or the haemoglobin level is less than 65g/L, parenteral iron should be substituted for oral iron. The regimen and dosage is provided in the manufacturer's product information sheet. Blood transfusions should be avoided, if possible, for obvious reasons.

Women who have severe anaemia should also be given folate, 5mg a day, as the severe anaemia may mask megaloblastic (folate-deficient) anaemia. The lower the haemoglobin level the greater the chance that the woman has megaloblastic anaemia. Megaloblastic anaemia may be suspected if more than 7% of neutrophils have five or more lobes, and confirmed by examining a bone marrow film for megaloblasts. Treatment consists of prescribing folate, 5–10mg daily by mouth, unless the woman has tropical sprue or coeliac disease, whereupon folate should be given parenterally. In addition, iron tablets should be prescribed.

SHOULD PROPHYLACTIC IRON BE GIVEN?

It is important to diagnose anaemia in pregnancy, as anaemic women have a higher mortality (3–5 times higher than for non-anaemic women) and the stillbirth rate is increased 6-fold. This raises the question: 'Should all pregnant women receive prophylactic iron tablets?' Tradition decrees that all women should be prescribed iron tablets, but the evidence is that most women fail to take them regularly because of nausea or constipation (which may or may not be due to the iron tablets). A healthy woman, whose haemoglobin is within the normal range and who eats a mixed diet, probably does not need to take additional iron, at least in the first half of pregnancy. A woman whose diet is less balanced, or who lives in a developing country, needs iron. The daily amount needed for a woman in the industrialized countries is 85mg of elemental iron, which can be obtained from any of the available

	Over period of pregnancy		Daily needs	
Week	**Net maternal needs[1] (mg)**	**Fetoplacental needs (mg)**	**Total daily need (mg)**	**Daily intake required[2] (mg)**
1–9	100	40	1.4	10–12
10–19	200	65	2.6	10–12
20–29	200	120	3.3	14–16
30–39	200	200	4.0	18–22

Fig. 16.1 Iron requirements in pregnancy

Notes

1. The net maternal needs are calculated from:

• Replacement of iron lost from epithelial cells 1mg/day.

• Increase in red cell mass and muscle development 1.6mg/day.

• Less savings due to amenorrhoea 0.6mg/day.

• Net daily needs 2.0 mg/day.

2. Assumes a daily utilization rate of 20–25% of dietary elemental iron.

Fig. 16.2 The diagnosis of anaemia in pregnancy	
Haemoglobin	<105g/L
Haemotocrit	<0.30
MCV	An MCV of <80fl indicates possible β-thalassaemia. If found, an estimation of haemoglobin A₂ and haemoglobin electrophoresis should be made.
MCH	<28pg
MCHC	<32g/dl
Serum ferritin	A level of 10–50μg/L indicates a strong possibility that anaemia will develop, whilst a level of <10μg/L indicates severe depletion of iron stores. In the latter case iron tablets should be prescribed, irrespective of the haemoglobin level. Some authorities estimate serum ferritin at 24, 30 and 36 weeks to ensure that iron deficiency does not occur.

iron preparations (none is better than any other); a woman in the non-industrialized countries needs 120–140mg a day, because of the increased severity of anaemia and the phytate in her diet which hinders absorption of iron. She should also take vitamin A (2.4mg) and 500μg of folate daily.

THALASSAEMIAS

The thalassaemias are a genetically determined group of blood disorders, characterized by a reduced production of one or more of the α- or β-chains of globin which make up haemoglobin. All forms of thalassaemia are inherited as an autosomal recessive trait. In α-thalassaemias, the α-chains accumulate and eventually precipitate causing severe anaemia (thalassaemia major or Cooley's anaemia). The β-thalasaemias may be either heretozygous, when they are symptomless, or homozygous, when they produce severe anaemia.

Thalassaemia in a woman who is anaemic in pregnancy can be excluded if the MCV is greater than 80fl. An MCV of less than 80fl indicates that haemoglobin electrophoresis should be performed. An HbA₂ greater than 3.5 indicates a β-thalassaemia trait.

If either α- or β-thalassaemia is diagnosed, the father of the child should have a full blood count and electrophoresis. If he is a carrier of the trait, genetic counselling should be obtained.

A pregnant woman carrying the thalassaemia trait has a 30% chance of becoming anaemic and a similar chance of developing urinary tract infection. Thalassaemia major in the fetus can be detected in the first quarter of pregnancy by chorionic villus sampling and, in the second quarter, by sampling fetal cord blood under ultrasonic guidance. If the tests are positive, termination of the pregnancy may be offered to the parents.

OTHER HAEMOGLOBINOPATHIES – SICKLE CELL ANAEMIA

In these cases a defective gene on the chromosome responsible for haemoglobin synthesis leads to the production of abnormal haemoglobin and an erthryocyte life of less than 15 days. The episodes of erthryocyte destruction may cause severe haemolytic anaemia and bone pains, because of infarction of the vessels supplying the bones.

The most common abnormal haemoglobin is haemoglobin S which causes sickle cell disease. The condition mainly affects Africans from East and West Africa.

All pregnant women suspected of carrying an abnormal haemoglobin should be given folate (15mg daily) routinely, and frequent haemoglobin estimations made. If the haemoglobin level falls below 60g/L, a direct or an exchange transfusion should be made. Infections, especially urinary tract infection, should be treated and prophylactic antibiotics given during childbirth and the puerperium. If a bone pain crisis occurs, heparin should be given and the haemoglobin measured every 2 hours; a fall of more than 2g indicates the need for an exchange transfusion.

Iso-immunization in pregnancy

Abnormal haemoglobinopathies predominantly affect Africans and southeast Asians; in contrast, rhesus iso-immunization mainly affects Caucasians and south Asians.

Rhesus iso-immunization is caused by a complex antigen, consisting of three pairs of alleles, occupying a locus on a chromosome. The antigen was discovered more than 50 years ago on erythrocytes of the rhesus monkey. One of these pairs, D, is likely to cause the majority of iso-immunization in humans. Eighty-five per cent of Caucasians have the D antigen, and are termed rhesus positive, whilst 15% are rhesus negative. If a woman who is rhesus negative conceives by a man who is rhesus positive, the fetus may be rhesus negative or positive depending on whether the man is heretozygous or homozygous for the rhesus antigen. In the case of a rhesus positive fetus, its blood cells may cross the placenta during pregnancy or, more commonly, during labour, in sufficient numbers to stimulate antibody production against the rhesus antigen in the mother. In the next pregnancy, if the fetus is again rhesus positive, the anti-D antibodies may cross the placenta from mother to fetus and attach to antigen sites on the surface of the fetal erythrocytes. In the presence of complement the antigen–antibody complex causes lysis of the fetal erythrocytes, which shows as haemolytic disease.

THE RHESUS PROBLEM

As rhesus iso-immunization occurs only if a rhesus negative mother is impregnated by a rhesus positive man (or has received a transfusion of rhesus positive blood which is an exceptionally rare occurrence today). All pregnant women should be tested to determine their rhesus group at the initial antenatal visit. If the woman is rhesus negative and there are no anti-Rh antibodies detected, she should be retested at 28 and 36 weeks' gestation.

If Rh antibodies are detected at a titre of 1:8 or greater, further assessment is made by amniocentesis and by testing a sample of amniotic fluid for the level of bilirubin, as this correlates fairly well with the degree of destruction of the fetal erythrocytes. In the absence of bilirubin, the absorption spectrum of amniotic fluid over the range of 360 to 630nmol is expressed as a straight line. The presence of albumin-bound bilirubin produces a deviation from this straight line, the degree of deviation relating to the severity of the erythrocyte haemolysis (Fig. 16.3).

In cases where the mother has previously given birth to a severely affected baby, the level of iso-agglutinins is tested earlier than the 24th week, and if found to be raised, fetal cord blood sampling and the measurement of the fetal haematocrit is performed, as amniocentesis is inaccurate before the 24th week of pregnancy.

The bilirubin peak is entered on to a graph (Fig. 16.4). If the level is in the high zone (or the high-to-mid zone on a second test), the baby is severely affected, may be hydropic if its haemoglobin is less than 40g/L and it may die in utero. If the pregnancy has advanced to 32 weeks the pregnancy should be terminated, usually by caesarean section. Earlier than 32 weeks, intra-uterine fetal transfusion should be made, either into the peritoneal cavity or into the umbilical vein under ultrasonic guidance. The latter procedure permits a sample of fetal blood to be checked for the severity of the anaemia and the amount of blood required to correct the anaemia to be assessed. It also produces a higher salvage rate.

If the level is in the mid zone, a second amniocentesis is performed 2–3 weeks later, treatment being based on this result. If the peak lies in the low zone, a second tap is made 3–4 weeks later.

PREVENTION OF RHESUS ISO-IMMUNIZATION

The following schema would solve the rhesus problem provided that no rhesus negative woman received a transfusion of rhesus positive blood:

- All rhesus negative, unsensitized women, who abort and require curettage, are given an injection of 50–125μg rhesus anti-D IgG within 72 hours of the abortion.
- All rhesus negative, unsensitized women (whose husband or partner is rhesus positive or has unknown rhesus status), who require chorionic villus sampling, amniocentesis, have an ectopic gestation, antepartum haemorrhage, abdominal trauma or who require an external cephalic version, are given rhesus anti-D IgG. The dose before the 20th week is 50μg; after 20 weeks it is 125μg.

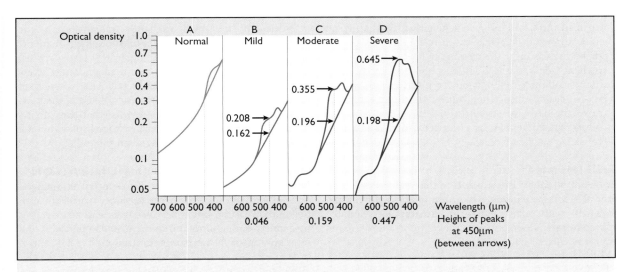

Fig. 16.3 Spectral absorption curves of amniotic fluid in (from left) normal late pregnancy; mild, moderate and severe haemolytic disease.

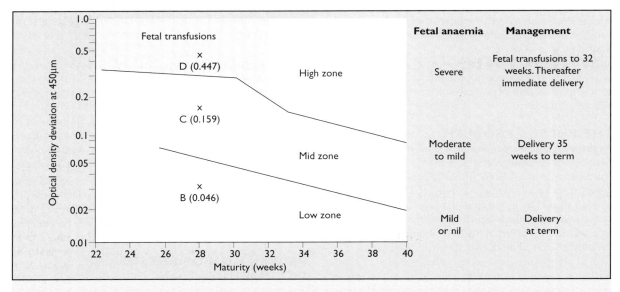

Fig. 16.4 *The relationship between the size of the amniotic fluid pigment peak at different stages of maturity, fetal anaemia and management. (The peak figures from Fig. 16.3 B, C and D are charted.)*

- All rhesus negative, unsensitized women, whose pregnancy progresses to the 28th week, receive an injection of 125μg rhesus anti-D IgG, repeated at 34 weeks, unless the father of the fetus is rhesus negative. This recommendation is controversial as only 1–2% of rhesus negative women are sensitized during pregnancy, but the amount of rhesus anti-D IgG required is increased at least 4-fold.

- All rhesus negative, unsensitized women, who give birth to a rhesus positive baby, are given an injection of 125μg rhesus anti-D IgG within 72 hours of the birth, if the Coombs' test is negative (indicating no circulating anti-D IgG). A test is made on the mother's blood to determine the number of fetal red blood cells present (Kleihauer test). A level of more than 80 fetal blood cells per 50 high-power fields equals a fetal transfusion of more than 5ml fetal blood. This indicates the need for an additional injection of rhesus anti-D IgG. The dose is 20μg/ml of fetal red blood cells.

THE INFANT

At birth, the infant is examined to determine the degree of fetal blood haemolysis. A very few infants are hydropic at birth, with ascites, pleural effusion and hepatosplenomegaly. Their outlook is very poor. Most infants appear normal or have mild jaundice.

Blood is taken for haemoglobin concentration, ABO and rhesus grouping, serum bilirubin assay and direct Coombs' test. The results will enable the neonatologist to decide if exchange transfusion is required. This is usually given within 10 hours of the birth. The objective is to restore the fetal blood haemoglobin level to 148g/L using rhesus negative, ABO-compatible blood.

Follow-up is essential as the infant may develop jaundice within 48 hours of birth (icterus gravis neonatorum). The infant's liver and spleen are enlarged and its serum bilirubin is greater than 210μmol/L.

Treatment consists of exchange transfusion. In the absence of these findings, serum bilirubin measurements are made at frequent intervals during the first 10 days of life, treatment being given depending on the level found. A few babies develop jaundice in the 2nd week of life, whereupon further haemolysis occurs (haemolytic disease of the newborn). The prognosis is good provided that the infant's haemoglobin and serum bilirubin levels are kept within the normal range. The baby is treated with phototherapy.

OTHER TYPES OF ISO-IMMUNIZATION

Few of the other irregular antibodies detected at antenatal screening cause problems to the neonate, apart from anti-Kell and anti-C iso-immunization, which are managed in pregnancy, during birth and in the neonatal period in the same way as for rhesus iso-immunization.

CHAPTER 17

Endocrine disorders in pregnancy

Diabetes mellitus

During pregnancy the placenta secretes substances that have an anti-insulin action, including human placental lactogen (hPL), progesterone, human chorionic gonado trophin (hCG) and cortisol. If the maternal beta islet cells are unable to produce the additional insulin required to counteract this effect, the woman will develop hyperglycaemia (gestational diabetes). Between 1.5 and 2.5% of pregnant women develop glucose intolerance during pregnancy.

As maternal glucose, but not insulin, can readily cross the placenta, the fetal pancreas will secrete additional insulin if there is maternal hyperglycaemia. This fetal hyperinsulinaemia can result in macrosomia, polycythaemia, impaired lung maturation, neonatal hypoglycaemia, jaundice, hypocalcaemia and hypomagnesaemia. Offspring may develop glucose intolerence in childhood and they are more prone to adult obesity.

Maternal hyperglycaemia, at the time of conception and during embryogenesis, can cause major fetal abnormalities (neural tube defects, cardiac abnormalities, skeletal abnormalities) and increase the risk of miscarriage.

DETECTION OF GESTATIONAL DIABETES

Routine screening of all pregnant women for hyperglycaemia is controversial and the diagnostic criteria that predict an adverse perinatal outcome are still being debated. The two most widely used tests are detailed in *Figure 17.1*.

If routine screening for hyperglycaemia during pregnancy is not undertaken, women who are at-risk should be tested using a non-fasting 75g glucose challenge test or an oral glucose tolerance test (see *Fig. 17.1*). Women who are more likely to develop gestational diabetes are those who: have a previous history of gestational diabetes; suffered an intra-uterine death late in pregnancy; have a close family member or members who are diabetic; are from an ethnic group with a high prevalence of Type II diabetes; are older than 30 years, have persistent glycosuria or there is fetal macrosomia.

MANAGEMENT OF DIABETES
Prepregnancy advice

Ideally, women who are known to be diabetic and women who have had gestational diabetes should be seen before they become pregnant. This consultation offers the opportunity

	Oral glucose load (g)	Plasma glucose level (mmol/L)			
		Fasting	**1 Hour**	**2 Hour**	**3 Hour**
Glucose challenge test (non-fasting) *	75		8.0		
	50		7.8		
Glucose tolerance test GTT (fasting) †	100 (O'Sullivan and Mahan criteria)	5.0	9.2	7.9 (2 or more values exceeded)	7.1
	75 (WHO Criteria)	<7.8		≥8.0	

Fig 17.1 The diagnosis of gestational diabetes

* If the plasma glucose exceeds these values GTT should be done

† If fasting ≥7.8 or 2 hour ≥11.1 then classified WHO diabetes

to explain to the woman the reasons for meticulously maintaining her blood glucose at normal levels before conception, and to ensure dietary advice has included taking folic acid to reduce the risk of neural tube defects. Each woman needs to be assessed for the presence of any complications associated with diabetes, such as diabetic retinopathy and nephropathy. Women who are taking oral hypoglycaemic agents should change to insulin therapy.

Pregnancy

In pregnancy there are certain principles of management:

- A multidisciplinary team, including an endocrinologist, a diabetic educator, a dietitian, a neonatologist and obstetrician, is desirable for management.
- Euglycaemia should be maintained throughout, with fasting blood glucose less than 6mmol/L and 2-hour postprandial blood glucose less than 7mmol/L.
- Ultrasound examination in the first 12 weeks of pregnancy provides accurate dating of the pregnancy, and ultrasound between 18 and 20 weeks of pregnancy allows exclusion of any major malformations and, around 34 weeks of pregnancy, permits assessment of fetal growth. Ultrasound scans may be performed more often if there is any suspicion of abnormal fetal growth.
- Fetal well-being is monitored with fetal movement counts, Doppler umbilical blood flow and cardiotocography (see Chapter 21, The at-risk fetus, for management of high-risk pregnancy).
- Optimal time for delivery is different for each case and is determined by the presence or absence of complications.
- The woman should be delivered in a hospital with neonatal facilities.

Maternal complications

Women with diabetes are more prone to pregnancy-induced hypertension (PIH), especially if any microvascular complications, urinary tract infections, polyhydramnios or candida vaginitis are present. Diabetic ketoacidosis must be avoided as it may cause fetal death. The incidence of the complications (*Fig. 17.2*) depends largely on the quality of the care of the diabetic woman before and during pregnancy.

Management of gestational diabetes

Most women with gestational diabetes can maintain euglycaemia by diet alone, but 10% or more may need insulin therapy. The same principles of management are used for women with diabetes prior to pregnancy as for those with diabetes arising during pregnancy. Fetal and maternal complications are less frequent in gestational diabetes and the risk of congenital abnormalities is not increased, as diabetes does not arise in early pregnancy.

TIMING OF DELIVERY

Most diabetic women, whose diabetes is well controlled, will be able to continue their pregnancy to full term. If metabolic control has been inadequate and polyhydramnios or fetal macrosomia is present, delivery is indicated by 38 weeks.

MANAGEMENT OF LABOUR

Labour can be induced in the usual way, and the fetus monitored as for any high-risk pregnancy. Blood glucose levels need to be monitored at frequent intervals and, if necessary, an infusion of short-acting insulin can be given to the woman. The fetus should be monitored throughout labour. During vaginal delivery shoulder dystocia should be anticipated.

An elective caesarean section for diabetic women who do not have complications is not indicated. A caesarean section may be performed if there is significant macrosomia or fetal distress, or if labour fails to progress satisfactorily.

As maternal insulin requirements quickly return to prepregnancy levels after delivery, monitoring of blood glucose levels is important.

THE NEWBORN BABY

Following delivery, the baby should be carefully assessed by a neonatologist (*Fig. 17.3*). Neonatal hypoglycaemia is usually prevented by oral glucose or breastfeeding within 1 hour of delivery. The blood glucose levels should be monitored for the following 2 days. If hypoglycaemia persists the baby may require enteral feeding or intravenous glucose or glucagon.

Babies of diabetic mothers who had difficulty controlling their blood glucose during pregnancy are likely to have poor temperature control, to feed slowly and to be jaundiced, hypocalaemic and hypomagnesaemia. If these babies are born before term, they are more likely to develop the respiratory distress syndrome because there is delayed resorption of lung fluid, which causes transient tachypnoea in the newborn baby.

Later in life these babies are at risk of developing abnormal glucose tolerance and obesity.

Fig. 17.2 The effects of diabetes mellitus on pregnancy

Condition	Risk (percentage of women affected)
Pregnancy-induced hypertension	10–20
Polyhydramnios	20–25
Bacteriuria	7–10
Congenital malformations	6
Perinatal mortality	20–100 per 1000

FOLLOW-UP OF WOMEN WHO HAVE HAD GESTATIONAL DIABETES

Follow-up is important as up to 50% of women with gestational diabetes may develop overt diabetes, usually Type II, and if this is detected early there is an opportunity to minimize the development of the complications of diabetes. Regular testing for hyperglycaemia should be performed, every 2 years if the GTT is normal, and every year if there is impaired glucose tolerance.

At these follow-up visits women who have had gestational diabetes can be encouraged to follow a diet appropriate for a diabetic, avoiding refined carbohydrates and ensuring adequate dietary fibre. Because of the risk of developing diabetes, the women should be advised to take the following measures: avoid becoming obese; take regular exercise; avoid cigarette smoking; and be checked annually for hypertension. These women should also be reminded that they have a 50% chance of developing gestational diabetes in a future pregnancy. If the woman is intending to become pregnant again, testing for hyperglycaemia immediately before conception is recommended. Otherwise, testing should be done early in pregnancy.

Thyroid disease

AUTO-IMMUNE HYPERTHYROIDISM (GRAVES' DISEASE)

Auto-immune hyperthyroidism (Graves' disease) may precede pregnancy or may arise in pregnancy because of the hypermetabolic state of the mother. In pregnancy, treatment with propylthiouracil is preferred as it does not readily cross the placenta. The objective is to maintain the free T_4 index in the normal range. Labour is usually uneventful. About 10% of neonates become thyrotoxic in the neonatal period because of the transplacental passage of thyroid-stimulating immunoglobulins. Affected babies can be identified during pregnancy by measuring the level of the long-acting thyroid stimulator–protector (LATS–P) in the maternal blood.

PARENCHYMATOUS (COLLOID) GOITRE

Although the mother's thyroid gland enlarges in pregnancy, it is uncommon for it to cause symptoms. The cause of the goitre is partly due to decreased absorption of iodine in the first half of pregnancy. A pregnant woman should take iodized table salt to prevent the fetus developing colloid goitre.

PRIMARY HYPOTHYROIDISM

This is an uncommon complication of pregnancy. In early pregnancy an increased need for thyroxine occurs that is associated with a rise in T_3 and T_4, which plateaus at about the 30th week. In women with hypothyroidism this rise cannot occur, and these women need more thyroxine than when not pregnant. The extra quantity needed can be estimated from the serum thyroid-stimulating hormone (TSH, or thyrotropin) level, a fall indicating a need for more thyroxine. In hypothyroid pregnant women, TSH should be measured at regular intervals and the dose of thyroxine adjusted, above the average daily dose of $100\mu g$, as required. The compliance of the patient should be ensured, as insufficient thyroxine may increase maternal and fetal morbidity.

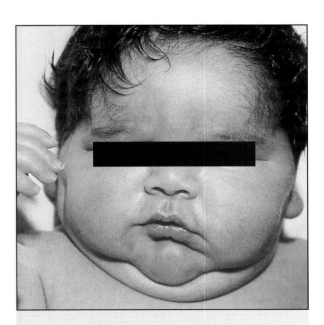

Fig. 17.3 Newborn baby of a diabetic mother.

CHAPTER 18

Infections during pregnancy

With the exception of poliomyelitis, pregnancy does not alter a woman's resistance to infection. The severity of any infection, however, correlates positively with its effect on the fetus. For example, the more severe the infection and the earlier in pregnancy it occurs, the greater is the risk of miscarriage or of intra-uterine death of the fetus.

Infections have an *indirect* and a *direct* effect on the fetus. The indirect effect operates by reducing the oxygenation of the placental blood, and by altering the nutrient exchange through the placenta. The direct effect depends on the ability of the invading organism to penetrate the placenta and infect the fetus. Viruses, being smaller than bacteria, are able to do this more easily. At first, the virus multiplies in the trophoblast and, subsequently, invades the fetus. Most viral infections do not affect the fetus unless the mother's infection is very severe. Three exceptions to this are rubella, cytomegalovirus and herpes simplex infections. The infections may cause congenital defects. The clinical effects of infections are microcephaly, congenital heart disease, eye damage (such as cataract), deafness, hepatosplenomegaly (with jaundice), purpura and, later in childhood, mental handicap.

As maternal antibodies cross the placenta, they offer the fetus a degree of immunity, except in the case of a primary infection. The fetus becomes immunologically competent from about the 14th week of pregnancy, but the efficacy of this protection is low until the second half of pregnancy.

Urinary tract infection

Urinary tract infection is the most disturbing of the bacterial infections. It occurs because the urinary tract dilates owing to the relaxation of the muscles of the ureter and the bladder in pregnancy with consequent urinary stasis.

ASYMPTOMATIC BACTERIURIA

The prevalence of asymptomatic bacteriuria (defined as more than 100,000 bacteria per ml of urine) in non-pregnant women is about 2%. In pregnancy it rises to 3–8% because of the physiological changes mentioned, and 30% of pregnant women who have asymptomatic bacteriuria will develop symptomatic urinary tract infection. Unless the infection is treated these women have a slightly higher chance of developing hypertension in pregnancy and twice the risk of delivering a low-birth-weight baby.

Because of this risk, many authorities recommend that all pregnant women are screened for asymptomatic bacteriuria in early pregnancy. A midstream specimen of urine is sent to a laboratory for culture. In 85% of cases *Escherichia coli* are isolated and, in the remainder, a variety of microorganisms are found. As the procedure is costly, other procedures, such as dip slides covered with a culture medium and reagent strips, have been developed and are reliable screening methods.

Treatment of asymptomatic bacteriuria consists of prescribing amoxycillin 3g or cephalexin 2g as a single dose or in appropriate doses for 5–7 days. Seven days after finishing the antibiotics, a midstream specimen of urine is re-examined. If the asymptomatic bacteriuria has not been eliminated, a longer course of antibiotics is prescribed. Regular follow-up urine cultures must be made, and recurrences treated.

PYELONEPHRITIS

As mentioned, about 30% of women who have untreated bacteriuria will develop pyelonephritis during pregnancy, as will 1% of women who do not have the condition.

The infection occurs when bacteria, growing in the stagnant urine, spread from the bladder to the ureter and then to the renal pelvis. Haematogenous infection is very uncommon. Pyelonephritis usually begins after the 20th week of pregnancy. In mild cases the woman complains of tiredness and urinary frequency and, occasionally, dysuria. More severe infections start suddenly with chills and rigors, fever, and pain over one or both renal areas. The patient may become rapidly dehydrated. The diagnosis is confirmed by examining a midstream specimen of urine, having excluded other causes of abdominal pain such as acute appendicitis and abruptio placentae.

Treatment consists of correcting the dehydration and prescribing appropriate antibiotics, having tested for bacterial sensitivity. In most cases, a cephalosporin or amoxycillin is appropriate initial treatment. As some women with pyelonephritis are nauseated, the antibiotic may have to be given intravenously. Follow-up examinations of a midstream urine culture at 2-week intervals for the remainder of the pregnancy should be instituted. Some authorities recommend prophylactic antibiotics for the duration of the pregnancy.

VAGINAL INFECTIONS

Vaginal infections during pregnancy due to *Candida* spp, *Trichomonas* and bacterial vaginosis are discussed on pages 260–261. The diagnosis and treatment are the same as in pregnancy.

GROUP B STREPTOCOCCUS

Colonies of Group B streptococci are harboured in the upper vagina of 6–30% of pregnant women.

If Group B streptococcal infection is present during labour the bacteria may colonize the neonate. Some studies suggest that half the babies born through an infected vagina are colonized, and 1–2% of them develop streptococcal infection.

Routine screening for Group B streptococcal infection, by taking a low vaginal swab between the 26th and 27th week of pregnancy and prescribing intrapartum parenteral ampicillin (1g every 6 hours until after delivery) to those women who are infected, is controversial. The public and the legal profession need to be educated that even with screening tests, some babies will be infected with Group B streptococcal infection. It is just as effective in reducing neonatal morbidity to treat only women who are in premature labour, whose membranes have been ruptured for more than 12 hours and women who have previously had an infected neonate.

GONORRHOEA

Depending on the population studied, between 1 and 6% of pregnant women are found to have gonorrhoea on culture studies using the Thayer-Martin medium. Many of these women have no symptoms. In symptomatic gonorrhoea, the woman complains of dysuria and a vaginal discharge which occurs within 5 days of sexual intercourse. If the symptoms suggest gonorrhoea or if the woman's sexual behaviour suggests that she may have gonorrhoea, cervical and urethral swabs should be taken and inoculated directly on to preheated plates of culture medium. In addition, vaginal swabs should be made for other vaginal infective organisms. The management of gonococcal infection is discussed on page 262.

SYPHILIS

The importance of syphilitic infection in pregnancy is that treponemes are able to penetrate the placenta after the 15th week of pregnancy and infect the fetus. If the fetus survives the initial infection, by the time of the birth it is in the second stage of syphilis.

For this reason every pregnant woman should be tested for syphilis using a reagin test [either the VDRL or the Rapid Plasma Reagin (RPR) test], although the incidence of syphilis in most areas is less than 0.1%. The test should be made at the first antenatal visit and, in the opinion of some authorities, repeated at the 30th week of pregnancy. False positives may occur, thus a woman who has had a positive screening test is investigated using a procedure which detects specific antitreponemal antibodies in her serum (e.g. the *Treponema pallidum* haemagglutination test; TPHA, the fluorescent treponemal antibody test; FTA-ABS, or the *T. pallidum* immobilization test, TPI).

The treatment is that described on page 258 for nonpregnant women. Follow-up serological tests are made monthly for 3 months; every 2 months for the next 6 months; and every 3 months for the next year.

As the signs of syphilis in a neonate are often equivocal and the serology is inaccurate, the infant of a woman who has been diagnosed as having syphilis whilst pregnant, and who has not had a complete course of treatment and follow-up, should be given a full course of antibiotic treatment (aqueous procaine penicillin 50,000U per kg body weight daily for 10 days).

TOXOPLASMOSIS

Toxoplasma gondii infects 3–6 pregnant women per 1000. In 90% there are no clinical signs. Infections acquired in pregnancy may lead to a miscarriage or congenital infection of the fetus, 1 fetus in 4 being affected. The eyes and the central nervous system may be severely damaged.

Screening tests for toxoplasma are available but are not cost-effective. If chosen they are best made before pregnancy, and seronegative women should be retested in each of the quarters of pregnancy.

Preventive measures taken by a pregnant women are more cost-effective. A pregnant woman should avoid touching cat faeces. She should avoid touching her eyes or mouth whilst handling raw meat, wash her hands after handling it and she should only eat well-cooked meat. The woman should wash vegetables and fruit thoroughly before eating them and, if a gardener, should wear gloves.

Viral infections

Six viral infections need some discussion.

RUBELLA

Rubella infection is widespread. By the age of 19 years, more than 85% of people have been infected and 9 out of 10 of those infected have lifelong immunity.

Should rubella occur in a non-immune woman in the first 14 weeks of pregnancy, viraemia and infection of the fetus are almost certain, and more than 40% of the infected fetuses will be damaged by the virus. The virus invades actively dividing cells and alters the genome. Infection in weeks 4–12 of pregnancy affects the lens of the eyes (causing cataract) or the ears (causing deafness). Infection between the 5th and 12th week damages the chambers of the heart. As well as causing damage to specific organs, rubella infection may cause widespread cellular damage leading to fetal growth restriction, thrombocytopenia, hepatosplenomegaly and vasculitis, and, in particular, renal artery stenosis.

These problems could be avoided if all women were immunized against rubella between the ages of 11 and 13 using a live attenuated strain of the virus (the RA 27/3 strain). Programmes to accomplish this have been developed in many countries.

A woman should be tested for rubella antibodies either when she decides to become pregnant or at the first pregnancy visit. The test used is the Single Radial Haemolysis Test (SRH test). If this test is positive with a titre greater than 15,000IU/L the woman is immune to rubella. A non-immune woman who is not pregnant may be offered vaccination but should avoid pregnancy for 3 months. If a pregnant woman is inadvertently vaccinated, the risk of the baby being infected is extremely small, no cases of congenital rubella syndrome have been reported in these circumstances.

A problem arises when a pregnant non-immune woman develops a rubelliform rash (as in half of women the rash is not due to rubella), or if the woman has been in contact with a case of rubella. A serological test should be made as soon as possible, preferably within 15 days of the appearance of the rash or the contact. An SRH test positive in a titre of more than 15,000 IU/L is evidence of immunity to rubella and the woman may be reassured that her baby is in no danger of being infected. A second SRH test is repeated in 21 days for confirmation. If the woman seroconverts, the problems of congenital infection should be discussed with her and a therapeutic abortion can be offered.

GENITAL HERPES

A general discussion on herpes simplex virus (HSV) can be found on page 257. In pregnancy HSV may cross the placental barrier to infect the fetus, and is more likely to be found in primary than in recurrent infections. Overall the risk is low, only 1 fetus per 1000 being infected. The risk is greater during childbirth, particularly if the mother has developed a recurrence of the condition or is shedding the virus from her cervix.

These findings suggest:

- A woman with a history of genital herpes need have no anxiety that her baby will be infected and may expect to be delivered vaginally, unless a recurrence of the infection or a new infection occurs during the pregnancy.
- If a first infection or a recurrence of genital herpes occurs during the pregnancy, but has healed by the time labour starts, the woman may give birth vaginally.
- If herpetic lesions are present when the membranes rupture or labour starts, a caesarean section should be performed to avoid the risk that the baby will acquire a herpetic infection during the passage through the birth canal.

The strategy of taking endocervical swabs for viral culture every 2 weeks from the 34th week of pregnancy in women can be abandoned, as positive HSV-infected swabs do not predict the risk of the infant being exposed to herpes infection during birth.

HEPATITIS B

Fewer than 0.5% of women in the developed nations are hepatitis B carriers, but, in contrast, up to 30% of migrants from parts of Africa and East and Southeast Asia have hepatitis B surface antigen (HB$_s$Ag) in their blood and are potentially infectious to healthcare workers, who may be infected by contact with blood and other body secretions. Many units now screen all pregnant women for hepatitis B. Precautions are taken when caring for such women in childbirth and most hospitals have developed appropriate protocols.

It is also known that the hepatitis B virus is readily transmitted to the baby, probably during the birth. Babies at particularly high risk are those whose mothers have HB$_c$Ag as well as HB$_s$Ag in their blood. If not treated, many of the babies will develop hepatocellular carcinoma when adult. This can be avoided, to a large extent, if babies at high risk are given hepatitis B immune globulin together with hepatitis B vaccine 10μg at birth, and two further injections of the vaccine at the ages of 1 and 6 months.

CYTOMEGALOVIRUS INFECTION (CMV)

Over half of all pregnant women show serological evidence of previous CMV infection. One per cent of women may become infected with CMV during pregnancy, most of whom are asymptomatic. The infection is associated with an increased perinatal mortality and 3–7% of the infants have congenital abnormalities.

Screening has proved to be of no value – there is no vaccine available.

HUMAN IMMUNODEFICIENCY VIRUS INFECTION (AIDS)

Although in Western countries most cases of HIV infection occur in homosexual or bisexual men, intravenous drug users who share needles are increasingly being infected, as are some heterosexual men and women who do not abuse drugs. In Sub Saharan Africa and South and Southeast Asia, many heterosexual women and men are HIV positive and the numbers are increasing. Infected women who become pregnant have a 20–40% risk of transmitting the virus to the fetus, and all infected fetuses will be antibody positive and develop AIDS. There is a strong argument that screening for HIV infection should be offered to all pregnant women, particularly as there is evidence that the use of antiviral drugs (such as zidovudine) can significantly reduce the risk of vertical transmission of the disease.

HIV infection has no adverse effect on pregnancy nor has the pregnancy any adverse effect on the progress of HIV infection. As the HIV infects the amniotic fluid as well as the women's blood, full infectious disease control precautions should be taken by attendant medical staff during labour and childbirth. Vaginal delivery may be anticipated and the place of caesarean section to prevent transmission of the fetus is controversial. Because of all the problems involved, women infected with HIV should be given the opportunity to choose to have an abortion rather than giving birth to a baby who may have HIV infection. If the woman chooses to continue the pregnancy she should be prescribed zidovudine from the 20th week of pregnancy and the infant should be given the drug. This regimen reduces the risk of vertical transmission of the virus to the fetus by two-thirds. Recent advances show that the addition of new viral protease inhibitors may have a further benefit. A major problem of this approach is that most pregnant women who have HIV-AIDS live in the poor countries where the cost of zidovudine is beyond their capacity to pay.

CHICKEN POX (VARICELLA)

Varicella infection is common, over 80% of pregnant women testing positive for IgG antibodies to the varicella zoster virus (VZV). Primary infection can result in serious complications for both mother and baby because, during pregnancy, the maternal immune system is less efficient. Pneumonia occurs in 10% of women and can result in death. If the infection occurs in the first trimester, 2–10% of the fetuses are infected and the viral vesicles can cause a wide spectrum of abnormalities including lung hypoplasia, microcephaly, cortical atrophy, cataracts, psychomotor retardation, convulsions and intra-uterine growth restriction. If the maternal infection becomes apparent 7 days before or 7 days after delivery, the baby is at risk of developing disseminated varicella infection, as maternal antibody production will not yet be adequate.

If there is doubt about the diagnosis or previous history of infection, maternal blood should be taken for anti-VZV, IgG and IgM antibodies. If there is a high risk of maternal or fetal complications, the mother should be given 12.5 units per kg of VZV immune globulin (VZIG) intramuscularly. For severe maternal infection, acyclovir 5–10mg/kg should be given every 8 hours. An infected infant may be given VZIG and acyclovir.

Infections in the tropics

HELMINTH INFESTATIONS – HOOKWORM DISEASE

Endemic infections by helminths are almost universal among rural dwellers in the tropics and subtropics, and the most serious of these is hookworm disease. Two types of hookworm are found, *Ancylostoma duodenale* and *Necator americanus*. In the gut the worms attach to the villi by suckers, and feed on blood obtained from the villi; after passing through their bodies, this blood is excreted into the lumen of the bowel. In studies in Malaysia in the 1950s, we found that the blood loss due to hookworm was found to relate closely to the hookworm load, and varied from 2 to 90ml per day. Hookworm infestation is a cause of iron deficiency anaemia, and this is particularly serious in pregnancy. Treatment consists of eliminating the worms by administering bephenium hydroxynaphthoate (Alcopar) in a dose of 5g daily for 3 days, and treating the anaemia with iron.

MALARIA

Exacerbation of malaria, or relapse in a partially immune woman, is particularly common during pregnancy, and each attack may precipitate abortion or the onset of premature labour. The fetus is protected by the placenta in most cases, although large numbers of immobilized parasites may be found in the placenta, particularly if the infection is by *Plasmodium falciparum*. Occasionally, in non-immune patients, congenital transmission of malaria occurs.

Pregnant women travelling to an area where malaria is endemic should take prophylactic antimalarial drugs. If the strains of *P. falciparum* in the area are chloroquine resistant, problems arise. The alternative drugs, Fansidar and Maloprim, affect folic acid synthesis and may induce a fatal Stevens–Johnson syndrome. They should be avoided. If the risk of chloroquine resistance is low, chloroquine and proguanil should be given. If the risk of chloroquine resistance is high, a pregnant woman should postpone her visit until she has given birth.

Any pregnant woman developing a high fever in a malarial area should be suspected of having the infection, and if this is confirmed by finding parasites in a thick blood film, treatment is given with chloroquine 600mg (base) initially, followed 8 hours later by 300mg, and 300mg daily for the next 3 days.

CHAPTER 19

Diseases of the placenta and membranes

Abnormal placentation

The shape of the definitive placenta is determined at the time the placenta forms, the variations found (*Fig. 19.1*) mostly having no clinical significance.

The umbilical cord may enter the placenta at its midpoint, may join it at an edge (*marginal insertion of the cord*) or the umbilical vessels may run some distance along the membranes (*velamentous insertion of the cord*). Should the vessels run across the cervix, they may be compressed by the fetal head during labour, or bleed causing fetal anaemia. In some cases the placenta is smaller than the chorionic plate and the trophoblast invades the decidua laterally more deeply, giving a ridged appearance on the placental surface (*placenta circumvallata*). In most cases this has no clinical significance but, occasionally, may be found in women who have antepartum or intrapartum haemorrhage. In other cases the placenta has an accessory lobe separated by membranes from the main placenta (*placenta succenturiata*).

In a few cases the trophoblastic invasion is not regulated by maternal immune defences and the myometrium is invaded causing *placenta accreta, increta or percreta*. *Haemangiomata* occur in 1% of placentae. In most cases they are small and of no clinical significance, but larger haemangiomata may be associated with polyhydramnios, antepartum haemorrhage or preterm labour.

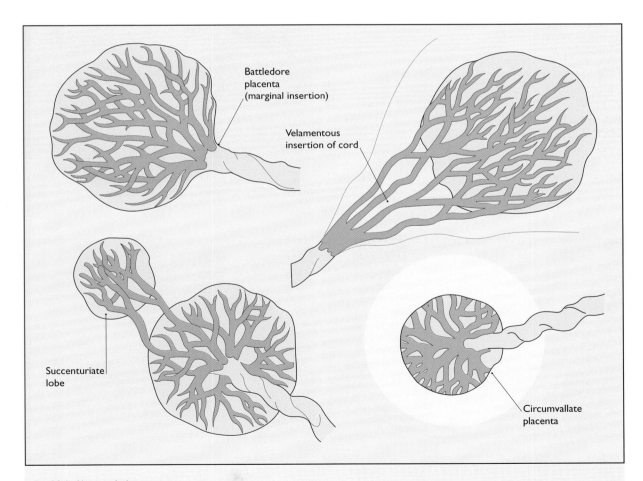

Battledore placenta (marginal insertion)

Velamentous insertion of cord

Succenturiate lobe

Circumvallate placenta

Fig. 19.1 Abnormal placentation.

Gestational trophoblastic disease

Gestational trophoblastic disease is uncommon. It is discussed here as it is potentially lethal, but with treatment a 90% cure rate is attainable. The disease occurs in two forms (*Fig. 19.2*).

HYDATIDIFORM MOLE

The tumour may have completely or partially replaced the placenta (*Fig. 19.3*). In the complete form, hydropic swelling and vesicle formation is associated with trophoblastic proliferation and a paucity or absence of blood vessels within the villi (*Fig. 19.4*). No fetus can be found. Five per cent of complete moles undergo malignant change.

In the partial form a fetus is present but areas of the placenta show the changes described for the complete mole. Partial moles become malignant less frequently (0.05%).

MALIGNANT TROPHOBLASTIC DISEASE

The tumour may be confined to the uterus (*invasive mole*) or spread via the bloodstream to distant organs (*choriocarcinoma*).

In the invasive mole the trophoblast-covered villi penetrate the myometrial fibres and may extend to other organs, the appearance of the villi remaining that of the benign tumour.

In choriocarcinoma (*Fig. 19.5*) the tumour is characterized by sheets of trophoblastic cells, both syncytio- and cytotrophoblast with few or no villi formed.

AETIOLOGY

Gestational trophoblastic disease is caused by a genetic disorder in which a spermatozoon enters an ovum which has lost its nucleus, or in which two sperms enter the ovum.

Fig. 19.2 Classification of trophoblastic neoplasms

Benign trophoblastic disease (hydatidiform mole)
Complete hydatidiform mole.
Partial hydatidiform mole.
Hydropic degeneration of the trophoblast.

Persistent trophoblastic disease (often malignant)
Apparently confined to the uterus (invasive mole).
Usually with extra-uterine spread (choriocarcinoma).

Fig. 19.3 Benign trophoblastic tumour (hydatidiform mole): gross specimen. Note the grape-like masses.

Fig. 19.4 Microphotograph of a benign trophoblastic tumour (hydatidiform mole), showing the distended villi and irregular trophoblastic proliferation.

Fig. 19.5 Choriocarcinoma.

In over 90% of complete moles only paternal genes are found and in 10% the mole is heterozygous. In contrast, partial moles usually have a triploid chromosomal constitution suggesting dispermy as the cause.

The development of gestational trophoblastic tumours is thought to be due to a defective maternal immune response to the invasion by the trophoblast. In consequence the villi become distended with nutrients. The primitive vasculature within each villus does not form properly with the result that the embryo starves, dies and is absorbed, whilst the trophoblast continues to thrive and, in certain circumstances, invades the maternal tissues.

The increased syncytiotrophoblast activity leads to an increased production of human chorionic gonadotrophin (hCG), chorionic thyrotrophin and progesterone. A fall in oestradiol secretion occurs, as oestradiol synthesis requires enzymes from the fetus, which does not exist. The raised hCG levels may induce the development of theca lutein cysts of the ovary.

DIAGNOSIS OF BENIGN GESTATIONAL TROPHOBLASTIC DISEASE

The first sign is bleeding per vaginam, which tends to persist. The bleeding may be followed fairly soon by uterine contractions and the expulsion of grape-like material. In other cases the tumour grows without symptoms. During this time examination will show the following features:

- The uterus is usually larger than expected from the gestational dates and is 'doughy' to the touch.
- Fetal heart sounds cannot be heard.
- Ultrasonic scanning shows a distinct speckled appearance (*Fig. 19.6*).
- If serum hCG is measured it is found to be unexpectedly high (*Fig. 19.7*).

Fig. 19.6 Characteristic vesicular pattern ('snowstorm') of a hydatidiform mole.

Treatment

If the patient is admitted expelling the tumour, no immediate treatment is needed unless the expulsion slows down, at which time a digital evacuation of the uterus is carried out. Blood is obtained for possible transfusion, as the expulsion is often accompanied by marked blood loss.

If the diagnosis is reached before the expulsion of any vesicles, the uterus may be evacuated using a suction curette or by the administration of prostaglandins to induce uterine contractions (this method has the disadvantage that it may lead to the intravascular dissemination of trophoblast). Gentle curettage may be performed later to remove any residual trophoblast. Some authorities give a single course of chemotherapy if they think that the woman presents with increased risk factors. If bleeding persists for more than 21 days a further curettage may be indicated.

Women over the age of 40 years, or women who have completed their family may prefer to have a hysterectomy, to avoid potential malignancy.

Follow-up

Follow-up is important as the disease persists in between 5 and 10% of cases, often developing a malignant form. Follow-up includes vaginal examinations at 2-weekly intervals to evaluate uterine involution and the presence, or absence, of theca lutein cysts. Alternatively, ultrasound examinations may be made at 2-weekly intervals. Human chorionic gonadotropin assays should be made according to a schedule (*Figs. 19.8* and *19.9*).

MALIGNANT GESTATIONAL TROPHOBLASTIC DISEASE

Malignancy follows a benign trophoblastic tumour in 1 in 10 cases, usually within 6 months of the expulsion of the benign tumour. It follows a spontaneous abortion in 1 in 5000 cases and a viable pregnancy in 1 in 50,000 cases.

Women who have had a benign gestational trophoblastic tumour are at greater risk of developing a malignancy if the woman:

- Is over the age of 40.
- Secretes large amounts of βhCG (more than 100,000IU/ml).
- Has theca lutein cyst(s) of more than 6cm diameter.

Malignant gestational trophoblastic disease is best managed at special centres, where meticulous follow-up is conducted. Treatment is by chemotherapy (*Fig. 19.10*) and follow-up is shown in *Figure 19.11*.

Abnormalities of the amniotic fluid

Amniotic fluid is secreted into the amniotic sac by the amniotic cells which lie over the placenta. The fluid is 99% water and increases in quantity during pregnancy. In the amniotic sac it is swallowed by the fetus. Most of the swallowed fluid is absorbed by the fetal intestinal villi and enters the fetal circulation. From the circulation most is exchanged in the placenta, but some is returned to the

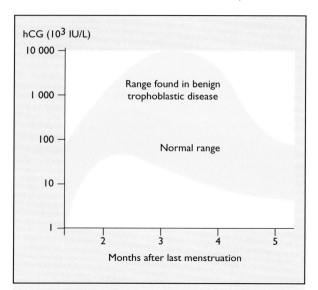

Fig. 19.7 *Chorionic gonadotrophin excretion in trophoblastic disease. The normal range is shown in pink; levels found in trophoblastic disease are shown in the in blue area.*

Fig. 19.9 *Hormone follow-up of benign trophoblastic disease (mean and 95% confidence limits).*

Fig. 19.8 *The follow-up of benign trophoblastic disease using a specific radio-immuno-assay*

1. Radio-immuno-assay of serum βhCG at 7–10 day intervals. If the level falls serially no drug treatment is needed. Complete disappearance of βhChG takes 12–14 weeks on average.

2. When βhCG level has been normal for 3 consecutive weeks, test monthly for 6 months.

3. If the assay shows normal βhCG levels for 6 consecutive months, follow-up can be discontinued.

4. During the follow-up period pregnancy should be avoided. Oral contraceptives may be prescribed.

5. If the serum βhCG level plateaus for more than 3 consecutive weeks, or rises, or if metastases are detected, treat with methotrexate or actinomycin D.

The fluid may accumulate rapidly (*acute polyhydramnios*), which causes considerable distress to the mother. She may develop dyspnoea, tachycardia, vomiting and severe abdominal pain. Treatment consists of removing amniotic fluid by amniocentesis, repeated if necessary. This has led to an improved outlook for the fetus.

The slow accumulation of amniotic fluid is more commonly found (*chronic polyhydramnios*). Symptoms similar to those of acute polyhydramnios may be experienced by the expectant mother and examination shows a distended uterus from which a fluid thrill can be obtained. Ultrasound scanning will confirm the diagnosis and identify the presence of either a multiple pregnancy or a fetal abnormality (in most cases).

Treatment

A patient who has a minor degree of polyhydramnios may be relieved by sedation at night. If the symptoms become worse between 30 and 35 weeks of pregnancy, an amniocentesis using a spinal needle to remove no more than 500ml at any one time (to reduce the onset of preterm labour) may be performed, although half the women go into labour as a result. After the 35th week labour may be induced by vaginal amniocentesis if the symptoms become worse, or if a gross fetal malformation is present. The liquor should be released slowly to prevent cord prolapse. Post-partum haemorrhage is likely and prophylactic oxytocin should be given.

amniotic sac by transudation through the fetal skin. In the last quarter of pregnancy fetal urination adds to the amniotic fluid.

POLYHYDRAMNIOS

Polyhydramnios is caused by increased secretion of amniotic fluid because of a large placenta, or by a fetal malformation which prevents the fetus swallowing the fluid or prevents the absorption of the fluid through the fetal intestinal villi. Examples of the former are multiple pregnancy and diabetes and, of the latter, anencephaly, spina bifida and atresia of the upper gastrointestinal tract.

Fig. 19.10 Chemotherapy in malignant trophoblastic disease		
Initial course	**Non-metastatic** mg/kg IM	**Metastatic** mg/kg IM
Methotrexate at 48-hour intervals for 4 doses.	1	1.5
Folinic acid (citrovorum factor) on alternate days, 24 hours after the injection of methotrexate.	0.1	0.15
Subsequent courses		
1. If response, ie a fall in the βhCG level <20%, repeat the regimen. 2. Without response, increase methotrexate by 0.5mg/kg and folinic acid by 0.05mg/kg. 3. If no response after two consecutive courses change to actinomycin D. 4. If no response to actinomycin D after two courses change to three chemotherapeutic drugs used in combination. Currently etoposide + methotrexate + cyclophosphamide (or vincristine) are recommended.		
Laboratory tests		
Full blood count, platelet count, SGOT on day 1 (before starting therapy) and days 3, 5, 7, 11, 15, 18, 21.		

Fig. 19.11 Principles of the management of malignant trophoblastic disease

1. During treatment the serum levels of the βhCG are assayed each week.

2. Provided that the βhCG level continues to fall after a course of chemotherapy, withhold further courses.

3. When the βhCG level is normal for 3 consecutive weeks, assay each month for 6 months.

4. If the βhCG level remains normal for 12 months, discontinue follow-up. Patients should avoid pregnancy throughout this period.

5. Repeat the course of chemotherapy if the βhCG level plateaus for more than 3 consecutive weeks, or rises, or if new metastases are detected.

6. If the βhCG level plateaus after 3 consecutive courses of chemotherapeutic agent, or if it rises during a course, change to another chemotherapeutic regimen.

The baby or babies should be examined carefully to detect fetal malformations including oesophageal and duodenal atresia.

OLIGOHYDRAMNIOS
Oligohydramnios is caused by defective liquor-secreting cells or, in late pregnancy, by renal tract malformations which prevent fetal urination; it also occurs in postdatism. If oligohydramnios occurs early in pregnancy abortion is usual. Should the pregnancy continue, amniotic bands may occur which may damage the fetus. Later in pregnancy, oligohydramnios may cause pulmonary hypoplasia pressure deformities such as wry neck,

altered shape of the skull or club foot, and the fetal skin is dry and leathery.

In labour the lack of amniotic fluid may lead to umbilical compression and fetal distress. Some obstetricians try to prevent this complication by the transcervical infusion of saline into the amniotic sac.

Abnormalities of the umbilical cord

A normal umbilical cord is 45–60cm long, but extremes of 2cm and 200cm have been recorded. The umbilical cord usually contains one vein and two arteries set in Wharton's jelly. In 1% of cords, only one artery is formed and this may be associated with congenital malformations. Long cords have no clinical significance unless they form a coil, or coils, around the fetal neck. A cord of normal length may be shortened by coiling around the fetus. During childbirth the cord may be pulled tight as the fetus descends, reducing the oxygen supply and, occasionally, causing fetal death. Knots, either true or false, may occur in the umbilical cord. True knots may lead to a reduced fetal circulation. False knots are accumulations of Wharton's jelly and have no clinical significance.

CHAPTER 20

Variations in the duration of pregnancy

The duration of human pregnancy averages 260 days from conception and 280 ± 14 days from the first day of the last menstrual period. In 5% of pregnancies the duration of pregnancy is curtailed and a preterm birth (less than 36 completed weeks) occurs. In 10% of cases the pregnancy is prolonged and the woman does not give birth until more than 41 weeks have been completed.

Curtailed pregnancy: preterm birth

There are some problems inherent in defining preterm birth as one which occurs before the 36th completed week of pregnancy. This is because the survival of the neonate depends not only on the duration of the pregnancy, but also on the birth weight of the baby.

By definition, a preterm baby born to a mother living in an industrialized country weighs less than 2500g. This includes two populations of babies: those who are really preterm and those whose growth has been restricted during the pregnancy (dysmature babies) but who are delivered after the 36th week of pregnancy.

Dysmature babies account for 6% of all babies born with a low birth weight (less than 2500g) and are at greater risk of dying.

Studies of preterm births show that curtailed pregnancy (preterm birth) may be associated with low social class, low maternal age, eating disorders leading to a low body weight (Body Mass Index less than 19), fetal abnormalities, multiple pregnancy and smoking. Preterm births may also be associated with medical complications, such as a history of abortion or stillbirth, uterine bleeding in pregnancy (threatened abortion, abruptio placentae and placenta praevia), hypertensive disorders and anaemia.

Recently, bacterial vaginosis (see page 261) has been implicated, which has been associated with an increase in preterm birth 2 to 3 times that compared with women who do not have bacterial vaginosis (15–20% compared with 6%). The question is: Should all women be screened and treated in the first half of pregnancy for bacterial vaginosis or only women with a history of previous preterm birth? Data are awaited.

It should also be noted that a large number of preterm births follows a spontaneous rupture of the membranes from unknown causes (Fig. 20.1).

PREVENTION OF PRETERM BIRTH

There are no effective ways of preventing preterm birth. Increased contact with health professionals to provide better social support (France), the prophylactic use of tocolytic agents such as terbutaline (Germany), uterine activity monitoring at home or in hospital (USA) or bed rest in early pregnancy have been tried and have not been shown to be effective.

Regular antenatal examinations will detect medical conditions complicating pregnancy and pregnancy-induced hypertension (PIH) at an early stage of their development but it is uncertain if this will reduce the incidence of preterm birth. Cervical cerclage increases the duration of pregnancy in women who have a diagnosis of incompetent cervix but not in other cases.

Preterm labour

The diagnosis of preterm labour must be made carefully or women who are having mild contractions, which do not cause cervical dilatation, will be included. The criteria for diagnosis are:
- The gestational period is less than 36 completed weeks.
- Uterine contractions, preferably recorded on a tocograph, occur every 5–10 minutes, last for at least 30 seconds and persist for at least 60 minutes.
- The cervix is more than 2.5cm dilated and more than 75% effaced.

Using these criteria, two-thirds of women presenting with presumed preterm labour will not be in labour. They need reassurance, not drug treatment.

A confirmatory test is to measure fetal fibronectin which, in cases of preterm labour, is released into cervical and vaginal secretions. A negative test means that it is very unlikely that the woman will deliver within 7 days (negative

Fig 20.1 Causes of curtailment of pregnancy and prematurity	
Cause	**Percentage**
No cause found (including premature rupture of the membrane)	35–45
Hypertensive disorders	18–30
Multiple pregnancy	12–18
Maternal disease	5–15
Abruptio placentae	5–7
Placenta praevia	3–4
Fetal malformations	1–2

predictive value approaches 100%). A positive test can occur in association with coitus, vaginal infection and examination and its specificity is low and positive predictions value 35–50 %. Its main benefit is to reduce the need to transfer women in possible preterm labour to tertiary units and/or commence tocolytic therapy.

If the criteria are met, the woman is in preterm labour. If the pregnancy is less than 35 completed weeks' gestation and the woman is not in a facility with a neonatal intensive care unit, she should have uterine contractions suppressed and be transferred as soon as possible to such a facility. If she has access to neonatal intensive care, the choice is to attempt to suppress uterine activity or to permit labour to proceed. In some third-level hospitals women who start preterm labour at or after the 34th week of gestation are permitted to proceed, as the premature infant can be competently cared for with no increase in perinatal mortality.

The greatest challenge is the management of a woman whose labour starts when the gestation period is less than 34 completed weeks.

MANAGEMENT OF PRETERM LABOUR OF LESS THAN 34 COMPLETED WEEKS

The major risk to the fetus is pulmonary immaturity. The principal objective of management is to enhance surfactant production in the fetal lungs to prevent hyaline membrane disease. The usefulness of bed rest to prevent premature rupture of membranes is uncertain. To be effective corticosteroids, two doses of 11.4mg betamethazone (celestone chronodose) 24 hours apart, must be given to the mother more than 24 hours and less than 10 days before birth. The corticosteroids also reduce the chance of intraventricular haemorrhage in these infants. After 34 weeks' gestation this treatment is no longer necessary as lung maturation is adequate. Once labour is established, tocolytic therapy can be administered (*Fig. 20.2*) to postpone delivery for at least 24 hours to allow for steroid-induced lung maturation to occur. This time can also permit the mother to be transferred to a hospital with neonatal intensive care facilities. The side effects of the tocolytics (especially the beta-agonists) mean that only some women are suitable to be treated with the drugs. These women include those in whom:

- The pregnancy is advanced to less than 35 weeks.
- There has been confirmation of preterm labour.
- The cervix is less than 5cm dilated.
- The patient is not hypertensive, has no cardiac disease, is not diabetic, does not have abruptio placentae and is not infected.
- The fetus is alive and no potentially lethal malformations have been detected by ultrasound scanning.

These exclusions mean that fewer than 15% of women in preterm labour can receive tocolytic drugs. The few

randomized trials of tocolytic drugs show that the only significant effect is to delay childbirth by a mean of 24 hours, although in a few instances, labour may be delayed for 2 weeks or more. The studies show that, statistically, the drugs do not reduce the frequency of delivery before the 37th week, the proportion of preterm babies born, or the incidence of membrane disease. It would appear that their main value is to enable a woman in preterm labour to be transferred to a hospital with a level-3 nursery.

The membranes should be kept intact for as long as possible and, when they rupture, a vaginal examination is made to exclude a prolapsed cord. If labour starts it may either be allowed to proceed or a caesarean section may be made. If vaginal delivery is chosen, and proceeds normally, an episiotomy should be made in the late second stage, because of the effect of pressure on the head of the premature infant. If there is a delay when the infant's head is in the pelvic outlet, a forceps delivery may be appropriate.

The place of caesarean section in the management of preterm labour is controversial. Most obstetricians believe that if labour starts when the pregnancy is 26–31 weeks' gestation, caesarean section should be performed if:

- The fetus does not present cephalically.
- There is associated antepartum haemorrhage.
- The labour fails to progress normally.
- Fetal distress develops.

While there can be little disagreement about these indications, the *routine* use of caesarean section to deliver babies weighing less than 1500g is controversial. In 1990, the US Institute of Child Health and Human Development examined the available data and concluded that routine caesarean section did not improve survival rates.

Prelabour rupture of the membranes

Prelabour (premature) rupture of the membranes may lead to the onset of preterm labour, with or without other causal factors. In most cases the baby is born within 7 days of the prelabour rupture. Rupture of the membranes after the 35th week is of no clinical significance, and if labour does not start quickly, it may be induced by the use of syntocinon (see page 194) depending on the state of the cervix. A woman whose cervix is 'not favourable' (see page 194), may prefer to delay induction for 48 to 72 hours in the anticipation that, during this time, the cervix will ripen and induction will be easier and more successful.

A recent (1996) multicentre study of 5000 women with prelabour rupture of the membranes, whose gestation was greater than 37 weeks, showed that there was no increase in the caesarean section rate or in infection whether or not induction, using oxytocics, or expectant treatment was chosen. The mother should be informed of the choices and her wishes accepted. If the woman is a carrier of Group B streptococcus she must be informed that there is an increased risk of neonatal morbidity.

The real problem occurs when the membranes rupture between the 26th and 35th week, as the longer the birth is delayed the more mature the baby becomes. Against this is the risk of ascending intra-uterine infection occurring. The woman should be admitted to or transferred to a hospital with a level-3 nursery. A high vaginal swab is also taken for bacteriological examination.

Regular assessments of maternal temperature and pulse are made to detect intra-uterine infection and observations are made to see if the amniotic fluid continues to leak. An ultrasound examination may be made to determine if oligo-hydramnios has occurred.

The use of prophylactic tocolytics has been suggested, but studies show them to be of little value. Prophylactic corticosteroids should be given as the risk that they will increase the chance of intra-uterine infection is less than their beneficial effect on fetal lung maturation.

The main dilemma is whether prophylactic antibiotics should be given to the mother. Although controlled trials of their use show no reduction in maternal infection before delivery or in neonatal infection (particularly pneumonia), many obstetricians give antibiotics prophylactically, either before labour or when labour starts. This applies, particularly, if Group B streptococci are grown in vaginal culture (see page 140).

Fig. 20.2 Tocolytic drugs in the management of preterm labour		
Drug	**Dose**	**Side effects**
Beta agonists		
Salbutamol	Infused at 4 g/min, increasing by 4 g/min every 20min until uterine contractions suppressed; dose maintained for 6 hours and then reduced. Oral salbutamol started 8mg 6-hourly for 5 days.	Tachycardia, palpitations, apprehension, anxiety. Increase in cardiac output. Pressure in the chest. Hypokalaemia.
Ritodrine	Infused at 50 g/min increased by 50 g every 10min until the contractions cease. Maximum dose 350 g/min. Run for 24 hours then oral ritrodine 10–20mg 2–6 hourly.	Pulmonary oedema and myocardial ischaemia in 5%. Fluid retention in all women.
Calcium channel blocker		
Nifedipine	10mg sublingually; repeated 20min later if contractions persist (max 40mg in first hour). If contractions cease, 20mg by mouth 4-6 hourly.	Limited experience but side effects said to be less than with beta agonists.
Note: Beta agonists and calcium channel blockers are relatively ineffective if the cervical dilatation is >5cm		
Maintenance of labour inhibition		
NSAIDs	This class of drugs is not effective in suppressing labour, but may have a place in maintaining inhibition of labour. Most experience has been with indomethacin. More data needed for evaluation.	May cause ductus arteriosus constriction. Inhibits platelet aggregation, especially in the fetus.
Nitric oxide donor: glyceryl trinitrate		
Nitric oxide donor; glyceryl trinitrate	50mg skin patches applied for 12 hours after cessation of contractions.	Headache in a few women

If antibiotics are not given and the mother develops signs of intra-uterine infection (chorioamnionitis), such as tachycardia, fever (higher than 38°C), leucocytosis and an offensive vaginal discharge, antibiotics should be prescribed and delivery expedited. In most cases the infection is poly-bacterial, with anaerobes and Group B streptococci predominating. Antibiotics are chosen that take these findings into account.

If labour does not start within 48 hours, the patient may ambulate, and provided her home conditions are suitable and she lives near the hospital, may go home. At home she should rest as much as possible, avoid sexual intercourse and return to hospital if she develops a fever or an offensive vaginal discharge.

Fetal maturity

As more women attend for antenatal care early in pregnancy and with the increasing use of ultrasound, the degree of maturity of the fetus is generally known to within 2 weeks. In a few cases, the woman does not seek medical attention until the fourth quarter of pregnancy, at which time the estimation of fetal maturity is less exact. If the fetal maturity is uncertain and labour starts prematurely, if an elective caesarean section is contemplated or if the pregnancy appears to have become postdate, it is helpful to know the stage of maturity of the fetus. Today the gestational age of the fetus can be determined satisfactorily using ultrasound to measure the length of the fetal femur (and if desired other fetal measurements), which has a good

correlation with fetal maturity; this does not indicate the maturity of the fetal lungs. In a mature fetus, hyaline membrane disease is unlikely to develop. Even if it does, neonatologists today have effective treatments. However, some obstetrical units still determine the lung maturity by the lecithin sphingomyelin (L/S) ratios. As pregnancy advances the L/S ratio increases (*Figs. 20.3* and *20.4*).

Post-term pregnancy or postdatism

In 10% of cases the pregnancy lasts for more than 42 weeks. In some cases there may be a genetic cause for postdatism, but for most the aetiology is not known. The diagnosis is established by scrutinizing the woman's antenatal record and confirmed, if needed, by an ultrasound examination in which the fetal abdominal circumference, the length of the femur and the length of the longest column of amniotic fluid are compared with nomogram data.

The risk of a post-term pregnancy is that the perinatal mortality rate increases, especially if the duration of the pregnancy exceeds 43 weeks. At least one-third of the increased mortality is due to the death of a malformed fetus.

MANAGEMENT

If the woman is an older primigravida, has a history of infertility or has PIH, diabetes mellitus or other pregnancy complications, the pregnancy should be terminated before it becomes post-term. In other cases three options are available and they should be discussed with the patient and her partner. These options are the induction of labour,

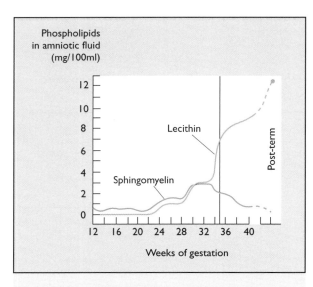

Fig. 20.3 Changes in the concentration of lecithin and sphingomyelin in amniotic fluid.

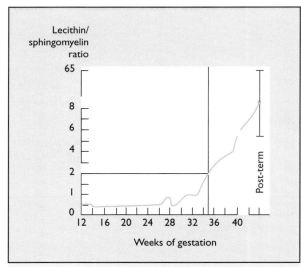

Fig. 20.4 Mean lecithin and sphingomyelin ratios during normal gestation.

to continue with the pregnancy or to perform an elective caesarean section. The induction of labour at 10 days post-term has been shown to be associated with lower rates of caesarean section and reduced neonatal morbidity and perinatal mortality.

If the option of continuing with the pregnancy in the expectation that labour will commence spontaneously is chosen, the welfare of the fetus must be monitored. The mother records fetal movements daily, non-stress cardiotocography is made twice weekly and ultrasound examinations are made to measure the volume of the amniotic fluid. A maximum vertical pool of amniotic fluid of less than 20mm is considered abnormal. Umbilical blood flow may also be measured. Abnormalities in these tests (see Chapter 21, The at-risk fetus) may indicate the need for induction of labour or caesarean section.

The at-risk fetus

The birth weight of an infant depends on its genetic growth potential, which may be restricted or enhanced by the growth support provided by the mother, the functional integrity of the placenta and the ability of the fetus to use the nutrients provided.

Most fetuses grow normally throughout pregnancy (see *Fig. 6.17, page 47*). Some fetuses are genetically programmed to have a low growth potential. They are healthy, but small at birth. Some fetuses have a genetic defect which reduces their growth potential and causes slow intra-uterine growth which may not become apparent until some time in the second half of pregnancy. Some fetuses grow normally initially, but in the last quarter of pregnancy their growth is restricted by alterations in the uteroplacental function. This has led to the use of descriptive term *placental dysfunction* or *placental insufficiency*.

Within genetically set limits, the actual fetal growth depends on:
- An adequate supply of nutrients (especially glucose) and oxygen from the mother.
- An adequate placental transfer of the nutrients, which depends on a good blood supply reaching the placenta.
- A good fetal circulation.
- Functioning fetal pancreatic beta cells, as insulin is the main regulator of fetal growth, provided that nutrients are available.

Of all these factors, an adequate blood supply reaching the placenta so that exchange of nutrients across the placenta can take place, seems the most important.

With this background the identified causes of fetal growth restriction can be defined (*Fig. 21.1*). The degree to which these causes affect fetal growth depends on the amount of placental functioning reserve, and so not all women having these complications will give birth to a growth-restricted fetus.

A growth-restricted fetus is more likely to develop metabolic disturbances, such as acidosis, hypoglycaemia, hypercapnia and erythroblastosis. If the disturbances are severe the fetus may die in the uterus. Less severe disturbances tend to become worse during labour, causing clinical or monitor-detected fetal distress, or the baby may be born with signs of severe hypoxia. Thus the fetus in an affected pregnancy is at greater risk of dying *in utero* or, if born alive, of needing resuscitation and possibly of being brain damaged (cerebral palsy). The pregnancy is high risk. Not all high-risk pregnancies have a growth-restricted fetus, but many do.

High-risk pregnancy

Women who have a high-risk pregnancy should be identified early, if this is possible, and given more intensive antenatal care, particularly after the 30th week of pregnancy. No reliable tests have been developed to identify high-risk pregnancies early, but an indication can be obtained by scoring as shown in *Figure 21.2*. A score of 4 or more will identify all growth-restricted (small-for-dates) babies, but the positive predictive value is only 34%. As mentioned, in some high-risk pregnancies the fetal growth rate is normal or, in the case of pregnancy in a diabetic woman, the baby may be large (macrosomic). In other words, a large number of normal-size-for-dates babies occur in high-risk pregnancies, and their morbidity and mortality is less than if the fetus is growth restricted.

A second method of detecting fetal growth restriction is to measure the symphysio–fundal height with a tape measure and refer to a chart (see *Fig. 6.16, page 46*).

A third test is to use ultrasound to determine the size of the fetus, the amniotic fluid volume and Doppler umbilical blood flow velocity measurements.

Tests for fetal well-being in high-risk pregnancies

Having identified that the pregnancy is high risk for the fetus, tests to determine fetal well-being should be started after the 30th week. In the past 10 years, biophysical tests to determine fetal well-being have superseded biochemical tests. The tests are:
- Fetal movement (fetal kick) counts.
- Cardiotocography.
- Serial ultrasound examinations.
- Doppler flow velocity wave forms.

None of these tests has a high positive predictive value, but each has a high negative predictive value.

A note of caution should be made. The authors of *Effective Care in Pregnancy and Childbirth* point out that, although the tests may provide 'a minimum level of care and attention in settings where these are adequate', in other settings their use may result in 'a variety of unwarranted interventions'. It should be added that unwarranted interventions may lead to an increase in obstetric interventions and possible medicolegal problems. The doctor may be 'damned if he does and damned if he does not'. It is essential that the doctor explains to the patient what is intended and why.

FETAL MOVEMENTS

The patient counts the number of times the fetus kicks until she has recorded 10 kicks. Usually this number of kicks occurs in a 3-hour period, but as fetuses have different patterns of activity, the woman may have to check the number of kicks during another 3-hour period that day. The test is performed three or more times a week. If the fetus fails to kick 10 times in a day, the patient should contact her doctor or hospital.

CARDIOTOCOGRAPHY –
THE NON-STRESS TEST

Cardiotocography (CTG) depends on the assumption that a healthy fetus will normally be more active than an at-risk

fetus and that its heart will respond to a uterine contraction by accelerating. An external cardiotocograph is applied to the woman's abdomen, as she sits in a reclining position (not on her back as this may result in erroneous findings). If spontaneous contractions do not occur over a 30-minute period, they may be provoked by nipple stimulation. The heart beat variations in relation to the contraction are recorded. If the fetus is lethargic, it may be stimulated to move by tapping the uterus gently. CTG is usually done in hospital but can be done at home using domiciliary fetal heart monitoring and a telephone link.

Four cardiotocographic patterns may occur. These are:
- Normal.
- Suboptimal.
- Decelerative.
- Preterminal.

A normal pattern indicates that the fetus is not at risk of dying in the next 7–10 days (Fig. 21.3). Such a fetus is termed reactive. If the suboptimal pattern is found the fetus is at slightly increased risk and the test should be repeated in 3–4 days. The decelerative pattern indicates that the test should be repeated the same day, unless conditions for delivery are suitable, in which case labour should be induced. The preterminal pattern indicates that the fetus is at considerable risk of dying in utero and should be delivered quickly (Fig. 21.4).

A problem with CTG is that normal patterns predict that the fetus is in no danger, but an abnormal pattern does not give an accurate prediction of fetal danger (Fig. 21.5).

SERIAL ULTRASOUND EXAMINATIONS

The growth of the fetus, as a measure of its health, may be monitored by examining it using real-time ultrasound at 2-weekly intervals. The fetal abdominal circumference and the longest column of amniotic fluid are measured. The relatively long interval between tests limits the value of ultrasonography in monitoring fetal well-being.

Fig. 21.1 Aetiological factors in fetal growth restriction (placental dysfunction)	
	Percentage
Maternal causes	
Hypertensive disorders	60
Prolonged pregnancy	5
Maternal diseases (especially eating disorders, renal disease and severe anaemia)	5
Fetal causes	10
Malformations, transplacental infections	
Multiple pregnancy	
Unknown	20

Fig. 21.2 At-risk fetus scoring system	
Variable	**Weighted value**
Previous birth of baby weighing ≤2500g, stillbirth or first week neonatal death	1
Blood pressure ≥140/90mmHg	1
History of renal disease, repeated urinary tract infection (UTI) or UTI in present pregnancy	1
Bleeding in current pregnancy	1
Weight gain >0.5kg in any week after 20 weeks	1
Decrease or no increase in girth	1
Smoking	2
Decrease or no increase in fundal height	3

Fig. 21.3 *Fetal heart acceleration during a uterine contraction (reactive).*

FETAL BLOOD FLOW VELOCITY

Uteroplacental and fetoplacental circulations are low-resistance systems in which the flow of blood towards the placenta continues throughout the cardiac cycle, causing wave forms of different types. If fetoplacental vascular resistance increases because of acute uteroplacental atherosclerosis, fetal disease or unknown causes, the wave forms are altered. In the umbilical artery the difference between the peak systolic flow (A) and end diastolic flow (B) can be measured (Fig. 21.6). The greater the A:B ratio the more likely it is that the fetus will be compromised, particularly if absent or reversed end-diastolic flow (AEDFV) or extreme S:D ratio is found. The finding identifies a major defect in fetoplacental perfusion associated with intra-uterine growth restriction (including cases of fetal aneuploidy) or pregnancy-induced hypertension clinically identified before the 34th gestational week.

Fetal blood flow velocity is a useful method of determining whether the placental function is insufficient and, hence, whether the well-being of the fetus is affected. It is a screening test and if abnormal should be followed by a CTG non-stress test. It should also be pointed out that if AEDVF is found, one in three of survivors will have major neurological sequelae.

Fig. 21.4 *Preterminal fetal heart rate pattern. Note marked reduction in short term variablility and repeated deceleration with Braxton-Hicks contractions.*

	Pattern			
	Normal	**Suboptimal**	**Decelerative**	**Preterminal**
Variation in baseline FHR (beats per min)	>10	>10	>5, <10	<5
Acceleration on fetal movement (over a 30–45min period)	At least 2 of 15bpm	At least 2 of 10bpm	At least one episode of acceleration (10bpm) every 20 min	None
Deceleration (in relation to Braxton Hicks contractions)	None	None	Variable	Late

Fig. 21.5 Patterns found on antepartum cardiotocography

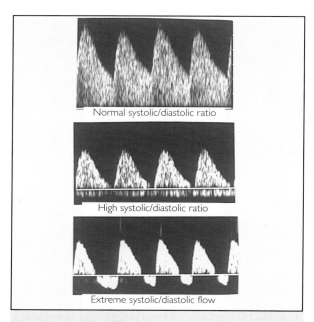

Fig. 21.6 Doppler umbilical blood patterns.

BIOPHYSICAL PROFILE

Some obstetric units, especially in the USA, believe that the at-risk status of a fetus can be detected with greater accuracy if a biophysical profile is obtained. This consists of monitoring fetal movements, breathing, tone and reactivity and amniotic fluid volume by real-time ultrasound. The procedure is costly and time consuming and, at present, there is no evidence that it is superior to non-stress testing.

A compromise may be to measure the fetal blood flow velocity in small-for-dates or premature fetuses and, if it is abnormal, to perform a CTG; and, in mature or postmature at-risk fetuses, to measure the liquor volume using ultrasound and to perform a CTG at intervals.

CORDIOCENTESIS (FETAL BLOOD SAMPLING)

This procedure has been suggested as it helps the clinician to make a better determination of the condition of the fetus, in selected patients, than with the other tests mentioned. It requires high technical skill and is not justified if the fetus is estimated to weigh more than 1500g.

Management of a high-risk pregnancy

Although fetal growth may be restricted at all stages of pregnancy (commonly in malformed fetuses), it is unusual for problems to arise before the 30th week of pregnancy. The effects of placental dysfunction are observable between the 30th and 35th week, and become more marked after that time. In three-quarters of cases the expectant mother has a clinical disorder.

There are no known preventive measures although a multicentre trial is taking place to determine if daily low doses of aspirin (75mg) will reduce the risk of the development of severe pregnancy-induced hypertension (PIH) and of fetal growth restriction among women who have previously had a compromised pregnancy.

All that can be done is to monitor the maternal disease if it is present, to detect deterioration and to check fetal well-being (Fig. 21.7). If the maternal condition worsens, for example PIH deteriorates or if the fetus appears likely to die *in utero*, the pregnancy should be terminated either by inducing labour or by caesarean section.

Monitoring the at-risk fetus in labour

When caesarean section is not chosen to perform an immediate delivery, the health of the mother and fetus should be monitored during the labour. The care of the woman in labour has been described in Chapter 9, Course and management of childbirth. In this section the care of the fetus will be described.

An at-risk fetus, particularly growth restricted, has fewer reserves on which it can draw for energy should placental gas and glucose transfer be reduced further during labour. Normally, the fetus converts glucose (released from glycogen stores) by anaerobic pathways into ketopyruvic acid and then, in the presence of oxygen, into carbon dioxide and water via the Krebs cycle. The process releases '30 high-energy bonds' per molecule of glucose. When the supply of oxygen is limited, the conversion cycle stops before the Krebs cycle is initiated and only the anaerobic cycle operates. Anaerobic glycosis releases far less energy, and leads to the accumulation of lactic acid in the fetal blood, causing acidaemia. In addition, if the fetus is growth restricted and has limited glycogen and fat stored, it is at great risk of developing acidaemia and may die.

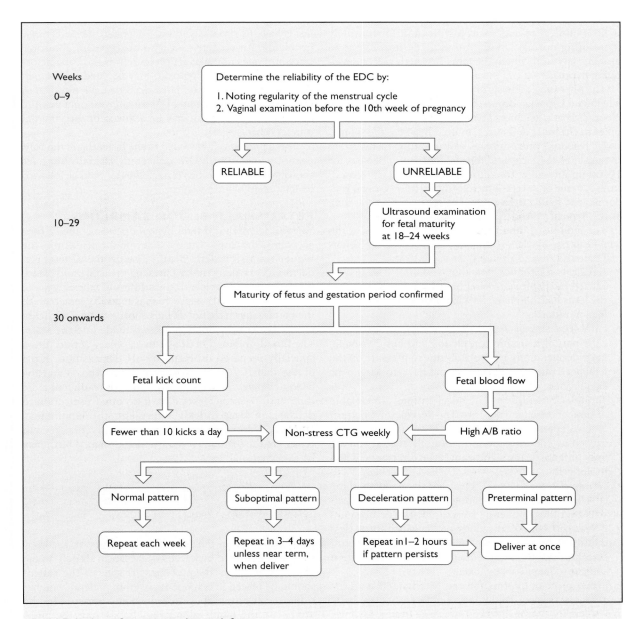

Fig. 21.7 A scheme for monitoring the at-risk fetus.

Fetuses which are at particular risk of developing hypoxia and acidaemia are those whose mother has had a pregnancy complication or those who have been compromised either before labour or during the birth process (Fig. 21.8).

During labour the well-being of the fetus may be monitored by listening to the fetal heart at regular intervals. A problem arising is that counting the fetal heart rate between contractions misses three-quarters of the early signs of fetal hypoxia (fetal distress).

This problem has been overcome by the development of fetal heart monitors (CTG machines), which monitor the fetal heart continuously throughout the labour. There is little clinical or statistical justification for routinely monitoring normal labour with a CTG. Its value is to monitor labour in which the fetus is at high risk of developing hypoxia.

The physiological basis of fetal heart monitoring is that when fetal hypoxia occurs, the altered composition of the blood causes a rise in sympathetic and vagal tone, which differ in character and effect. In mild hypoxia, the sympathetic response predominates with resulting tachycardia; the onset of the tachycardia is delayed and it persists for 10–30 minutes after the cause of the hypoxia has ceased. In moderate or severe hypoxia, the vagal response predominates. Bradycardia is rapid in onset and lasts as long as the hypoxic episode and then disappears rapidly.

The fetal heart monitor records these changes in the fetal heart rate in relation to uterine contraction. The abnormal patterns are shown in *Fig. 21.9*:

- *Persistent tachycardia* (more than 160bpm). This may be caused by maternal or fetal pyrexia and indicates that the fetus has mild hypoxia which requires more careful fetal monitoring.
- *Early decelerations* (Type 1 dips). The dip occurs in the early part of a uterine contraction and has a V-shape. Early decelerations are probably due to pressure on the fetal head during a contraction and have no prognostic significance.
- *Variable decelerations.* The decelerations are variable in time of onset and severity. The deceleration pattern is U-shaped. Variable decelerations are probably caused by compression of the umbilical cord and are only prognostically significant if the dip is severe and prolonged.
- *Late decelerations* (Type 2 dips). The deceleration of the fetal heart rate starts late during the contraction and persists after the contraction has ceased. The deceleration is V-shaped. Late decelerations, particularly if severe (less than 100 bpm) indicate impairment of the utero-placental blood flow, a reduction in fetal oxygenation and consequent fetal hypoxia.

A further piece of information can be obtained from the heart monitor tracing, i.e.this is beat-to-beat variation (baseline variability). Normally the beat-to-beat heart rate shows variations of more than 5bpm, leading to a wavy line on the trace. The diminution, or absence, of b*eat-to-beat variation* indicates some degree of fetal hazard.

If, in addition to abnormal fetal heart tracings, the fetus passes thick, green meconium, the probability of severe fetal hypoxia is increased.

BENEFITS AND PROBLEMS OF FETAL HEART MONITORING

Fetal heart monitors are available in most obstetric units and it is believed that their use 'saves' 1–2 infants per 1000 births. However, there are problems with their use and these include the fact that the interpretation of the trace may be difficult and, although the sensitivity of the test is high, its specificity is low. There also are medicolegal problems. An obstetrician who observes an abnormal trace and does not take action to deliver the baby before it dies from possible hypoxia, may be sued by the parents should the baby be born dead or have physical or mental damage; whilst an obstetrician who operates and delivers a healthy baby may be accused of carrying out unnecessary surgery.

These problems add weight to the belief that if the baby cannot expeditiously be delivered vaginally, a trace showing late decelerations (Type 2 dips) should be followed by fetal scalp blood sampling.

FETAL SCALP BLOOD SAMPLING

You will recall that if fetal hypoxia persists, after a time acidaemia develops. The more severe the acidaemia, the higher the risk of fetal death. The degree of fetal acidaemia can be detected by sampling the fetal scalp blood. A tubular speculum is introduced through the cervix and pressed on the fetal scalp, which is made hyperaemic. (If the membranes have not already ruptured, they are deliberately broken.) A small incision is made into the scalp. The blood obtained is drawn by capillary action into a specially prepared tube and its pH is measured. A pH of less than 7.20 indicates severe fetal hypoxia and the need to deliver the baby expeditiously. A reading of more than 7.20–7.25 suggests that, if no other indication to deliver the fetus quickly is present, the labour may continue whilst maintaining close surveillance and repeating the scalp pH if indicated and vaginal birth may be expected.

Management of monitor-detected fetal distress

If the patient is in the second stage of labour, the baby should be delivered by forceps or caesarean section. In the first stage of labour the problems are greater. The patient should be placed in a different position, preferably on her side or well propped up to reduce any pressure by the uterus on the major blood vessels; she may be given oxygen via a face mask, although the benefit of this has

Fig. 21.8 *Fetuses at high risk of developing intrapartum hypoxia and acidaemia*

Maternal factors

Hypertensive diseases in pregnancy
Diabetes
Multiple pregnancy
Severe anaemia
Severe malnutrition

Placental factors

Abruptio placentae

Fetal factors

Growth restriction (small for dates)
Malpresentations
Cord complications
Clinical 'fetal distress'*

*Clinical fetal distress is diagnosed if the fetal heart rate is >160 but <110 beats per minute sustained for 5 minutes or meconium stained liquor is seen.

not been proven. If an oxytocin infusion causes very strong uterine contractions, the drip should be slowed or stopped.

After these actions have been taken, the monitor tracing is observed to see if the fetal heart pattern reverts to normal. If it does not the baby must be delivered.

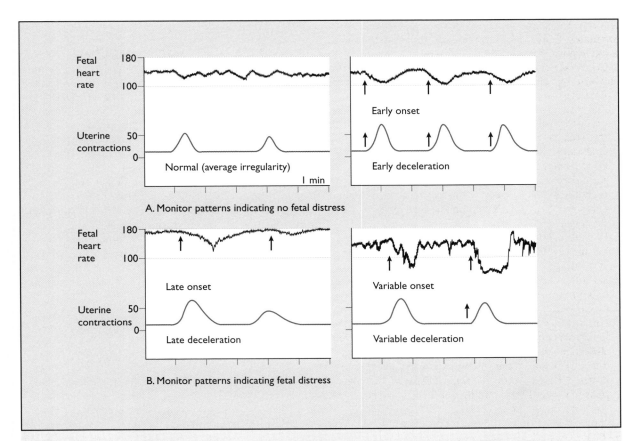

Fig. 21.9 *Abnormal fetal heart patterns in labour. (Arrows indicate the time of commencement of the uterine contraction.)*

CHAPTER 22

Abnormal fetal presentations

Abnormal presentations include, in order of frequency, occipito-posterior presentations, breech presentations, face presentations, transverse presentations and brow presentations.

Occipito-posterior presentations

In about 10% of pregnancies, the fetal head enters the maternal pelvis with its occiput in one of the posterior segments of the pelvis (see *Fig. 9.5*, page 75). In most cases the pelvic architecture is normal, but in a few it is classified as long oval (see *Fig. 23.13*, page 183).

The diagnosis may be made on abdominal palpation when the fetal back is felt in one of the mother's flanks, the fetal heart being loudest here (*Fig. 22.1*). In labour, vaginal examination provides more information, the occiput and the anterior fontanelle being identified (*Fig. 22.2*).

During labour, the fetal head is forced deeper into the pelvis, and usually flexes on the fetal neck. Once full dilatation of the cervix has occurred its progress may be in one of three ways (see *Fig. 22.2*):

Fig. 22.1 Occipito-posterior position – abdominal findings.

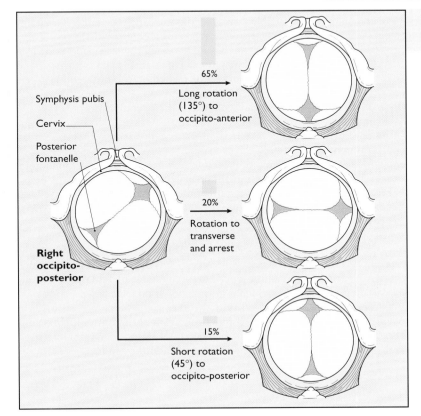

Fig. 22.2 Possible modes of rotation of the head.

Symphysis pubis

Cervix

Posterior fontanelle

Right occipito-posterior

65%
Long rotation (135°) to occipito-anterior

20%
Rotation to transverse and arrest

15%
Short rotation (45°) to occipito-posterior

- In 65% of cases the head rotates through 135° so that the occiput lies behind the symphysis pubis.
- In 20% of cases rotation of the fetal head ceases and it becomes arrested in a transverse diameter of the pelvis.
- In 15% of cases the fetal head rotates posteriorly.

Thus, in most cases, the fetal head undergoes a long or a short rotation (Fig. 22.3).

MANAGEMENT OF OCCIPITO-POSTERIOR PRESENTATIONS

There is no management before labour starts. Once begun, the duration of labour tends to be longer in occipito-posterior positions, and the mother requires more support, analgesia and hydration. Progress is monitored using a partogram. The descent of the head, and its position, are checked regularly. Any marked delay in the first stage of labour leads to prolonged labour (see page 180) and a decision has to be made whether to continue or to perform a caesarean section. Delay in the second stage of labour of longer than 1.5–2 hours' duration indicates the need for help to deliver the baby. If the fetal head undergoes the long rotation a spontaneous vaginal delivery may be expected. This occurs in 65% of cases. If the fetal head undergoes the short rotation and descends to the pelvic floor in the posterior position, the infant may be born spontaneously (8% of all cases) or may need to be helped by forceps (7%). On the other hand, the fetus may not descend much beyond the ischial spines and a manual rotation and forceps delivery, Kjelland's forceps delivery or vacuum extraction may be necessary (see Chapter 23, Abnormal labour [dystocia] and prolonged labour). These procedures are also required if the fetal head arrests in a transverse diameter of the pelvis. Between 5 and 10% of babies who are occipito-posterior are delivered by caesarean section.

Breech presentations

The frequency of breech presentation falls as pregnancy advances. At the 30th week of pregnancy 15% of fetuses present as a breech; by the 35th week the proportion has fallen to 6% and, by term, only 3% present as a breech. Most of these babies spontaneously turn to become cephalic. If the presentation is still a breech at the 37th week, many obstetricians attempt a cephalic version, which is described on page 202. Version is easier if the breech has flexed legs, one of the three types of breech presentation (Fig. 22.4).

The presentation of the fetus is of no clinical importance before the 32nd–35th week. At this stage of pregnancy, the diagnosis of a breech presentation is made by finding, on palpation, that the lower pole of the uterus is occupied by a soft, irregular mass and that, in the fundal area, a firm, smooth, rounded mass is present which bounces between the fingers if gently pushed. On auscultation the fetal heart beat is loudest above the umbilicus. If any doubt exists after palpation and a vaginal examination, an ultrasound image will clarify the diagnosis, and will exclude fetal malformations.

The fetus may be left as a breech or an external cephalic version may be attempted at 36–37 weeks of gestation, depending on local custom.

PROBLEMS WITH BREECH PRESENTATIONS

Few problems occur during pregnancy, although some expectant mothers complain of pressure beneath the diaphragm. Since breech births frequently require operative delivery, there is an increased risk to the fetus, which is minimized by skilled attention and decision making. In the absence of any other complications of pregnancy, preterm breech births (weight less than 2500g) carry a mortality of 12%, as do large postmature babies (weight more than 3500g). Mature fetuses whose weight is in the normal range have a mortality of 1%.

The main causes of morbidity are intracranial haemorrhage, asphyxia and fracture of the humerus, femur or clavicle.

MANAGEMENT OF BREECH BIRTHS
Elective caesarean section at term

Because of the risks mentioned, an increasing number of breech presentations at term are being delivered, electively, by caesarean section. In some institutions the caesarean section rate is greater than 60%; the average rate is about 30%.

The arguments in favour of caesarean section are:
- Possible damage to the fetus and the perinatal mortality is less than that following a vaginal birth.
- Couples are having fewer children, demand a 'perfect' child and may sue if a 'damaged' child is born.
- 30–40% of trials of vaginal breech birth end as a caesarean birth.
- Caesarean section is a safe operation.
  Counter-arguments are:
- The maternal morbidity is greater after caesarean section.
- 5–15% of breech fetuses have a congenital malformation, and might be better delivered vaginally.
- Some expectant mothers prefer to attempt to give birth vaginally.

Vaginal breech birth

The success of the vaginal birth of a breech depends on the relative size of the breech and the maternal pelvis (which may require a pelvimetry to establish) and the skill of the doctor, which in turn depends on experience.

To understand the management of breech birth, a description of the mechanism of the birth of a breech is needed. This is shown in the sequence of illustrations (Figs. 22.5–22.14) and is described in the captions.

Long rotation

a The uterus and fetal axis move forward, and the head flexes as it is forced down into the pelvis

b Early second stage. The occiput has reached the pelvic floor. Anterior rotation now begins and the head flexes still more

c Anterior rotation is occurring through 135°

d Anterior rotation is complete and the remainder of the delivery is as for an occipito-anterior position

Short rotation

e The uterus and fetal axis move forward and the head enters the pelvis

f The head fails to flex and descends into the pelvis in the posterior position

g The occiput rotating backwards through 45° when it reaches the pelvic floor to lie in the hollow of the sacrum

h Birth of the head occurs by further flexion to permit the occiput to crown and escape over the perineum. Then by extension, the brow, nose, face and chin appear from behind the symphysis

Fig. 22.3 Occipito-posterior. Long rotation (a–d); short rotation (e–h).

Fig. 22.4 Types of breech presentation. (a) Breech with extended legs (frank); (b) breech with flexed legs (complete); (c) footling.

Fig. 22.5 The breech is presenting as a right sacro-anterior. The bitrochanteric diameter of the buttocks has entered the pelvis in the transverse diameter of the pelvic brim. With full dilatation of the cervix, the buttocks descend deeply into the pelvis.

Fig. 22.6 When the buttocks reach the pelvic floor, the pelvic 'gutter' causes the buttocks to rotate internally so that the bitrochanteric diameter lies in the anterior-posterior diameter of the pelvic outlet.

Fig. 22.7 The anterior buttock appears at the vulva. With further uterine contractions the buttocks distend the vaginal outlet. Lateral flexion of the fetal trunk takes place and the shoulders rotate so that they may enter the pelvis. At this stage the attending doctor or nurse–midwife has donned gown and gloves and is prepared to aid the delivery.

Fig. 22.8 If the buttocks make no advance during the next several contractions, an episiotomy is made and the buttocks are born by groin traction.

Fig. 22.9 The buttocks have been born and the shoulders have entered the pelvis in its transverse diameter. This causes the external rotation of the buttocks so that the fetal back becomes uppermost.

Fig. 22.10 If the fetus has extended legs, the attendant may have to slip a hand along the anterior leg of the fetus and deliver it by flexion and abduction, so that the rest of the birth may proceed.

Fig. 22.11 The fetal shoulders have reached the pelvic 'gutter' and have rotated internally so that the bis-achromial diameter lies in the antero-posterior diameter of the outlet. Simultaneously, the buttocks have rotated anteriorly through 90°. The fetal head is now entering the pelvic brim, its sagittal suture lying in the brim's transverse diameter. Descent into the pelvis occurs with flexion of the fetal head.

Fig. 22.12 The baby has been born to beyond its umbilicus. A loop of umbilical cord is pulled down to make sure that it is not holding back the birth. Gentle traction downwards and backwards is made by the attendant, so that the anterior shoulder and arm are born. The baby is now lifted upwards in a circle so that the posterior shoulder and arm may be born. Sometimes one arm is extended and has to be dislodged downwards. The procedure requires skill otherwise a fractured clavicle or humerus may result. Once the anterior arm has been born, the baby's body and the posterior arm are freed in a similar manner.

Fig. 22.13 (a) The baby hangs unsupported from the mother's vulva. The doctor applies slight suprapubic pressure to encourage further flexion of the head. When the nape of the baby's neck has appeared, the attendant holds the baby by the feet and swings it upwards through an arc. (b) This manoeuvre, by using the lower border of the sacrum, pulls the head down and rotates it through the pelvic outlet so that the chin, nose and forehead appear.

a

b

Fig. 22.14 An alternative is to deliver the fetal head by forceps.

AN ALGORITHM FOR THE MANAGEMENT OF BREECH PRESENTATIONS

In *Figure 22.15* an algorithm for the management of breech presentations is given. Not included is breech extraction. In breech extraction the baby is delivered by the doctor. The main use of breech extraction is for the birth of a second twin, or if the breech is impacted in the midpelvic cavity. Unless the obstetrician is very skilled, caesarean section is safer.

Transverse lies, oblique lies and shoulder presentations

Shoulder presentations, unstable lie, transverse lie and oblique lie may be detected in late pregnancy. These conditions occur in 1 in 200 births, usually among multiparous women. The aetiology is varied. They may occur in a lax multiparous uterus with no other complication of pregnancy, but may be associated with polyhydramnios, placenta praevia or a uterine malformation (page 279). An ultrasound examination is helpful in excluding placenta praevia.

The diagnosis is made by finding a broad asymmetrical uterus with a firm, ballotable round head in one iliac fossa, and a softer mass in the other (*Fig. 22.16*).

MANAGEMENT IN PREGNANCY

When placenta praevia has been excluded, a gentle cephalic version may be attempted, but in many cases the fetus returns after some time to its previous presentation. If the lie remains unstable, the expectant mother should be advised to report to hospital immediately labour starts or, if the social conditions are unfavourable, may be admitted to hospital to await labour. In some cases the presentation is corrected to cephalic and the head is held over the brim. The membranes are then ruptured and the head pressed into the pelvis as the liquor amnii is released.

Another choice is to perform an elective caesarean section.

MANAGEMENT IN LABOUR

If the shoulder presentation is not detected until labour has been established, caesarean section is the preferred option, although the manoeuvre of guiding the fetal head to lie above the pelvic brim and rupturing the membranes has some advocates.

Face presentations

Face presentation occurs in 1 in 500 births, usually by chance, but in 15% of cases the baby is anencephalic, or has a tumour of the neck or shortening of the neck muscles.

Face presentation is rarely diagnosed before labour, and even then may be missed until a face with swollen, distorted lips appears at the vulva. Abdominal palpation may reveal a peculiar S-shaped fetus with feet on the opposite side to the prominent occiput. The fetal head has not usually entered the pelvis (*Fig. 22.17*).

Vaginal examination during labour may clarify the presentation (*Fig. 22.18*), but in late labour, when much facial oedema has occurred, a breech may be misdiagnosed.

MECHANISM AND MANAGEMENT OF LABOUR

In most cases the face enters the transverse diameter of the pelvis with the fetal chin in a mento-transverse position. Descent into the pelvis is delayed until late in the first stage or the second stage of labour (*Fig. 22.19*). Rotation usually occurs anteriorly so that the chin lies behind the pubis, and delivery occurs spontaneously by flexion of the head or may be aided by forceps. In a few cases the fetal chin rotates posteriorly, impacting the fetal head and preventing vaginal delivery. The impacted fetal head may be rotated using Kjelland's forceps or, preferably, the fetus may be delivered by caesarean section.

Brow presentations

Brow is the most unfavourable and the least common (1 in 1500 births) of all malpositions and malpresentations. It

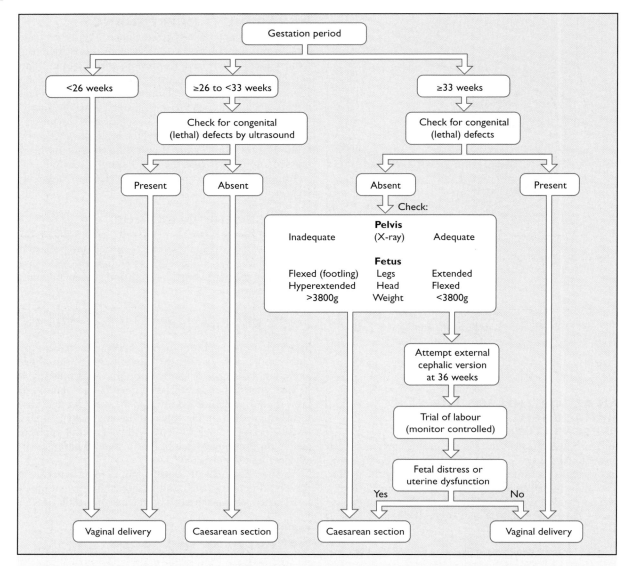

Fig. 22.15 *Management of breech presentations. If detected at 36 weeks confirm gestation period by checking date of last menstrual period, visits during pregnancy and ultrasound examination. Attempt external cephalic version (ECV) without anaesthesia, ? using tocolytics and real-time ultrasound. If ECV fails wait for labour.*

may occur during late pregnancy (when it usually converts into a cephalic presentation). An ultrasound examination should be made to exclude fetal malformations, particularly hydrocephaly.

The patient should be seen each week to check the presentation and told to come into hospital as soon as contractions start or the membranes rupture.

In labour, brow presentation is diagnosed when the fetal head is high and a sulcus can be identified between the head and the back.

Treatment consists of performing a caesarean section, unless the baby is grossly abnormal or dead, when a destructive operation may be chosen (see page 202).

Multiple pregnancy

Multiple pregnancy occurs when two or more ova are released and fertilized (dizygotic) or when a single fertilized ovum divides early to form two identical embryos at the inner cell mass stage or earlier (monozygotic). The incidence of twins is 1 in 90 pregnancies and that of triplets is 1 in 90 × 90 (8100) pregnancies. Since the introduction of assisted reproductive technology, the incidence of multiple pregnancies has increased. Ultrasound examination in early pregnancy has also identified more twins but in half of those identified one fetus dies and disappears before the second half of pregnancy, the so-called vanishing twin.

Fig. 22.16 Transverse lie.

Fig. 22.17 Abdominal palpation in face presentation.

Fig. 22.18 Touch picture of the face.

Fig. 22.19 Diagram of engagement. In the face presentation engagement occurs late as the parietal prominences do not enter the brim until the face has reached the pelvic floor.

In dizygotic multiple pregnancy, each fetus is a separate individual with its own placenta, amnion and chorion. In monozygotic multiple pregnancy, the two fetuses have a single placenta and chorion, but each twin has its own amniotic sac. As there is vascular communication between the two parts of the placenta it is not unusual for one twin to obtain a reduced supply of nutrients and grow more slowly than the other. Occasionally one fetus dies early in pregnancy, becoming mummified (fetus papyraceous).

Because of the greater demands for nutrients, a fetus in a multiple pregnancy tends to be smaller than a singleton fetus, as its growth *in utero* is slower (*Fig. 22.20*).

DIAGNOSIS OF MULTIPLE PREGNANCY

Few multiple pregnancies are diagnosed in the first half of pregnancy except by ultrasound scanning. In the second half of pregnancy, a multiple pregnancy can be suspected if:

- The abdominal girth and uterine size are greater than expected from the period of amenorrhoea.
- Palpation shows an excess of fetal parts, and two fetal heads can be detected.

Multiple pregnancy is confirmed by an ultrasound examination (*Fig. 22.21*).

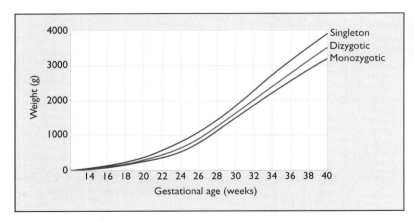

Fig. 22.20 The intra-uterine growth of multiple and single pregnancies as assessed by ultrasound fetometry.

Fig. 22.21 Multiple pregnancy. Transverse scan at 32 weeks – two heads visible.

MANAGEMENT OF MULTIPLE PREGNANCY

Compared with a singleton pregnancy, a multiple pregnancy is likely to be associated with more pregnancy complications (Fig. 22.22). For this reason the expectant mother requires additional antenatal care. She should be seen at 2-weekly intervals from the time of diagnosis. Maternal anaemia should be sought and treated, and there is a strong argument for insisting that the patient takes folic acid 5mg and an iron salt each day. When a woman carrying twins goes into preterm labour, the decision whether to deliver the twins by caesarean section or to attempt a vaginal birth has to be made. A problem is that in 20% of twin pregnancies, the weight of one twin is 20% less than that of the other. There is no consensus about the safest method to use.

A woman carrying a multiple pregnancy has an increased blood volume and an extra burden on her cardiovascular system. Traditionally, the doctor recommends that an expectant mother carrying a multiple pregnancy takes extra rest, for example 2 hours in the afternoon, supposedly to reduce the risk of PIH and preterm labour. There

are no accurate data to support this belief, and the woman should be given the opportunity to make up her own mind.

It is common practice to monitor fetal growth by ultrasound every 2–3 weeks from the 30th week. If growth ceases and/or Doppler blood flow indices are abnormal delivery is expedited.

Higher multiple pregnancies

Since the development of assisted reproductive technology, the prevalence of multiple pregnancies has increased. A number of these will be triplets or higher. The perinatal mortality of these fetuses and neonates is high. To manage this problem, selective termination of some or all fetuses, by intracardiac injection, has been used. This has led to medical and legal problems which have not been resolved.

MANAGEMENT IN LABOUR

The position of the leading fetus should be checked on admission. In a twin pregnancy, both fetuses present as cephalic in 45% of cases; as cephalic and breech in 25%; and as breech and cephalic or breech and breech in 10%

Fig. 22.22 *Complications of pregnancy in singleton and multiple pregnancies*

Complication	Singleton (%)	Multiple (%)
Pregnancy induced hypertension	5	15
Anaemia	3–5	15
Polyhydramnios	<2	>5
Preterm labour (birth before 37th week)	<5	>25
Perinatal mortality	0.9	5.6

each. If the first twin presents transversely, caesarean section is the preferable approach. In other cases a vaginal birth may be expected. The management of the labour is conducted in the way already described (Chapter 9, Course and management of childbirth). When the membranes rupture a vaginal examination is made to check if the umbilical cord has prolapsed.

The first baby is usually born without difficulty, if necessary following an episiotomy. Immediately following the birth, the doctor makes an abdominal examination to determine the lie and presentation of the second twin. If it is transverse, the doctor may attempt external version to bring the fetus into a longitudinal position. A vaginal examination is then made to confirm the presentation and, if it is longitudinal, the second amniotic sac is artificially ruptured. The fetal presenting part is led into the pelvis. A second twin which remains in the transverse presentation should be delivered either by caesarean section or by internal podalic version, depending on the skill of the obstetrician.

Following the birth of the first twin, uterine contractions may diminish for a few minutes. If they do not return soon, an intravenous oxytocin infusion may be set up. The birth of the second twin is usually uncomplicated, but postpartum haemorrhage may be expected and should be anticipated by managing the third stage actively.

RISK TO MOTHER AND FETUSES

There is no increased risk to a mother who has received appropriate antenatal care. The risk to a fetus of a multiple pregnancy is higher than to a singleton, mainly because of the increased incidence of preterm birth. The perinatal mortality of twin births is 50 per 1000, five times that of a singleton birth. The death of one of the twins during the birth, or the neonatal period, presents the parents with unique problems, as they have to adjust to having one living baby who no longer has a same-age sibling.

PSYCHOLOGICAL EFFECTS OF TWINS ON THE PARENTS

The knowledge that she is carrying twins may have a considerable psychological effect on the mother and her partner, and the attending health professional needs to help and counsel the couple. If the multiple pregnancy has been diagnosed in the early weeks of pregnancy by ultrasound scanning, the first matter to be discussed is the problem of the 'vanishing twin'. After the 20th week of pregnancy the woman and her partner should be made aware that there is a higher chance of developing complications during the pregnancy, which may require admission to hospital, and may lead to a premature birth. If the woman already has a child, or children, her absence from the home may require help from partner or relatives, and studies have shown that she has an increased chance of developing depression in late pregnancy. She also has a greater chance that the birth will be by caesarean section, which may cause anxiety and the issue should be discussed.

In the postnatal period, the demands of caring for two small babies adds to the problem of adjusting to parenthood (see page 98), and usually means that the couple have little time to be with each other to enhance their general and their sexual relationship. In the period after childbirth, more women who have given birth to twins report anxiety and depression and often need support and help. Women report that discussion of these matters during pregnancy and the availability of support both during and after pregnancy reduce the 'stress' of having twins. Fortunately, in the community there are self-help groups whose support and counselling are invaluable. However, the doctor or nurse attending the woman during and after pregnancy should be aware of the problems and of the need to talk with the woman and her partner.

Prolapse of the umbilical cord

Although prolapse of the umbilical cord is not a malpresentation, it is more likely to occur when there is a fetal malpresentation or position. For this reason it is included in this chapter. Prolapse of the umbilical cord occurs in 1 in 300 deliveries. The cord may be contained within the forewaters, when it is said to be presenting, or may have prolapsed to lie in front of the fetal presenting part after the membranes have ruptured (Fig. 22.23).

AETIOLOGY

The umbilical cord is more likely to prolapse if anything prevents the snug application of the presenting part in the lower uterine segment or its descent into the maternal pelvis. For this reason, fetal malpresentations and positions, cephalopelvic disproportion and preterm births are more likely to be associated with cord prolapse. The cord may also prolapse at amniotomy, during version of the fetus and in other obstetric manipulations.

DIAGNOSIS

Presentation of the umbilical cord is rarely diagnosed. When prolapse of the cord occurs after the membranes have ruptured, it can be detected by a vaginal examination. This should be made in all cases of preterm labour or if a fetal malpresentation or position is present. If the cord is felt on the vaginal examination, its pulsations should be sought and the fetal heart sounds checked to determine if they are within the normal range or show tachycardia or bradycardia.

MANAGEMENT

The management of prolapsed cord depends on the condition of the fetus and the degree of cervical dilatation. If the fetus is dead, its birth may be awaited. If the fetus is alive and the cervix is not fully dilated, a caesarean section is safest for the baby. Whilst arranging for the section, it may help to relieve pressure on the cord by placing the woman in the knee-chest position. The umbilical cord should be replaced into the vagina to reduce the risk of cold causing spasm of the umbilical vessels.

If the cervix is fully dilated, and the fetal head or breech is deep in the pelvis, a forceps delivery or breech extraction may be performed if an experienced obstetrician is present.

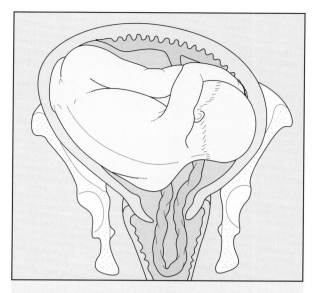

Fig. 22.23 Prolapse of the umbilical cord.

CHAPTER 23

Abnormal labour (dystocia) and prolonged labour

If the duration of labour exceeds the accepted norm, or if intervention has to be made either before or during labour, the condition is defined as dystocia. Dystocia may result from:

- 'Faults' in fetus.
- An abnormal size or shape of the pelvis.
- Inefficient uterine contractions.

These matters are discussed in this chapter.

'Faults' in the fetus (the passenger)

The presentation of the fetus may cause prolongation of labour (for example an occipito-posterior position), as may the size of the fetus. A large fetus (weight more than 4000g) may not be able to be born vaginally easily even if the pelvis is of normal size. Some genetically programmed mothers habitually produce large babies, as do some diabetic mothers. Some babies have congenital defects which may make vaginal births difficult or impossible, for example a fetus who has hydrocephaly or a tumour of the neck or abdomen. A fault in the fetus may be anticipated if an abdominal examination in late pregnancy reveals a large fetus whose head has not entered the maternal pelvis. The diagnosis can be established by an ultrasound examination.

Abnormal shape or size of the pelvis (the passages)

The ideal obstetric pelvis is described on page 55. If any of the two main diameters, particularly those of the pelvic brim, is reduced by 2cm or more the pelvis is considered to be contracted. The shape of the pelvis may also be affected for example the sacral curve may be replaced by a straight sacrum, or the pelvis may have been damaged by a serious accident. Pelvic abnormalities are classified and described on pages 183–186.

In many cases an abnormal size or shape of the pelvis is detected in primigravidae by determining the woman's height (women less than 150cm in height may have a small pelvis) and by making a pelvic examination at the 36–38th week of pregnancy, particularly if the biparietal diameter of the fetal head has not entered the maternal pelvis. If the woman has previously given birth and there is concern about her ability to deliver vaginally, the doctor should scrutinize her obstetric history and assess if the fetal head is able to enter the pelvis, by pressing on it in a downwards and backwards direction, or by performing the examination shown in *Figure 6.25* (see page 50).

If the doctor has any doubt, after these investigations, about the capacity of the pelvis to permit the fetus to be delivered vaginally, X-ray pelvimetry or computerized tomograph (CT) pelvimetry (*Fig. 23.1*) may be carried out. In developed countries, pelvimetry is not often needed nowadays. The reason is that better maternal nutrition during childhood has led to a substantial reduction in the incidence of contracted pelvis and it has become realized that, provided that the pelvis is not too small or the fetus too large, the quality of the uterine contractions is the final arbiter of a successful vaginal delivery. However, CT pelvimetry may be of importance in determining if a breech presentation should be delivered by caesarean section or the woman should have a trial of labour.

In the developing nations pelvimetry, preferably by CT scan (if available), still has a place to enable the obstetrician to make a decision about a vaginal delivery, but this prognosis is not particularly accurate, as different observers attach different prognostic values to the measurements and the shape of the pelvis. For example, if the anteroposterior diameter of the pelvic brim is less than 9cm, nearly all obstetricians will perform a caesarean section; whilst if the anteroposterior diameter is between 9cm and 10.5cm, an obstetrician may attempt a trial of labour, provided the woman is agreeable, unless the sacrum is straight, when a caesarean section will be performed. If the anteroposterior diameter is more than 10.5cm a vaginal delivery will be anticipated, unless the fetal head is very large.

Fig. 23.1 Computerized tomograph (CT) scan of the pelvis.

Cephalopelvic disproportion

Apart from the quality of the uterine contractions, the main issue with regard to vaginal birth is the size of the fetus *relative* to the size of the maternal pelvis; thus the concept of cephalopelvic disproportion (CPD) has arisen. The term cephalopelvic is used rather than fetopelvic as any presentation other than cephalic would be treated by caesarean section.

In cases of CPD, if the fetal head has not entered the pelvic brim by term, a caesarean section is likely to be performed because of risks to the fetus should labour proceed. On the other hand, if the fetal head has entered the pelvic brim the choice is between an elective caesarean section and a trial of labour. The decision depends on the woman's preference and the doctor's experience. For example, a woman over the age of 35, or one who has had a long history of infertility will generally be delivered by caesarean section, as will women with medical complications.

If a trial of labour is attempted, the patient should be told that she has about a 30% chance that she will require a forceps delivery and a 30% chance that the trial will be abandoned and a caesarean section will be performed.

In a trial of labour the aim is to determine what the woman can accomplish, not how much she can endure. As operative delivery is likely, an intravenous infusion should be established and no food permitted by mouth. The progress of the labour is monitored using the partogram, particular attention being paid to the speed of the descent of the fetal head and the dilatation of the cervix. A vaginal examination is made when the membranes rupture, to exclude cord prolapse. Special attention is paid to the woman's response to the trial. The trial should be abandoned if:

- There is no increase in cervical dilatation over a period of 4 hours (or 2 hours after rupture of the membranes) in spite of strong uterine contractions.
- Fetal distress develops.
- Full dilatation of the cervix is not achieved within 12 hours of labour.

Abnormalities of uterine action

Labour will only progress normally if the contractile wave is propagated over the entire uterus in a triple descending gradient of activity (see page 66).

If the normal pattern of uterine activity fails to occur, the progress of labour will be abnormal, usually prolonged. Until the 1940s, prolonged labour was considered to be caused by 'uterine inertia'. Research since then shows that several patterns of uterine activity may lead to delay in the birth of the child. The patterns are designated inefficient uterine activity and are divided into subgroups of abnormal uterine activity (*Fig. 23.2*). In some cases of labour the reverse occurs and the uterus is overactive, leading to a precipitate birth.

Changes in the management of labour in recent years, with the increasing use of epidural anaesthesia and of caesarean section, have rendered the description of the patterns of uterine activity less useful. They are worth recording, however, as they form the physiological basis of the modern classification.

INEFFICIENT UTERINE ACTIVITY

The two main types of inefficient uterine activity are:
- Hypoactive uterine activity.
- Hyperactive incoordinate activity, which includes incoordinate uterine activity, 'colicky' uterus and constriction ring dystocia.

It is difficult to determine exactly how often labour is complicated by inefficient uterine activity, but the most reliable estimates suggest that this condition is predominantly found among primigravidae, affecting 4–6% of such labours; and about 1% of all labours.

Aetiology

The aetiology of inefficient uterine action is not clear. In some cases cephalopelvic disproportion is present; in others, psychological factors are postulated as uterine dysfunction is predominantly a disorder of primigravid labours which is not repeated in a subsequent labour.

TYPES OF ABNORMAL UTERINE ACTION

Hypoactive states (uterine inertia)

The uterine resting tone is low and the intensity of the contraction is reduced, with the result that only a feeble contractile wave is propagated (*Fig. 23.3*). The contractions occur at longer intervals than usual and do not cause the patient much distress.

Hyperactive incoordinate states (incoordinate uterine action)

In normal labour the perception of pain is usually only reached when the uterine tone exceeds 25 torr. In hyperactive, incoordinate uterine activity the resting uterine tone is increased; in consequence the pain threshold is reached

---

Fig. 23.2 *Classification of abnormal uterine activity*
Inefficient uterine activity
Hypoactive states
Hyperactive, incoordinate states
Hyperactive lower uterine segment
Colicky uterus
Constriction ring dystocia
Cervical dystocia
Over-efficient uterine activity
Precipitate labour
Tetanic uterine activity

earlier during the contraction and the pain persists for longer (*Fig. 23.4*). In spite of the strong contractions, cervical dilatation is slow, because the triple gradient is reversed (*Fig. 23.5*).

If the patient has not been given an epidural anaesthetic, she will complain of severe backache, which increases during each contraction when the pain radiates into her lower abdomen.

Two variations of hyperactive uterine activity may occur. Both are uncommon today and are the result of action not being taken to relieve the problem. They are colicky uterus and constriction ring dystocia. In colicky uterus, various parts of the uterus contract independently and the pain of the contraction is generalized and severe. Constriction ring dystocia occurs when an annular spasm arises at the junction between the upper uterine segment and the lower uterine segment, usually late in the first stage of labour or early in the second stage. It may follow the injudicious use of oxytocin or intra-uterine manipulations.

THE MODERN CLASSIFICATION OF INEFFICIENT UTERINE ACTIVITY

As the clinical diagnosis of the two main types of inefficient uterine activity depends on the patient's perception of the severity of the pain, its distribution and the findings on uterine palpation, the increasing use of epidural anaesthesia has limited the value of the classification.

With the introduction of the partogram, a different classification has been developed (*Fig. 23.6*).

- *Prolonged latent (quiet) phase*. The duration of the latent phase of labour is increased. In most cases the pattern of uterine activity shows hypoactivity.
- *Prolonged active phase*. This can be equated to the hyperactive incoordinate state of uterine activity, usually involving a hyperactive uterine lower segment (ie a reverse gradient of uterine activity).
- *Secondary arrest of cervical dilatation*. This pattern can be equated to incoordinate uterine activity or to the end result of obstruction to the birth in a primigravida.

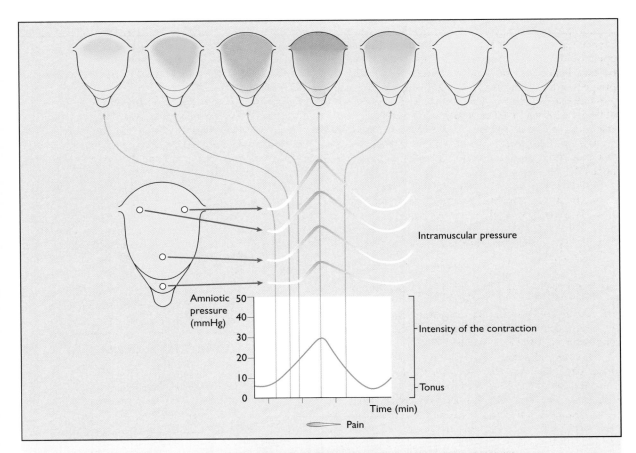

Fig. 23.3 *Hypoactive uterus. Note that the intensity of the contraction is diminished and the tone lowered slightly.*

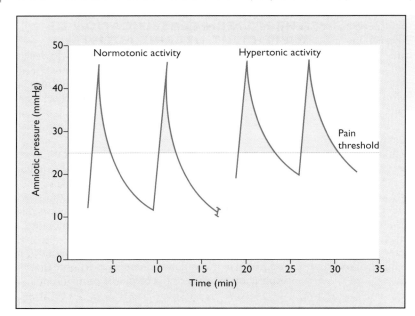

Fig. 23.4 Pain in incoordinate uterine action. Because the resting tone is raised, the pain threshold is reached earlier in the contraction, and remains above the threshold for longer.

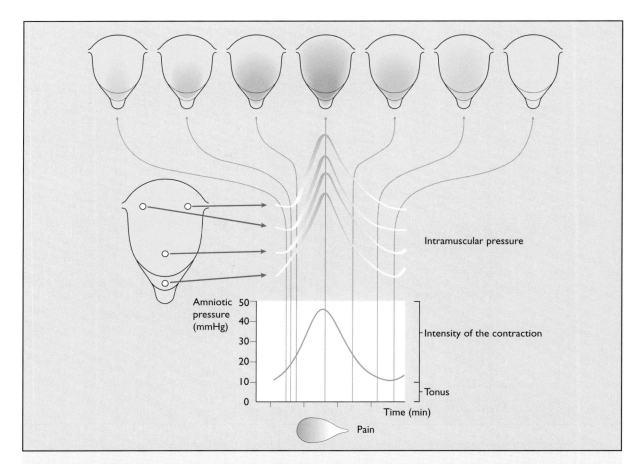

Fig. 23.5 Hyperactive lower uterine segment, with reversal of the normal gradients of activity. In this case the uterine tone is still normal but the cervix fails to dilate.

MANAGEMENT OF INEFFICIENT UTERINE ACTIVITY

Before any specific treatment is considered the course of the labour so far must be reviewed by scrutinizing the partogram, to identify, if possible, the abnormality of uterine action. The physical and psychological condition of the patient must be assessed. Dehydration and ketoacidosis should be sought and if present corrected by infusing 500ml of Hartmann's solution rapidly. After this, Hartmann's solution is alternated with 5% glucose infused at a rate of 50–100ml/h. Fluids by mouth are avoided.

Specific treatment
Prolonged latent phase

Having established that there is no major degree of CPD and that the woman is prepared to continue with the labour, two approaches are possible. In the first, no treatment beyond reassurance is given and the onset of the active phase is awaited. The alternative is to rupture the membranes and to set up a dilute oxytocin infusion which is increased incrementally (see page 194). Abdominal palpation and a vaginal examination are made at 2-hourly intervals. There are no reliable data to show that the invasive approach shortens the duration of labour significantly.

Prolonged active phase

If CPD is excluded and the woman's condition is good, the membranes are deliberately ruptured, if they are still intact, and a dilute oxytocin infusion is set up, the rate of which is increased incrementally. Progress of labour is monitored as in the management of the prolonged latent phase. Failure of the cervix to dilate by more than 2cm over a 4-hour period may be an indication for caesarean section.

Secondary arrest of the active stage

In this pattern of uterine activity it is essential to exclude CPD. If the woman does not have an epidural anaesthetic, this should be established and a dilute oxytocin infusion set up. (If it is not possible to provide epidural anaesthesia, an alternative is to sedate the woman with an intravenous infusion containing pethidine 300mg and diazepam 10mg in normal saline. The rate of the infusion is adjusted so that the woman sleeps between uterine contractions.) Monitoring the progress of labour is essential, and preparations for caesarean section are made if the cervix has not dilated by more than 2cm over a 4-hour period.

OUTCOME OF LABOUR

The outcome of labour treated in the above way has been reported in several studies of which a representative is shown in *Figure 23.7*. Since the date of that study the

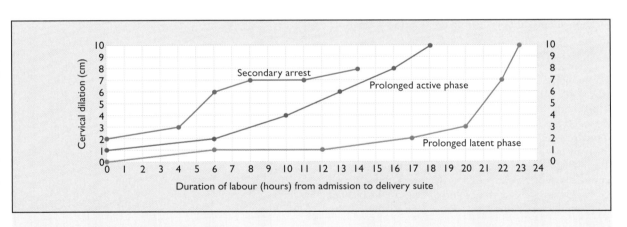

Fig. 23.6 Abnormal patterns of cervical dilatation.

Fig. 23.7 Classification of abnormal uterine activity and method of delivery in 684 British primigravidae

Pattern	All cases (%)	Outcome (%)		
		Spontaneous	Forceps	Caesarean
Normal pattern	65–70	80	18	2
Prolonged latent phase	2–5	75	10	15
Prolonged active phase	20–30	55	30	15
Secondary arrest	5–10	40	35	25

proportion of women delivered by caesarean section has increased but this has not led to a reduction in the perinatal mortality or morbidity, which is low.

Uterine over-efficiency

PRECIPITATE LABOUR

The birth occurs within 2 hours of the contractions starting. The contractions are intense and frequent. The problems are that the baby may be born in an inappropriate place without adequate care; may be anoxic *in utero* because of the frequent, intense contractions; may suffer intracranial haemorrhage during its rapid descent through the birth canal; or may be injured by falling on the floor.

Management

If the baby has been born before the arrival of a medical attendant, mother and baby should be examined for any injury.

Since precipitate birth tends to recur, in her next pregnancy consideration should be given to admitting the mother to hospital just before the estimated date of birth and inducing labour by artificial rupture of the membranes when the cervix is favourable.

TETANIC UTERINE ACTIVITY

This follows the uncontrolled use of oxytocin. The treatment consists of stopping the oxytocin infusion. This complication should not occur in today's obstetric practice.

Shoulder girdle dystocia

Occasionally, following a trial of labour or when a large baby was not diagnosed before labour, the fetal head may be born but the shoulders cannot be delivered. The delay occurs because the bis-achromial diameter of the fetus fails to rotate to enter the transverse diameter of the pelvic brim. The baby must be delivered quickly or it will die (*Fig. 23.8*). Shoulder girdle dystocia occurs rarely and the delivery requires considerable experience: damage to the lower genital tract is a usual occurrence and damage to the baby not uncommon. Most often the damage is to the brachial plexus, or a fractured clavicle or humerus occurs.

Prolonged labour

By convention, a labour which has lasted more than 12 hours after the woman has been admitted to hospital in labour, is considered to be prolonged. Between 5 and 8% of labours are classified as prolonged; and the incidence is twice as common among primigravidae than among multigravidae. Cepholopelvic disproportion and inefficient uterine action are the usual causes of prolonged labour, but in a few cases no cause can be identified.

Forty years ago, labour was defined as being prolonged if it had lasted for more than 48 hours. Labours of this length were associated with increased maternal morbidity.

During these labours dehydration often occurred, infection was not uncommon and the risk of postpartum haemorrhage was increased. These problems should not arise in the developed countries today, but they still occur in some developing countries. Perinatal morbidity and mortality also increase in prolonged labour. The main causes are pneumonia following intra-uterine infection, increased fetal acidaemia, and trauma from an operative delivery.

Earlier intervention has reduced or eliminated these problems, but care must be taken to monitor women in labour to ensure they do not become dehydrated, ketoacidotic or infected. If the woman is anxious and distressed this should be attended to by reassurance and explanation of the progress of the labour.

Fig. 23.8 Shoulder girdle dystocia. (a) The anterior shoulder is brought into the pelvis by backward traction; (b) the posterior shoulder is brought lower in the pelvis by anterior traction.

Psychological effects of dystocia and prolonged labour

The memory of a difficult labour, attended by unsympathetic, uncommunicative medical personnel and terminated by an operative delivery, may leave a scar on the woman's mind deeper than the scar on her abdomen or perineum.

The woman and her partner need explanation and reassurance. Most couples are anxious to know if the next childbirth will be as difficult and painful as the last one. As inefficient uterine action is the only identified cause in many cases of prolonged labour, and as this is less likely to occur in a subsequent labour, the woman can be given some reassurance. When she becomes pregnant again, the doctor or nurse responsible for her antenatal care needs to listen to her concerns, to reduce her anxieties and to communicate with her, so that she reaches labour in a positive frame of mind. The use of adequate anaesthesia should be discussed and the patient given the choice of having an epidural anaesthetic if she so wishes.

Obstructed labour

Obstructed labour is the end result of a poorly managed or neglected labour, in which CPD or a shoulder presentation has not been detected early and timely intervention effected.

During an obstructed labour, uterine contractions attempt to overcome the obstruction. In a first labour, the uterus contracts strongly for a while and then, failing to overcome the obstruction, becomes hypoactive, developing secondary arrest. In contrast, if the obstruction occurs in a subsequent labour, the uterus continues to contract strongly in an attempt to push the fetus through the maternal pelvis.

With each contraction there is some myometrial shortening (retraction), the upper uterine segment becoming progressively thicker and shorter, and the lower segment of the uterus becoming progressively stretched and thinner. The junction between the two segments becomes obvious, forming a pathological retraction ring – Bandl's ring (Fig. 23.9). The pathological retraction ring may be confused with a distended urinary bladder, but the oblique line is diagnostic. The patient becomes dehydrated, with a coated tongue and dry lips. She has tachycardia and concentrated urine. She faces the risk of ruptured uterus at any time.

Treatment is urgent. The dehydration should be corrected rapidly and a caesarean section performed under antibiotic cover as soon as possible, even if the fetus is dead.

Rupture of the uterus

The end result of obstructed labour, unless intervention is made, is rupture of the uterus. Rupture may also occur in late pregnancy when it may follow trauma to the uterus, or derive from a caesarean scar. In labour, as well as following an obstructed labour (Fig. 23.10), rupture of the uterus may be caused by the inappropriate use of oxytocics and the dehiscence of a caesarean section scar.

In modern obstetric practice, the most common cause of uterine rupture is caesarean scar. Three per cent of classic scars rupture, most of them during labour, which is the reason for performing an elective caesarean section on a woman who has a classic caesarean scar. Rupture of a lower segment caesarean scar is less common, 0.25% rupturing, mostly during labour.

In cases of uterine rupture following trauma or obstructed labour, the rupture usually involves one or other lateral wall and extends into the upper uterine segment (Fig. 23.11).

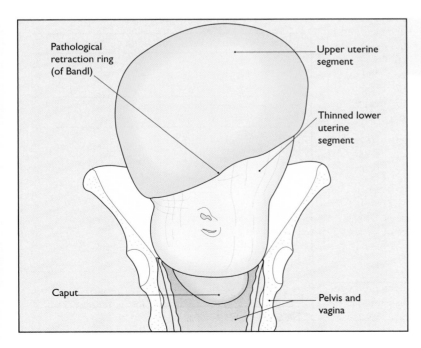

Fig. 23.9 Threatened rupture of the uterus in a case of cephalopelvic disproportion and obstructed labour.

Pathological retraction ring (of Bandl)

Upper uterine segment

Thinned lower uterine segment

Caput

Pelvis and vagina

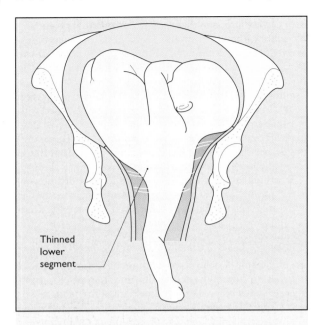

Fig. 23.10 Threatened rupture of the uterus in a neglected shoulder presentation.

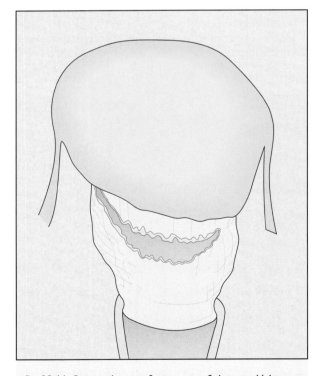

Fig. 23.11 Ruptured uterus, from a case of obstructed labour.

Rupture of a lower segment caesarean scar is usually quiet. Slight vaginal bleeding may occur and the patient complains of pain which becomes constant. The patient's pulse begins to rise and shock supervenes in some cases. In some patients no symptoms or signs occur and the ruptured uterus is only detected by routine intra-uterine palpation following the birth.

TREATMENT
Rupture following obstructed labour or trauma generally requires hysterectomy, although, in a few cases, the uterine tear can be sutured. Rupture of a caesarean scar generally can be sutured.

Classification of pelvic abnormalities

In the developed nations of the world, contracted pelvis has diminished as a cause of dystocia. However, among the less privileged groups in the rich nations and among the urban poor in the developing nations, contracted pelvis still occurs and may lead to a difficult labour. Of the many classifications of pelvic abnormalities available, that suggested by Baird is one of the most helpful. Studies by his group in Aberdeen found that nutritional influences in infancy and childhood were the major factors in causing minor alterations from the normal, whilst gross alterations were due to disease or injury. The classification is based on brim size and shape, as it has been found that midpelvic or outlet contraction is rare if the brim shape and size are normal (*Fig. 23.12*). There is one

Fig. 23.12 Pelvic classification (after Baird)
Pelves with normal shape and bone development
(Measurements usually normal, may be small)
Round ('gynaecoid')
Long oval ('anthropoid')
Pelves with abnormality of shape and bone development
(Measurements usually decreased)
Defects of nutrition and environment
Minor defects: Triangular brim ('android')
Flat brim ('platypelloid')
Major defects: Rachitic
Osteomalacic
Disease or injury
Spinal (kyphosis, scoliosis, spondylolisthesis)
Pelvic (tumours, fractures, caries)
Limbs (poliomyelitis in childhood, congenital
dislocation of the hip)
Congenital malformations
Naegele's pelvis and Robert's pelvis
High assimilation pelvis
Midpelvic contraction

exception to this: tall, thin girls, whose growth has spurted during puberty, may have midpelvic narrowing with no brim contraction.

PELVES WITH NORMAL SHAPE AND BONE DEVELOPMENT

The *round* brim is obstetrically ideal (*Fig. 23.13*) and in the developed countries is found in 70% of women whose

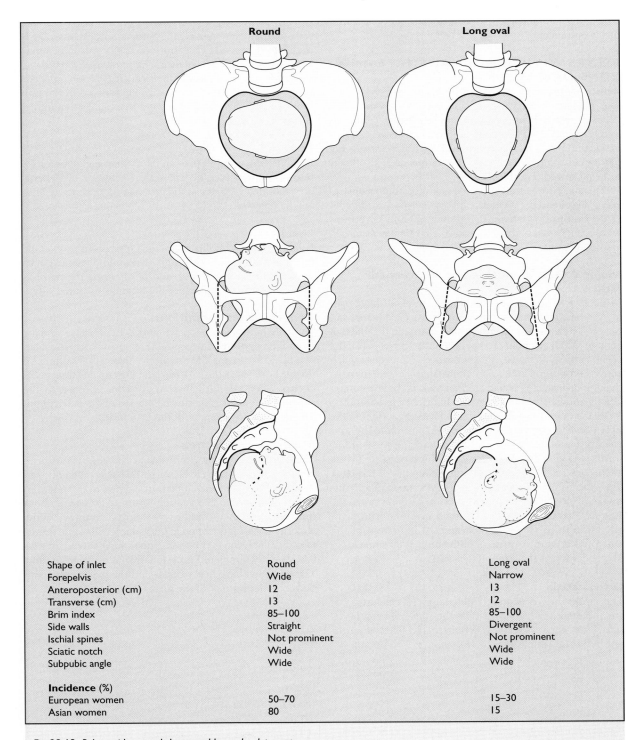

	Round	Long oval
Shape of inlet	Round	Long oval
Forepelvis	Wide	Narrow
Anteroposterior (cm)	12	13
Transverse (cm)	13	12
Brim index	85–100	85–100
Side walls	Straight	Divergent
Ischial spines	Not prominent	Not prominent
Sciatic notch	Wide	Wide
Subpubic angle	Wide	Wide
Incidence (%)		
European women	50–70	15–30
Asian women	80	15

Fig. 23.13 Pelves with normal shape and bone development.

height exceeds 163cm, dropping to 55% in women less than 153cm tall. The factor of height does not apply in Asian countries, where the overall incidence of the round pelvis is more than 80%.

The *long oval* brim (see *Fig. 23.13*) is relatively uncommon and is found in about 15% of women; in Asia the incidence is smaller.

PELVES WITH ABNORMAL SHAPE AND BONE DEVELOPMENT
Minor defects of nutrition or environment

The *triangular* brim, with some degree of funnelling of the pelvis, is relatively uncommon, and in a British study was found in only 2% of women. It appears to have a higher incidence among women from southern Europe, but is not particularly common in Asia. The midpelvis is also likely to be narrowed (*Fig. 23.14*).

The *flat* brim is the commonest minor abnormality of pelvic shape and the incidence increases from less than 5% in tall European women to more than 30% in Europeans whose height is less than 150cm. It is even more common among Africans.

Major defects of nutrition or environment
Rickets

In the past 40 years most developed countries have paid increasing attention to social and preventive medicine, and rickets – a disease of poor nutrition, particularly a lack of vitamin D and calcium – has largely disappeared. Since the developing countries have an abundance of sunshine (which converts ergosterol in the skin into vitamin D) and, in most, the drinking water is rich in calcium, rickets is not common among children, although protein deficiency is common.

In a young child suffering from rickets the weight of the upper body presses down through the spine on to the softened pelvic bones. The sacral promontory is pushed forwards and downwards, whilst the sacrum itself pivots backwards. At the same time, the ligaments of the back draw the spinous process medially and the ilia flare outwards, as do the ischial tuberosities. In extreme cases, the softened acetabulae may be forced inwards. The main alteration in pelvic shape is a marked reduction of the anteroposterior measurement of the brim, with some irregular widening of the cavity (*Fig. 23.15*).

Osteomalacia

This is due to an acquired deficiency of calcium and, encountered in adult life, causes the same deformities as rickets but is rare, except in certain inland parts of northern India and China (*Fig. 23.16*).

Disease or injury
Spinal

Kyphosis of the lower dorsal or lumbar region that started in childhood, may alter the shape of the brim of the pelvis, as the weight of the body pushes the upper part of the sacrum backwards and the lower part forwards. The side walls of the pelvis converge forming a funnel. In scoliosis the altered pressure distribution on the soft bones may cause bays on each side of the sacral promontory, rendering the shape of the brim asymmetrical (*Fig. 23.17*). Spondylolisthesis, which means the slipping forward of the fifth lumbar vertebra to project beyond the sacral promontory, is rare (*Fig. 23.18*).

Pelvic

Osteomata may develop, or an injury may lead to excessive bone formation over the site of the fracture. If all patients are examined vaginally at the first visit these abnormalities will be detected.

Limbs

Poliomyelitis in childhood, or congenital dislocation of the hip, may cause pelvic deformity. The child puts most of its weight on the stronger leg, and on this side the pelvis is pressed in, with flattening of the brim on the same side.

Congenital malformations

These include Naegele's pelvis and Robert's pelvis and are due to the defective development of one or both sacral lateral masses, causing the sacrum to fuse with the ilium on one or both sides (*Fig. 23.19*). The *high assimilation pelvis* occurs when the fifth lumbar vertebra is fused to the sacrum, thus increasing the inclination of the pelvic brim. This hinders engagement of the fetal head.

Midpelvic contraction

The incidence of this condition in the absence of brim abnormality is difficult to estimate. As has been mentioned the condition is found in certain women over 163cm in height, who have had a sudden 'spurt' of growth at about the time of puberty. Another type of woman in whom the abnormality is found, often in association with some degree of triangular brim, is the short, squat, hirsute woman who is frequently obese and occasionally has reduced fertility. These women have heavy bones and the pelvic cavity and outlet resembles that of the male.

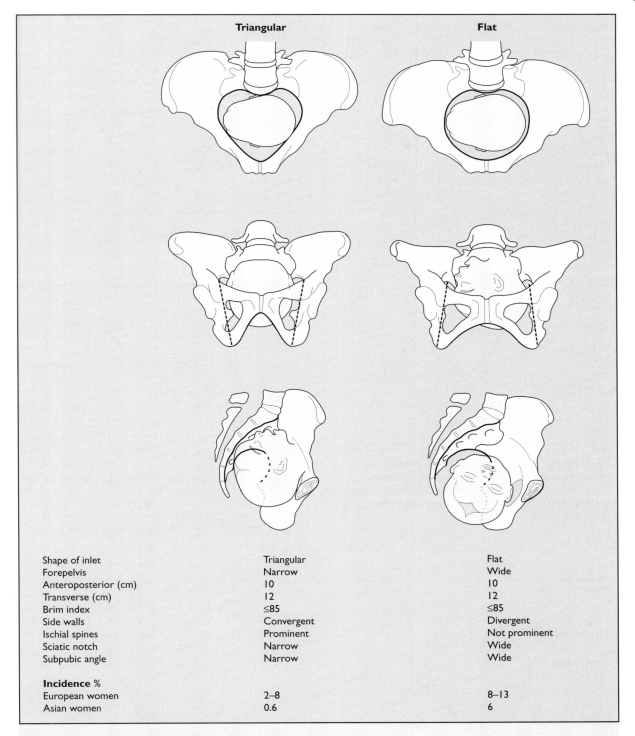

	Triangular	Flat
Shape of inlet	Triangular	Flat
Forepelvis	Narrow	Wide
Anteroposterior (cm)	10	10
Transverse (cm)	12	12
Brim index	≤85	≤85
Side walls	Convergent	Divergent
Ischial spines	Prominent	Not prominent
Sciatic notch	Narrow	Wide
Subpubic angle	Narrow	Wide
Incidence %		
European women	2–8	8–13
Asian women	0.6	6

Fig. 23.14 Pelves with abnormal shape and bone development.

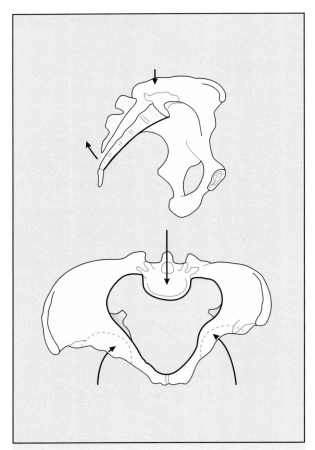

Fig. 23.15 The rachitic pelvis. Tracing from a radiograph showing the anteroposterior diameter of 8cm, the widest transverse diameter of 11.7cm and a brim index of 69. The arrows show how pressure on the softened bones alters the shape of the pelvis.

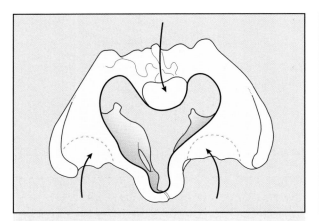

Fig. 23.16 Osteomalacic pelvis. The arrows show how pressure deforms the softened bones.

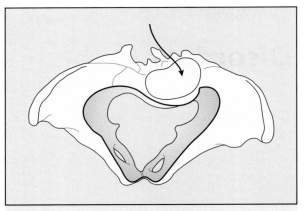

Fig. 23.17 Scoliosis and kyphosis.

Fig. 23.18 Spondylolisthesis; tracing from the radiograph showing the subluxation of the fifth lumbar vertebra upon the sacrum. The diagnosis can only be made by radiography.

Fig. 23.19 Naegele's pelvis. Note the absence of the sacral ala.

CHAPTER 24

Disorders in the puerperium

During the puerperium four main problems may arise. These are:
- Postpartum haemorrhage.
- Puerperal infection.
- Thromboembolism.
- Postpartum depression.

Postpartum haemorrhage

Primary postpartum haemorrhage is a blood loss per vaginum of more than 500ml in the first 24 hours after birth. Secondary postpartum haemorrhage is defined as abnormal bleeding from 24 hours after birth until 6 weeks postpartum.

PRIMARY POSTPARTUM HAEMORRHAGE (PPH)

Better obstetric care and the appropriate use of oxytocic drugs after birth has reduced the incidence and the severity of PPH to less than 4%.

Aetiology

In normal labour following the birth of the baby, a blood loss of 200–600ml of blood occurs before myometrial retraction supplemented by strong uterine contractions. This causes shortening and kinking of the uterine blood vessels and a retraction of the placental bed. These changes prevent further blood loss (*Fig. 24.1*). Some discussion arises as to whether this traditional quantity of blood loss is an underestimate, when blood loss is measured accurately. Provided the blood loss is less than 800ml, the woman should have no problems.

If the uterus does not contract effectively (atonic uterus) or if placental remnants prevent good placental site retraction, haemorrhage may occur ('an empty contracted uterus does not bleed!'). These two causes account for 80% of cases of PPH.

In 20% of cases the cause is a laceration of the genital tract, usually of the vagina or cervix, but rarely following uterine rupture (see page 181). In a few instances PPH follows a blood coagulation defect, such as may occur following abruptio placentae.

PPH is more likely to occur following a prolonged labour; overdistension of the uterus (multiple pregnancy or polyhydramnios); antepartum haemorrhage; and deep general anaesthesia. In these cases action is taken to prevent PPH; either prophylactic oxytocics are given following the birth or, if the third stage is managed traditionally, 'fundal fiddling' is avoided. If an oxytocic is not routinely administered, the PPH rate is quadrupled to 16%.

Diagnosis

The diagnosis is usually obvious, excessive blood loss occurring before the placenta has been delivered (third stage bleeding), or following its expulsion. After the delivery of the placenta, blood may clot inside the uterus and not be expelled causing the fundus to rise in the abdomen and, if a contraction is rubbed up, the uterus contracts and blood clots are expelled. The bleeding tends to be intermittent, as the uterus contracts periodically.

Fig. 24.1 'Living tourniquet' of contracted uterine muscle. (a) Uterine muscle fibres relaxed. (b) Contraction of muscle fibres restrict blood flow through the uterine vessels.

Management

PPH must be dealt with expeditiously, as it is a cause of maternal death. The management differs depending on whether the placenta is still in the uterus or if it has been expelled.

Third stage bleeding (placenta in the uterus)

Two stages are involved:

- A contraction is rubbed up and fundal pressure combined with controlled cord traction is generated with the aim of delivering the placenta. If bleeding continues in spite of a contracted uterus, the lower vaginal tract should be inspected to see if there is any damage.
- If the placenta cannot be delivered or if, when it is delivered, inspection shows that it is incomplete, the uterine cavity must be explored. Unless the patient already has an epidural anaesthetic, a general anaesthetic is given and manual removal of the placenta is effected by inserting a gloved hand into the uterine cavity and controlling its actions with the other hand placed on the fundus (*Fig. 24.2*). The umbilical cord is followed to its insertion and the lower placental edge is identified. With the palm of the intra-uterine hand facing the uterine cavity, the doctor separates the placenta from its attachments with a sawing motion. When the placenta has been completely detached, the remainder of the uterine cavity is explored for further placental remnants and damage. This completed, the placenta is grasped by the hand in the uterus and the membranes are pulled out of the birth canal, whilst the external hand massages the fundus. The placenta is inspected carefully to ensure that it is complete. Ergometrine 0.5mg is then injected intravenously and 0.5mg is given intramuscularly.

True postpartum haemorrhage (placenta expelled)

Several stages are involved:

- Check the placenta to determine if it is complete.
- Massage the uterus with a slow, rotary movement.
- Set up an infusion of Hartmann's solution and give 0.25mg of ergometrine intravenously or Syntocin by continuous infusion (10IU in 500ml Hartmann's solution). Alternatives are syntometrine or misoprostol 600μg. As syntometrine is contraindicated if the mother has hypertension, misoprostol may be preferred. In cases of severe PPH (a loss estimated at over 1000ml) due to a hypotonic uterus, an intramuscular or intramyometrial injection of carboprost (15-methyl-PGF$_{2\alpha}$) 25mg repeated after 5 minutes if there is no response.
- If the blood loss is more than 1000ml, a blood transfusion may be needed.
- Check blood samples for coagulation defects and, if present, treat.
- If bleeding continues in spite of firm uterine contractions induced by the oxytocics mentioned, inspect the genital tract for lacerations.
- If bleeding persists, try bimanual compression of the uterus (*Fig. 24.3*). This is painful to the patient and tiring to the obstetrician.
- If bleeding persists, internal iliac artery ligation or hysterectomy may have to be performed.

Fig. 24.2 Manual removal of the placenta.

Fig. 24.3 Bimanual compression of the uterus.

SECONDARY POSTPARTUM HAEMORRHAGE

The most common causes of secondary postpartum haemorrhage are:

- Poor epithelialization of the placental site (80% of cases).
- A retained placental fragment and/or blood clots.

An ultrasound scan of the uterus will identify placental tissue or clots. The uterus may be bulky and tender and the cervix open. The initial treatment is to give ergometrine 0.5mg intramuscularly, repeated if needed; and antibiotics are given to control any infection present. Curettage is only needed if placental tissue or clots are found in the uterus by ultrasound scanning or if bleeding persists in spite of the oxytocics.

Puerperal infection

Puerperal infection (puerperal pyrexia) is defined as a rise in temperature to 38°C or over, maintained for 24 hours or recurring during the period from the end of the 1st to the end of the 10th day after childbirth or abortion. In recent years, because of better obstetric care, better hygiene and better control of infection within the hospital, the incidence of puerperal pyrexia has fallen to 1–3% of all births or abortions.

The infection may be genital or non-genital. The main causes and the probable infecting agent are shown in *Figure 24.4*.

SITE AND SPREAD OF THE INFECTION

Most cases of puerperal infection arising in the genital tract are ascending infections from the vagina or cervix which infect the placental bed. Spread from here is either into the parametrium or, via the uterine cavity, to the Fallopian tubes and, in some cases, onwards to cause pelvic peritonitis.

The severity of the infection depends on the virulence of the infective agent and the patient's immune response.

DIAGNOSIS

Any woman who develops puerperal pyrexia should be investigated and may require to be isolated. The breasts are examined for signs of mastitis and a midstream urine specimen is examined to exclude urinary tract infection. An abdominal examination may reveal a tender, bulky uterus. The lower genital tract is inspected for infected lacerations, tears or episiotomy wound. A high vaginal swab is made for bacteriological examination, and the lochia smelt for an offensive odour.

TREATMENT

Treatment consists of giving broad spectrum antibiotics appropriate for the infecting agent and metronidazole for 5 days. As the preferred antibiotic depends on the institution and on local knowledge, the hospital infection disease control officer should be consulted, whether the woman is in hospital or is being treated by her general practitioner at home.

Thromboembolism

Thrombosis of a vein may occur in pregnancy (see page 130) or, more commonly, in the puerperium, usually between day 5 and 15 of the puerperium. With better obstetric care and early ambulation, fewer women nowadays develop thromboembolic disorders in the puerperium. The incidence is less than 1 per 1000 births. The condition is more likely to occur among women who are overweight or over the age of 35 years or who have had a caesarean section.

The thrombotic process usually starts in the deep veins of the lower leg but may extend into the femoral or pelvic

Fig. 24.4 The main bacterial causes of infection in the puerperium	
Genital infection	**Proportion (%)**
Potential pathogens which normally inhabit the vagina:	
Anaerobic streptococci	65–85
Anaerobic Gram-negative bacilli	5
Haemolytic streptococci (other than group A)	1
Bacteria introduced from adjacent viscera:	
E. coli	5–15
Cl. welchii	Rare
Bacteria introduced from distant organs or from outside:	
Staphylococci	5–15
Streptococcus haemolyticus (group A)	3
Mycoplasma hominis	Rare
Non-genital infection	
Urinary tract infection:	
E. coli	
Breast infection:	
Staphylococci (mainly from the baby)	

veins before being detected, or may arise *de novo* in the pelvic veins. If these veins are involved, pulmonary embolism may occur. Pulmonary embolism affects one puerperal woman in 6000 births in most developed Western nations, and one affected woman in five dies.

DIAGNOSIS OF DEEP VEIN THROMBOSIS (DVT)

The clinical signs are the presence of a low-grade pyrexia, a raised pulse rate and a feeling of uneasiness. The clinical signs are a poor guide to the diagnosis of DVT and do not give any indication whether the thrombus is stationary, lysing or progressing. If the calf muscles are examined and are found to be tender and painful on firm palpation, DVT may be suspected. The diagnosis should be confirmed by compression ultrasound scanning, preferably using colour-enhanced Doppler imaging, in which the tibial and femoral veins are imaged in longitudinal and lateral planes and the lumen of each vein is inspected.

DIAGNOSIS OF PULMONARY EMBOLISM

The woman complains of dyspnoea and, later, pleural pain. Cyanosis may develop. Examination of the chest may reveal a friction rub. A lung scan will confirm the clinical diagnosis. It should be made urgently as two-thirds of the number of women dying from pulmonary embolus do so within 2–4 hours.

TREATMENT
DVT

Heparin is given by an intravenous infusion pump (20,000U in 500ml normal saline at 25ml/h). This provides 25,000U per day. The rate is adjusted to provide a blood heparin concentration of 0.6–1.0U/ml, as assessed by the active partial thromboplastin time (APTT). Heparin is continued for 5 days. Warfarin is started at the same time as the heparin, which is continued until warfarin has prolonged the prothrombin time (international normalized ratio) to 2.5–3.5. Warfarin is continued for 6–12 weeks in cases of proven DVT and for 12–24 weeks in cases of pulmonary embolism.

The patient remains in bed with her leg elevated until fully heparinized and until the limb ceases to be tender. She may then walk about but should wear a properly fitted elastic stocking.

Pulmonary embolism

A bolus of heparin 25,000U is given intravenously and followed by an infusion as in the treatment of DVT. The idea of the heparin bolus is to reverse the bronchoconstriction and vasoconstriction which follows the release of serotonin from platelets. An alternative is to give streptokinase. Pulmonary embolism is so serious that expert help should be obtained.

LONG-TERM CONSQUENCES OF DVT

The long-term follow-up of women who have DVT in pregnancy or the puerperium, which is adequately treated, shows that, after a median time of 10 years, only 25% of the women are without symptoms of deep vein insufficiency. Half of the women have a swollen leg, 40% have leg cramps, 25% leg discoloration and 4% leg ulceration.

Postpartum psychiatric problems

Three psychiatric conditions affect women after childbirth: third day blues, postpartum depression and postpartum psychosis.

THIRD DAY BLUES

Between 50 and 70% of mothers become emotionally labile and irritable, with episodes of crying, and feel miserable. The cause is not known. The symptoms start between the 3rd and 5th day after the birth of the baby. The emotional lability usually lasts for less than a week but may persist for a month. This is discussed on pages 98–99.

POSTNATAL DEPRESSION

Between 8 and 12% of women develop clinically diagnosed depression in the first 5 months after childbirth, and twice that number have psychometric evidence of depression. Women at increased risk are:

- Those who are under the age of 16 when giving birth.
- Those who have a family history or a personal history of depression.
- Those who have had depression diagnosed during the pregnancy.
- Those who lacked experience in parenting when a child or an adolescent (for example, having no siblings to care for).
- Those who had an unstable or abusive family during childhood and adolescence.
- Those who lacked positive support from husband or partner during and after pregnancy.
- Those who do not have a near relative or friend who could care for the baby from time to time.
- Possibly those who had negative experiences in their contact with health professionals during the pregnancy (for example, inadequate communication and information).
- Those who have experienced a complicated pregnancy (for example, PIH, placenta praevia, preterm birth, multiple birth).

In other words, women are more likely to develop postnatal depression if they are socially and emotionally isolated or have had recent stressful life events.

There is no persuasive information, however, that postnatal depression is related to any hormonal or biochemical change or to any nutritional deficiency.

It is likely that women who develop postnatal depression may develop problems in maternal–infant relationships and adverse effects on infant cognitive development may occur. Because of potential problems to the mother and infant, signs of postnatal depression should be sought early and help provided.

Women developing postnatal depression show the symptoms of ordinary depressive illness, although fatigue, irritability and anxiety are more common than in most clinically depressed women. Some psychiatrists recommend that all women presenting at a postnatal clinic 6–8 weeks after the birth, should be screened using the Edinburgh Postnatal Depression Scale.

Management

The woman needs support and encouragement initially, not drugs. The doctor should listen to what she is saying, help her resolve her anxieties and conflicts about her ability to be a parent and arrange for assistance in caring for the baby so that she may have 'time out'. In some cases, admission to hospital for a few days for support and group therapy may help; in others antidepressants should be prescribed. In more severe depression a psychiatric consultation should be obtained. Parents should be reassured that if the mother takes antidepressant drugs for the recommended 4 months or so, the medications will have no effect on the neurological development or intelligence of her child.

If hospital treatment is needed, admission should be to a 'Mother and Baby' unit if one is available, rather than to a psychiatric ward. It is important that the treatment is given early as women whose postnatal depression lasts for more than 4 months are more likely to have depressive episodes in a subsequent pregnancy and at other times.

POSTNATAL PSYCHOSIS

Between 1 and 3 per 1000 women develop postnatal psychosis, usually manic or depressive illness, but occasionally a schizophrenic episode. The illness starts abruptly between the 5th and 15th day of the puerperium. In the beginning, the woman is confused, anxious, perplexed, restless and sad. Delusions (that the baby has died or is deformed) or hallucinations develop rapidly and the melancholia deepens.

Management

Admission to hospital is essential, preferably with the baby so the woman's delusions may decrease. This throws a considerable strain on the staff who have to make sure that the baby will not be harmed. Psychotropic drugs are given, haloperidol being currently preferred. Most women respond well and relatively quickly. About 15% develop the illness in a subsequent pregnancy, and one woman in three develops a non-puerperal psychosis.

CHAPTER 25

Obstetric operations

Induction of labour

Induction of labour may be required to 'rescue' the fetus from a potentially hazardous intra-uterine environment in late pregnancy for a variety of reasons or because continuation of the pregnancy is dangerous to the expectant mother.

The method adopted depends on:
- The duration of the pregnancy.
- The condition of the cervix (ie favourable or unfavourable) (*Fig. 25.1*).
- The position of the fetal head in relation to the pelvis.

The highest rate of success, (ie that the induction is followed by a vaginal birth within 24 hours) occurs in a woman whose cervix is favourable and whose Bishop score is 5 or more (*Fig. 25.2*).

If the chances of success are evaluated as low, the doctor may recommend caesarean section.

TECHNIQUES OF INDUCING LABOUR

Labour may be induced by drugs or by the surgical technique of amniotomy, which is also known as artificial rupture of the membranes (ARM).

Induction of labour using drugs

Two methods are available: the use of prostaglandins and the use of oxytocin.

Prostaglandins

Four prostaglandins with different properties are available.
- PGE_1 (gemeprost, Cervigem) is available in pessary form or as an intracervical injection system. It is the preferred prostaglandin for the termination of pregnancy and for the induction of labour in the third quarter. It should be avoided in the fourth quarter of pregnancy as cases of uterine hypertonicity have been reported.
- PGE_2 is available as a gel or in pessary form and may be introduced intravaginally or intracervically. The gel appears to be more effective and is associated with a lower risk of producing uterine hypertonicity. PGE_2 softens the cervical connective tissue and relaxes cervical muscle fibres, 'ripening' the cervix. PGE_2 may stimulate the production of $PGF_{2\alpha}$, which will induce uterine contractions. PGE_2 produces cervical ripening when the cervical (Bishop) score is less than 5 and therefore amniotomy is contraindicated. PGE_2 is available in a prefilled syringe, in a dose of 1–2mg, which is introduced into the posterior vaginal fornix. The patient's pulse rate, fetal heart and uterine activity are monitored for 30 minutes after which time she may walk about if she wishes, providing that the pregnancy is not at high risk. If labour is not established within 6 hours a further dose is administered. Some obstetricians perform ARM at this time if the cervix is favourable.
- Misoprostol, a synthetic PGE_1 analogue is as effective as PGE_2 or gemeprost in inducing labour. It is stable, cheap and easily stored. It can also be used to ripen the cervix in late pregnancy. The dose of misoprostol for labour induction is 25–50µg given 3-hourly for a maximum of 8 doses. This dose is chosen to reduce the risk of excessive uterine activity.
- $PGF_{2\alpha}$ is available as a vaginal gel or as an intravenous infusion. Its main place is in the augmentation of uterine contractions.

| Soft, effacing. External os admits one finger | Soft, long, closed. Whole canal admits one finger | Firm, long, closed. External os will not admit one finger | Firm, short. External os admits one finger. Internal os rigid |

95% favourable   Efficiency rate   65% unfavourable

Fig. 25.1 The relationship between the condition of the cervix and success rate of surgical induction.

	Scoring rating			
Factor	**0**	**1**	**2**	**3**
Cervix				
Length (cm)	>4	>2	1–2	<1
Dilatation (cm)	<1	<2	2–3	>4
Consistency	Firm	'Average'	Soft	Soft
Position	Posterior	Other (mid, anterior)	Other	Other
Fetal head				
Position relative to Ischial spines (cm)	–3	–2	–1 or 0	+1 or more

Fig. 25.2 A method of cervical 'scoring' (Bishop score)

Some patients receiving prostaglandins may have side effects, mainly nausea, vomiting or diarrhoea, but these are unusual in the doses recommended.

Oxytocin (syntocinon)
Oxytocin should always be administered by intravenous infusion, preferably using an infusion pump. Used alone, 50% of women will be in labour within 12 hours. Induction is more effective if preceded by prostaglandin PGE_2 vaginal pessaries or following amniotomy.

The infusion rate is increased by 5mU per minute every 20 minutes until contractions lasting longer than 60 seconds recur at 3–5 minute intervals. The maximum concentration used is 60mU per minute. Because of the risk of water intoxication and possible neonatal jaundice, the quantity of fluid infused should not exceed 1500ml in 10 hours.

Surgical induction of labour (amniotomy)
Surgical induction of labour (amniotomy) is more effective if the cervix is favourable (Bishop score 5+). The patient is put in the dorsal or lithotomy position and the vagina swabbed with antiseptic. Two of the doctor's fingers are inserted to reach the cervix and, if practicable, one is inserted through the cervix to 'sweep' the membranes. An amnihook, or a Kocher forceps, is introduced along the intravaginal fingers and the membranes below the fetal head (the forewaters) are broken with the instrument.

The problems following amniotomy are:
* Prolapse of the umbilical cord (0.5% of cases).
* Infection, if the induction–delivery interval is more than 24 hours.
* Haemorrhage, which is usually slight.
* Postpartum haemorrhage (relative risk doubled compared with no induction of labour).

* Neonatal hyperbilirubinaemia (bilirubin greater than 250μmol/L), which appears to be related to the maximum dose and duration of an oxytocin infusion following amniotomy.

A suggested schema (flow chart) for the induction of labour is shown in *Figure 25.3*.

As can be seen from the flow chart, if the cervix is 'unfavourable' (ie a low Bishop score), the drugs mentioned may be used to ripen the cervix so that surgical induction, if needed, will be more effective. In the flow chart PGE_2 is featured but the other prostaglandins listed above are equally effective.

Augmentation of labour

In cases where the quality of the uterine contractions is poor (see page 176), their strength may be augmented by performing ARM and if necessary by setting up an incremental oxytocic infusion, or by both methods. A few obstetricians use $PGF_{2\alpha}$ vaginal pessary form in preference to oxytocin infusion.

Instrumental delivery

In the second stage of labour situations may arise wherein it becomes necessary to deliver the baby. These indications are:
* *Delay in the birth of the baby* when the second stage of labour has exceeded 1.5 hours or the fetal head has been delayed on the perineum for mo re than 30 minutes. The delay usually occurs because:
  1. The fetal head has not rotated and is arrested in the transverse diameter of the midpelvic cavity (deep transverse arrest of the head).

2. The head has rotated into the posterior position in the midcavity or in the lower pelvic strait (posterior arrest of the head).
3. A minor degree of cephalopelvic disproportion is present.
4. The uterine contractions have become weaker.

- *The fetus shows signs of distress* (ie bradycardia or the passage of meconium).
- *The mother has become distressed*, either physically or mentally, in the second stage of labour.
- *The mother has an existing obstetric condition or a medical one* (eg pregnancy-induced hypertension, chronic hypertension, cardiac disease) which may deteriorate during the expulsive stage of labour.
- *To aid in the delivery of the aftercoming head in a breech presentation*.

METHODS AND CONDITIONS OF INSTRUMENTAL DELIVERY

The incidence of instrumental delivery varies from between 5 and 12% of all deliveries. Two methods are available. The first, delivery by obstetric forceps, was introduced 400 years ago; the second, delivery by vacuum extraction, was introduced 40 years ago. The method used depends on the hospital protocol and on the preference of the obstetrician.

The conditions for instrumental delivery are:

- The greatest diameter of the fetal head must have passed the pelvic brim.
- The cervix must be fully dilated.
- The membranes must have ruptured and the bladder must be empty.
- The patient must receive adequate anaesthesia or analgesia. Women requiring a vacuum extraction or a low forceps require a perineal nerve block at the very least. Women requiring a midforceps delivery should have an epidural block, a pudendal nerve block or a general anaesthetic.

OBSTETRIC FORCEPS

From crude beginnings the obstetric forceps has developed into a precision instrument, which must be used with great skill to avoid damage to the woman or her fetus. More than

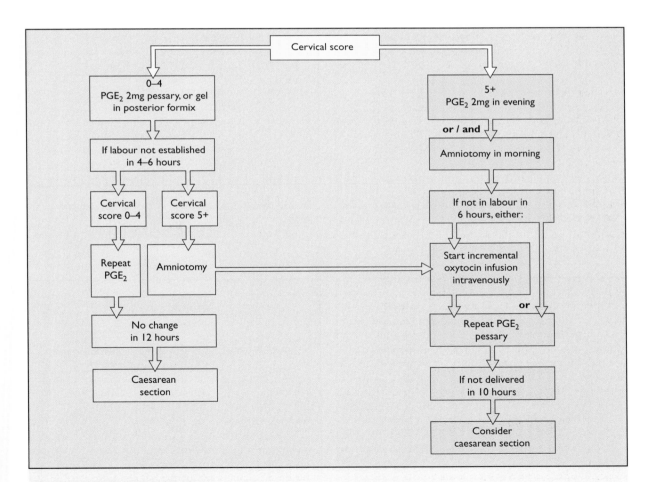

Fig. 25.3 Induction of labour flow chart.

four-fifths of forceps deliveries are by low or outlet forceps, which are relatively safe.

Types of forceps deliveries

As shown in *Figure 25.4*, the station of the fetal head is used to describe the type of forceps delivery.

- High forceps are no longer performed because of the high risk of causing serious fetal and maternal damage. Delivery should be by caesarean section.
- Midforceps. The forceps blades are applied to the sides of the fetal head, whose biparietal diameter has entered the pelvis but has not advanced much beyond the ischial spines. Usually the occiput lies in one or other transverse diameter of the maternal pelvis.
- Low forceps. The forceps blades are applied to the sides of the fetal head, whose biparietal diameter has advanced to or beyond the ischial tuberosities and has rotated so that the sagittal suture lies in the anteroposterior diameter of the maternal pelvis.
- Outlet forceps. The fetal head distends the vaginal introitus, but the perineum is holding it back.

The *short-shanked forceps* is used for low or outlet forceps procedures (see *Fig. 25.5*). The *long-shanked forceps* is used for midforceps delivery after manually rotating the fetal head if it is arrested in the transverse diameter of the pelvis (see *Fig. 25.6*) they are also suitable for low or outlet deliveries. *Kjelland's forceps* has a sliding lock and can be used to rotate the fetal head and deliver it (see *Fig. 25.7*).

All forceps compress the fetal head to some extent and apply traction to effect the birth.

Technique of forceps delivery

The technique of forceps delivery is shown in *Figures 25.8–25.16.*

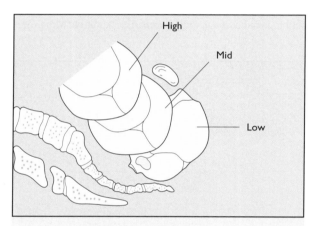

Fig. 25.4 Types of forceps deliveries – showing the station of the head when the forceps is applied.

Fig. 25.5 Wrigley's forceps (scale ×2 that of Figs. 26.5 and 26.6).

Fig. 25.6 Simpson's obstetric forceps.

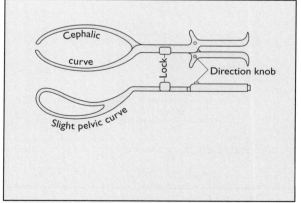

Fig. 25.7 Kjelland's forceps.

Low or outlet forceps
The use of these is described in *Figures 25.8–25.11*.

Midforceps
The technique for applying the long-shanked curved forceps is the same as that used to apply the short-shanked forceps. As the forceps blades have to be introduced further into the vagina, great care must be exercised to avoid damaging the vaginal wall and to ensure that the forceps blades are correctly applied along the sides of the fetal head.

Because the head has to be pulled through the pelvic curve, the mother should be positioned correctly, with her legs in stirrups and her buttocks projecting over the end of

Fig. 25.8 The assembled forceps are held in front of the woman's vulva, with the pelvic curve uppermost. The left blade is introduced, without force, into the vagina between the fetal head and the vaginal wall, which is protected by the doctor's fingers; the blade is steered to lie along the left side of the baby's head.

Fig. 25.9 When correctly applied the shank will press on the mother's perineum.

Fig. 25.10 The right blade is introduced in a similar manner and the two blades are assembled in the lock. If they do not fit easily into the lock, there is a malapplication and, if they cannot be made to adjust easily, the forceps is removed and the procedure is repeated.

Fig 25.11 The forceps is held as shown and the baby's head is delivered in a smooth curve using controlled traction, preferably during a uterine contraction. An episiotomy is often needed to prevent a perineal tear.

Fig. 25.12 Position of the patient for midforceps delivery.

Fig. 25.13 Direction of traction in forceps delivery. In midforceps delivery (1) the initial direction of pull is downwards, in low forceps (2) horizontal and in outlet forceps (3) slightly upwards.

Fig. 25.14 The mechanics of forceps delivery. Midforceps: with axis traction the force is resolved and the pull is in the axis of the birth canal.

the bed (see *Fig. 25.12*). This is because the pull required to deliver the baby has to be downwards initially and then curving upwards (see *Fig. 25.13*). Some obstetricians use the axis traction device but skill is required to use it properly (see *Fig. 25.14*).

If the baby's head is arrested in the transverse diameter of the midpelvis, manual rotation may be attempted (see *Fig. 25.15*) followed by midforceps delivery. Alternatively Kjelland's forceps may be used or a caesarean section performed.

Fig. 25.15 Manual rotation of the head from a left occipito-posterior position. (a) The left hand is placed on the abdomen and pulls the right shoulder of the baby towards the mother's right side. Simultaneously, the right hand, in supination, holds the head by its biparietal diameter and rotates it through 180° to a position of pronation. (b) The occiput becomes anterior at the end of the manoeuvre.

Kjelland's forceps

This instrument is used to rotate a head arrested in the transverse diameter of the midpelvis. It requires considerable skill and the woman should be delivered in an operating theatre so that, if any difficulty is experienced, a caesarean section can be done immediately.

The forceps is held in front of the woman's vulva and positioned so that the dot on the shoulders of the instrument points to the side of the pelvis where the baby's occiput lies. The remainder of the application of Kjelland's forceps is shown in *Figure 25.16*. Usually a wide episiotomy is made as perineal damage is almost inevitable. Alternative

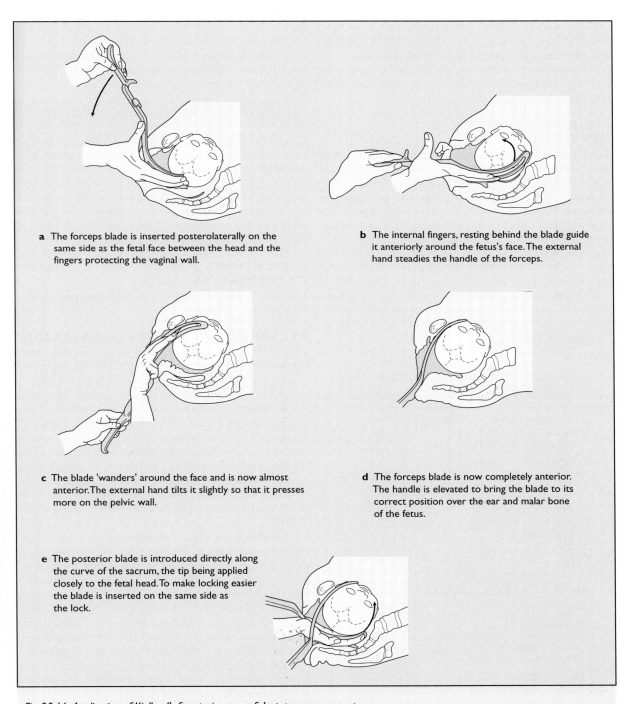

a The forceps blade is inserted posterolaterally on the same side as the fetal face between the head and the fingers protecting the vaginal wall.

b The internal fingers, resting behind the blade guide it anteriorly around the fetus's face. The external hand steadies the handle of the forceps.

c The blade 'wanders' around the face and is now almost anterior. The external hand tilts it slightly so that it presses more on the pelvic wall.

d The forceps blade is now completely anterior. The handle is elevated to bring the blade to its correct position over the ear and malar bone of the fetus.

e The posterior blade is introduced directly along the curve of the sacrum, the tip being applied closely to the fetal head. To make locking easier the blade is inserted on the same side as the lock.

Fig. 25.16 Application of Kjelland's forceps in cases of deep transverse arrest.

methods of delivery are vacuum extraction, manual rotation of the fetal head and forceps delivery, or caesarean section.

Dangers of a difficult forceps delivery

The vagina and cervix may be damaged, causing haemorrhage. Following a midforceps delivery, the entire vagina should be inspected with good illumination, and lacerations looked for and sutured.

The dangers to the fetus are trauma, compression of the brain and tentorial tearing caused by too strong compression and traction. Fracture of the fetal skull and facial paresis may occur if the forceps has been incorrectly applied and compresses the nerve as the nerve emerges in front of the mastoid process.

VACUUM EXTRACTOR OR VENTOUSE

The vacuum extractor, or ventouse, consists of a cup, either metal or plastic (the 'soft cup') which has a chain and a handle. The cup is attached to a tube which connects with the suction apparatus. The cup is positioned over the occipital region of the fetal head and is held firmly against the scalp whilst a vacuum is slowly built up. This sucks some of the scalp into the cup, forming a firm attachment. Once a vacuum of $0.8kg/cm^2$ is obtained, the perimeter of the cup is checked to ensure that no vaginal tissue is included and traction is applied by pulling the handle at right angles to the pelvic curve, concurrently with a uterine contraction. Skilled operators use the vacuum extractor to deliver the fetus, whether the head is fully rotated or has arrested in the transverse position.

The advantages of the vacuum extractor are that vaginal and perineal damage is less than that following a forceps delivery, and the patient usually needs less analgesia or anaesthesia.

The disadvantages of the vacuum extractor are that the delivery is slower, the ventouse may slip off the fetal head, the baby develops a circumscribed caput (a chignon), which usually subsides within 48 hours, and the baby may have scalp lacerations. There is also a greater chance that the baby will become jaundiced. The ventouse cannot be used to aid the delivery of the aftercoming head of a breech presentation or if the baby is preterm. Between 3 and 9% of births are effected using a vacuum extractor.

Caesarean section

Caesarean section means that the baby is removed from an intact uterus by abdominal operation. In many developed countries the caesarean section rate has risen from 5%, 30 years ago, to over 15%. The increase is due, in part to fashion, in part to fear of litigation if a perfect baby is not born and, in part to the changing pattern of conception – women are delaying the conception of their first child and are limiting the number of children they have.

INDICATIONS FOR CAESAREAN SECTION

These have broadened in recent years and are listed in *Figure 25.17*.

TECHNIQUE OF CAESAREAN SECTION

There are two types of caesarean section. In the first, a transverse incision is made through the stretched lower uterine segment. In the second – the classic section – a vertical incision is made through the myometrium. The classic section is now rarely used, except when the lower uterine segment is excessively vascular, cannot be reached because of extensive adhesions, or if the fetus presents as a transverse lie, with an impacted shoulder. Caesarean hysterectomy may be required if intractable bleeding occurs, for placenta accreta or if the uterus has ruptured.

The operative technique is shown in *Figure 25.18*. As blood loss is unpredictable, crossmatched blood should be available.

Postoperative care is no different from any other abdominal operation. Early ambulation is encouraged, especially since, in some hospitals, the neonate is kept in the nursery for 24–48 hours. Maternal morbidity varies between 3 and 12% depending on the reason for the caesarean section. Endometritis accounts for two-thirds of morbidity. For this reason, prophylactic antibiotics are routinely given during the operation. Women at higher risk of developing thromboembolism are prescribed prophylactic anticoagulants.

Caesarean section is a very safe operation, the overall mortality rate being about 0.4 per 1000 sections and 0.1 per 1000 sections performed electively.

Fig. 25.17 Indications for caesarean section

- Failure of labour to progress (dystocia)
  abnormal uterine action
  cephalopelvic disproportion
- Malpresentation or malpositions
  breech
  face and brow
  transverse lie
  occipito-posterior
  prolapse of umbilical cord
  multiple pregnancy
- Antepartum haemorrhage
  abrupto placentae
  placenta praevia
- Hypertensive disease in pregnancy
- Diabetes mellitus
- Fetal conditions
  fetal distress
  iso-immunization
  very low birth weight
- Older primigravidae
- Failed induction of labour
- Repeat caesarean section

VAGINAL BIRTH AFTER PREVIOUS CAESAREAN SECTION

When a caesarean section is performed for a non-recurrent condition, the next baby may be born vaginally or by caesarean section depending on the wishes of the woman and the advice of the obstetrician. Studies from countries outside North America show that nearly half the women who had a previous caesarean section deliver their next baby vaginally. In North America less than one-third deliver vaginally.

Fig. 25.18 The technique of caesarean section. (a) and (b) The loose peritoneum covering the lower uterine segment is divided and pushed down. (c) The exposed muscle of the lower segment is incised so that the membranes bulge into the wound. The incision may be extended with a knife, or the muscle fibres separated with the fingers. (d) The membranes are ruptured and the head delivered using a forceps blade as an inclined plane, counter pressure being exerted on the fundus. (e) The placenta has been expelled and the wound sutured in layers. Great care must be taken at the angles.

If a woman chooses a vaginal birth after a caesarean section (VBAC), the birth should take place in a well-equipped hospital staffed by experienced obstetricians. The reason for this is that the trial of vaginal delivery is terminated by caesarean section in one-fifth of all cases, 0.25% of women suffering a ruptured uterus.

If an elective caesarean section is chosen, the maturity of the fetus must be established so that the operation is performed when the gestation period is greater than 38 weeks to obtain the lowest neonatal respiratory morbidity.

Version

External cephalic version may be chosen when a fetus presenting as a breech has not turned cephalically by the 37th week of pregnancy. Before attempting the version the doctor must be sure that the pelvis has normal dimensions and that the placenta is not praevia. The mother should not have hypertension or a multiple pregnancy.

Some doctors give a tocolytic drug intravenously before the attempt, and a few perform external version with the woman anaesthetized. The version is performed gently. The breech is mobilized and the version attempted by lifting it with one hand and pushing the fetal head down with the other (Fig. 25.19). The fetal heart rate is either monitored continuously or every 2 minutes during, and for 30 minutes after, the version. If the fetal heart rate falls below 90bpm during the version, the attempt is abandoned.

Problems associated with version are uncommon. They include rupture of the membranes, cord entanglement around a limb of the fetus and the onset of premature labour.

Internal podalic version, in which the doctor's hand is introduced into the uterus to grasp a limb and pull it through a fully dilated cervix, is rarely performed today. It may find use in cases of the delayed birth of a second twin, which is lying transversely in the uterus, but caesarean section is safer in most cases.

Destructive operations on the fetus

There is very little place for these procedures in modern obstetric practice. An exception may be when a hydrocephalic fetus has died during labour. In this case the head is perforated with a perforator and the fluid allowed to drain, making the fetus easier to deliver.

Fig. 25.19 External version. The obstetrician has lifted the buttocks out of the pelvis; his right thumb controls the baby's head and the direction in which the child is moved encourages flexion.

CHAPTER 26

The epidemiology of obstetrics

The quality of obstetric care in a country can be measured by the maternal and the perinatal mortality rates. The death of a woman in pregnancy or childbirth is one of the greatest tragedies which can befall a family.

Maternal mortality

A maternal death is defined by the International Federation of Obstetricians and Gynaecologists (FIGO) as 'the death of any woman dying whilst pregnant or within one year of the termination of the pregnancy, from any cause related to or aggravated by the pregnancy or its management but not from accidental or incidental causes'. The maternal mortality rate is the number of such deaths per 100,000 maternities.

In most developed countries, the maternal death rate remained about the same from 1850 to 1934 when it began falling. In the period before the mid-1930s it was about 500 per 100,000; by the mid-1980s it had fallen, in many industrialized countries, to less than 10 per 100,000 maternities (*Fig. 26.1*). The initial fall was due to the control of infections by better obstetric care and the introduction of antibiotics. The second factor was that most women availed themselves of good-quality antenatal care, which enabled complications to be detected early and treatment to be offered, usually in well-equipped hospitals, staffed by trained medical attendants. Blood became increasingly and quickly available from blood banks, which considerably reduced the deaths due to haemorrhage. Sociological changes have also occurred in the past 60 years: fewer women now have more than 3 children, and most have their pregnancies before the age of 35. Higher parity and advancing age increase the risk of maternal death.

In the developing countries, the maternal mortality rate is much higher. In sub-Saharan Africa it averages 600 per 100,000 live births; in south Asia, 500 per 100,000 births; in southeast Asia and Latin America 300 per 100,000 live births. The reasons for these high maternal mortality rates are: frequent pregnancies, with short intervals between them; the resort to unsafe abortion performed in unhygienic surroundings; a relative lack of prenatal care and a lack of the perception of its value by poorly educated and poorly informed women; a lack of access to skilled medical help; and a lack of Government support to make changes to the status, education and empowerment of women.

CAUSES OF MATERNAL DEATH

Several developed countries publish the results of confidential enquiries into maternal deaths at intervals of about 3 years. In these reports the causes of the deaths are analysed and suggestions are made which might prevent such deaths occurring.

These reports have been published in the UK since 1952 and in Australia since 1965. In 1990, a report was published analysing all maternal deaths which had occurred in the USA between 1979 and 1986. Study of these reports shows that the main causes of maternal death are similar in the three countries. In *Figure 26.2* the most common causes of death are shown. In *Figure 26.3* the decline in the major causes of maternal death in England and Wales is shown. Maternal deaths can be reduced further, particularly those associated with anaesthesia, ectopic gestation and pulmonary embolism.

Perinatal mortality

The death of a fetus *in utero* or its death in the neonatal period causes much distress to the parents and is a measure of the quality of obstetric care.

Before perinatal mortality can be discussed, some terms need to be clarified. In 1979, the World Health Organisation (WHO) published some international definitions.

• *Live birth* is the complete expulsion or extraction from its mother of a product of conception, irrespective of the duration of the pregnancy, which, after such separation, breathes or shows any evidence of life such as beating of the heart, pulsation of the umbilical cord or definite

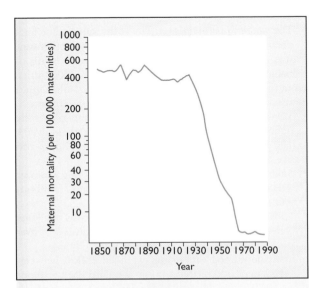

Fig. 26.1 *The secular trend of maternal mortality in Australia and the United Kingdom.*

Fig. 26.2 Most common causes of maternal deaths (Australia, England and Wales, and USA)		
Cause	Deaths (%)	Proportion avoidable (%)
Hypertensive disease of pregnancy	10–25	50
Pulmonary embolism	5–20	30
Abortion	5–10	25
Ectopic gestation	5–15	20
Haemorrhage	5–15	50
Sepsis	5–10	30
Cardiorespiratory (including anaesthetic)	5–15	30

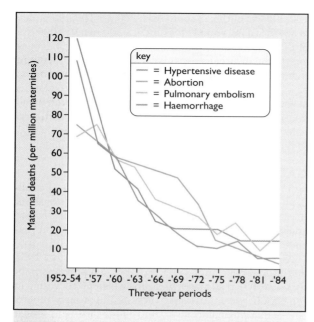

Fig. 26.3 Main causes of maternal death directly due to pregnancy or childbirth (England and Wales, 1952–84) per 1,000,000 maternities.

movement of the voluntary muscles: whether or not the umbilical cord has been cut or the placenta is attached, each product of such a birth is considered live born.

• *Fetal death* is death prior to the complete expulsion or extraction from its mother of a product of conception, irrespective of the duration of pregnancy; the death is indicated by the fact that after such separation the fetus does not breathe or show other evidence of life, such as beating of the heart, pulsation of the umbilical cord, or definite movement of voluntary muscles.

• *Early fetal deaths* equate to abortions, and *intermediate fetal deaths* are those occurring between the 22nd and 27th completed gestational weeks, the fetus weighing 500–999g (also called stillbirth).

• *Late fetal death* is fetal death at 28 completed weeks of gestation and over. The fetus usually weighs 1000g or more (also called stillbirth).

In 1975, the following definitions recommended by the WHO, were accepted by the FIGO:

• *Neonatal deaths* are deaths of live born infants occurring before 28 completed days of life. Neonatal deaths can be divided into two groups: *early neonatal* deaths and *late neonatal* deaths.

• *Early neonatal*, or *postnatal death*, is the death of a live born baby in the first 7 completed days (168 hours) of life.

• *Late neonatal death* is the death of a live born infant after 7 completed days but before 28 completed days of life.

Two definitions of perinatal mortality are therefore possible: the extended perinatal mortality rate (PMR); and the basic, or standard, PMR.

• The *extended perinatal mortality* is the sum of all fetal deaths (excluding pregnancies terminating before the 22nd week of pregnancy in which the conceptus weighed less than 500g) and all neonatal deaths per 1000 births.

• The *standard perinatal mortality* is the sum of late fetal deaths and early neonatal deaths, or, put in another way, it is the number of stillbirths and first week deaths of babies weighing 1000g or more at birth per 1000 births.

From these data mortality rates can be inferred and should be used for the purposes of international comparison.

• *Standard PMR*. The ratio of stillborn infants plus early neonatal deaths of infants weighing 1000g and over × 1000, *divided* by the total births of infants stillborn and live born weighing 1000g and over.

• *Stillbirth rate*. Stillborn infants weighing 1000g and over × 1000, *divided* by the total births of infants (stillborn and live born) weighing 1000g and over.

• *Early neonatal death rate*. Early neonatal deaths of infants weighing 1000g or more at birth × 1000, *divided* by live-born infants weighing 1000g and over.

In many developed nations the extended PMR is between 7 and 12 per 1000 births, and the standard PMR is about 9 per 1000 births. In the few developing countries which have been able to publish reasonably reliable data the standard PMR is between 35 and 55 per 1000 births.

SOCIAL FACTORS AFFECTING THE PMR

The most exact information about the effect of sociological factors on the PMR is obtained from the British Perinatal Mortality Surveys published in 1958 and 1970. All births occurring during 1 week and all singleton stillbirths and neonatal deaths over a 3-month period were surveyed. The findings were that:

- The lower the social class the higher the standard PMR, which rose from 7.5 per 1000 in social class 1 to 26.8 per 1000 in social classes IV and V.
- The mother's age affected the PMR. It was highest among the infants of mothers younger than 17 years and older than 35 years.
- Women who did not avail themselves of antenatal care had 5–10 times the mean PMR.
- The management of the labour affected the PMR. One-third of the perinatal deaths were due to intrapartum anoxia alone or associated with birth trauma. In some cases, the intrapartum anoxia was a sequel to antepartum conditions, the fetus entering labour in poor health; in other cases, mismanagement of labour or the misuse of forceps damaged the baby, which was either stillborn or died in the early neonatal period.

ANALYSIS OF PERINATAL MORTALITY

Knowledge of the precise cause of death of the fetus or neonate is not always helpful as only immediate causes of death are entered. For this reason a clinicopathological classification was devised by Professor Dugald Baird in the 1950s (Fig. 26.4). This classification is based on why the baby became ill and died rather than the pathological cause of death. It enables health professionals to identify correctable problems. An analysis based on surveys in New South Wales and Scotland, carried out in the early 1980s, is shown in Figure 26.5. The recorded standard PMR in New South Wales was 11.0 and, in Scotland 14.0. Since that date there has been a decline of perinatal mortality in both countries, but the proportionality of the causes remains the same.

REDUCTION OF PERINATAL MORTALITY

Many of the measures which have been effective in reducing maternal deaths are effective in reducing perinatal deaths. In addition, the provision of well-equipped, well-staffed neonatal intensive care units (NICUs) will enable a number of low birth weight babies to survive and grow.

Fig. 26.4 Standard perinatal mortality by clinico-pathological classification showing mothers likely to have the highest risk. (Information from Perinatal Problems, Chapter 12, by Sir Dugald Baird and A.M. Thompson; and Perinatal Mortality Committee Reports, The Women's Hospital, Crown Street, Sydney).

Causes of death	High-risk mothers
1. Unexplained, low birth weight (25–30% of all)	Low socio-economic status Reduced height In all social classes, highest in women under 17 and over 35 Para 4 or more Cigarette smoking
2. Antepartum haemorrhage (10–15% of all)	Para 4 or more Low socio-economic status

3. Fetal malformations (20–30% of all)
    a. CNS
 	
    b. Other
	
	Increase with diminishing socio-economic status; poor nutrition
	Primiparity, especially in primiparae under the age of 20
	Increase with increasing parity and age

4. Maternal disease (3–5% of all)	Increase with increasing maternal age; no effect from parity
5. Pregnancy-induced hypertension (6–10% of all)	Primiparae Women over 30 History of the condition in a previous pregnancy
6. Mechanical/trauma (3–5% of all)	Primiparity, especially if aged 30 or more Short stature Para 4 or more (inadequate obstetric care)
7. Unexplained, normal birth weight (10–20% of all)	Primiparae, especially aged 30 or more Para 4 or more Post-term (ie 42 weeks' gestation) especially in older primigravidae
8. Iso-immunization (<1% of all)	Increasing parity
9. Infections (1–4% of all)	None discerned apart from ?increasing age

Fig. 26.5 *Comparison of the clinicopathological classification of perinatal deaths in New South Wales and Scotland*

	NSW 1979 (proportional %)	**Scotland 1977–81** (proportional %)
Environmental		
Unexplained, low birth weight	25.1	33.4
Antepartum haemorrhage	10.4	12.1
Congenital anomaly	20.6	24.1
Maternal disorder	5.5	4.1
Obstetric		
Unexplained, normal birth weight	19.1	7.2
Pregnancy-induced hypertension	7.2	8.4
Mechanical/trauma	4.7	3.6
Iso-immunization	1.8	1.3
Infection/miscellaneous	5.6	2.2
	n = 866	n = 3781
Standard perinatal mortality rate	11.03	14.0
Births in period	78,502	270,581

PSYCHOLOGICAL EFFECT ON THE PARENTS OF FETAL OR NEONATAL LOSS

The loss of a fetus or of a neonate usually causes a considerable grief reaction in the mother, including post-partum depression. The father is also affected. The more mature the fetus or neonate at the time of death the greater is the grief reaction. The grief reaction is reduced if the parents touch and hold the infant for as long as they wish, if keepsakes are available including a lock of hair and a photograph, and if a health professional is readily available if the parents want more information. If the couple are contemplating a further pregnancy, conception should probably be delayed for about 6 months to permit the couple to overcome their grief.

CHAPTER 27

The newborn infant

Following birth the neonate undergoes several physiological changes so that it can adapt to extra-uterine life. Two main changes affect respiration and cardiovascular function.

First breaths

The several control systems that regulate breathing are already present in fetal life. Most of them only operate in fetal active states, such as REM sleep. In quiet sleep, long periods without breathing occur.

At birth there is a need to ensure a continued supply of oxygen and the removal of carbon dioxide. Breathing is augmented by an elevated carbon dioxide. Soon after birth, hypoxia causes a transient increase, then a reduction, in breathing efforts.

Nonspecific stimuli such as pain, cold, light and, possibly, the release of adrenaline in late labour, lead to stimulation of breathing.

In most infants, the first breathing efforts occur within 30 seconds of birth and are forceful enough to overcome the high resistance of the liquid in the airways and to inflate the lungs. In immature and abnormal infants the breathing efforts may be reduced.

Changes in the pattern of blood circulation

The second change is the redirection of the blood flow following the cessation of the high blood flow through the umbilical arteries which perfused the placental villi, and a lowering of the large volume of blood returning through the umbilical vein and the vena cava. The venous pressure in the vena cava falls and the ductus venosus closes. The lungs expand with the first breath and the pulmonary vascular resistance falls abruptly. The infant's systemic blood pressure rises slightly at the same time, which results in a temporary reversal in the direction of the blood flowing through the ductus arteriosus. As the infant breathes, the oxygen tension in the blood rises and the muscular walls of the ductus contract, the passage of blood through it ceasing. At the same time, the pressure in the right atrium falls. There is a simultaneous increase in the blood flow through the lungs. This blood enters and increases the pressure in the left atrium. Because of the changes in pressure between the two atria, the foramen ovale closes.

With the closure of the ductus venosus, the foramen ovale and the ductus arteriosus, the adult pattern of circulation of the blood is established (*Fig. 27.1*; compare with *Fig. 4.2*, page 29).

Changes in liver function

After the cardiovascular changes have taken place the infant's liver is perfused with a larger quantity of blood. The infant's liver can convert glucose into glycogen as efficiently as an adult liver, but some of its enzymatic functions are immature. The most important is its ability to conjugate bilirubin. In consequence, a mild physiological jaundice may occur in the first 6 days of life.

Most of the glycogen stored in the liver is laid down in the last 8 weeks of intra-uterine life. This is now mobilized for the energy needs of the first few days of life. Preterm babies have smaller liver glycogen stores and may develop hypoglycaemia. After a few days of life, the neonate obtains energy from food and by oxidizing fats stored in adipose tissue.

Temperature control

At birth, vasoconstriction of the skin vessels preserves body heat, but temperature maintenance is relatively difficult because of the relatively large surface area of a newborn infant. The body temperature of many newborn infants falls by 1.5°C immediately after the birth, because of rapid heat loss from the wet skin, but returns to normal within a few hours. A mature infant will have laid down fat in brown adipose tissue and can utilize this for heat production without shivering. Preterm babies have less brown fat and may become hypothermic.

Because of the instability of temperature control, neonates should be wrapped properly in cold climates, but in hot climates too much wrapping should be avoided.

Hypoxia in pregnancy and in the newborn

Most babies establish respiration rapidly and easily. A few infants are hypoxic at birth and require resuscitation. Any condition occurring during late pregnancy or labour which reduces the oxygen available to the fetus will predispose it to neonatal hypoxia. These conditions have been mentioned when discussing the at-risk fetus in pregnancy and labour (see page 155).

If severe fetal hypoxia develops in pregnancy, the fetus may die *in utero* or may be born with acidaemia and hypercapnia as well as hypoxia (asphyxia). A blood pH of less than 7.10 may lead to reflex pulmonary vasoconstriction which further impairs gas exchange. Hypoxia, on the other hand, increases the base deficit. Both of these changes increase the risk to the fetus of neurological damage. In such cases, resuscitation is urgently needed at birth.

The severity of hypoxia around the time of birth, and its effect on the subsequent development of the infant, can be measured by the Apgar scoring system (*Fig. 27.2*) or by the pH of umbilical artery blood. Both are useful in managing the immediate problem but are relatively poor indicators of long-term outcome.

The basic resuscitation of the newborn has been described on page 82 (see *Fig. 9.17*). The first column of *Figure 9.17* equates to a 1-minute Apgar score of 7–10. The second column to an Apgar score 4–6, whilst the third

column equates to an Apgar score of 0–3. The most important step in resuscitation is administering oxygen with intermittent positive pressure respiration. If the infant does not respond and remains bradycardic, the circulation should be supported by external cardiac massage (*Fig. 27.3*) and, possibly, endotracheal adrenaline. In addition, acidosis can be corrected with sodium bicarbonate (5ml/kg body weight) infusion via the umbilical vein. A 5-minute Apgar of less than 6 should be followed by measurements of umbilical blood gases and pH and treatment given to adjust the findings if necessary.

Fossa
ovalis

Ligamentum
teres

Lateral umbilical
ligaments

Ligamentum
arteriosum

Ligamentum
venosum

Fig. 27.1 Normal circulation in the newborn.

Fig. 27.2 Apgar scoring method for evaluating the infant (from Apgar and associates)			
	Score		
Sign	**0**	**1**	**2**
Colour	Blue; pale	Body pink; extremities blue	Completely pink
Respiratory effort	Absent	Weak cry; hypoventilation	Good; strong cry
Muscle tone	Limp	Some flexion of extremities	Active motion; extremities well flexed
Reflex irritability (response to stimulation of sole of foot)	No response	Grimace	Cry
Heart rate	Absent	Slow (<100)	Fast (>100)

Fig. 27.3 Closed cardiac massage. Intermittent pressure is applied over the middle-third of the sternum (which is pressed down about half an inch) with two fingers. The heart is compressed between the rib cage and the vertebral column and blood is expelled into the great vessel. For clarity the endotracheal tube has been omitted in the drawing.

Respiratory distress syndrome (hyaline membrane disease)

Hyaline membrane disease is caused by a relative lack of surfactant in the alveoli. Surfactant determines the stability of the lung after birth, and lowers the surface tension in the alveoli, ensuring a normal residual volume of air and the capacity for gas exchange. In the absence of surfactant, the alveoli become airless at the end of each breath and their ability to expand against the forces of surface tension is decreased. The consequent relative hypoxia causes pulmonary vasoconstriction and hinders the closure of the foramen ovale and the ductus arteriosus, which in turn reduces the pulmonary blood flow, with increasing respiratory and metabolic acidosis.

Hyaline membrane disease affects 0.5–1.0% of all neonates. It is uncommon if the baby weighs more than 2500g at birth, but affects 10% of premature infants, and is particularly damaging to infants weighing less than 1500g at birth.

DIAGNOSIS AND TREATMENT
Within a few hours of birth the infant's respiratory rate increases, with nasal flaring, expiratory grunting and sternal or intercostal retraction. The infant may be cyanosed and limp. The diagnosis is confirmed by radiology which shows ground glass shadowing. In 80% of cases the disease is only moderately severe, but in 20% the infant is seriously ill.

A neonatologist must be consulted and the infant admitted to a neonatal intensive care unit. The principles of treatment are:

- To keep the infant warm in an incubator adjusted to the neutral thermal range.
- To provide oxygen to obtain an arterial blood saturation of 95%, or a tension of 60–80mmHg by monitoring blood gases frequently.
- To provide assisted ventilation if needed.
- To avoid retinal damage by uncontrolled use of oxygen.
- To ensure that the baby is adequately nourished with fluid and energy, by giving an intravenous infusion of a glucose electrolyte solution, or breast milk by a nasogastric tube.
- To give either natural or synthetic surfactant in cases that require mechanical ventilation. The installation of surfactant into the infant's trachea reduces the severity of hyaline membrane disease, and its complications such as pneumothorax, and halves the mortality.

The mortality from hyaline membrane disease varies from 15 to 50% depending on the weight of the neonate, the severity of the disease and the skill of the medical and nursing staff.

Birth injuries

With increasingly good obstetric care during childbirth, birth injuries are becoming less common and less severe. Only those injuries most likely to occur will be discussed. In all cases, the injury must be explained to the parents and the treatment and prognosis discussed.

CRANIAL INJURIES
Caput succedanum
Caput succedanum is due to pressure on the fetal scalp when the head is being pushed deeply into the pelvis and the venous return from the scalp is impeded. The oedematous swelling covers a large area of scalp. Treatment is not required and the caput disappears within a few days.

Cephalohaematoma
Cephalohaematoma occurs following trauma by the obstetric forceps or the ventouse. The periosteum is dragged from the underlying parietal bone and subperiosteal haemorrhage occurs. The swelling is limited to the shape of the bone and is fluctuant initially, after which the rim becomes hard. The haematoma remains for 2–3 weeks and then is slowly absorbed.

Intracranial haemorrhage
Intracranial haemorrhage may be subdural or intraventricular. Both are uncommon. *Subdural haemorrhage* follows the misapplication of forceps. The infant, if born alive, is shocked and shows little response to resuscitation. *Intraventricular haemorrhage* is found, most often, among preterm infants and is related to worsening hypoxia. Most cases are diagnosed within 72 hours of birth, when the

infant's condition deteriorates suddenly. This condition is diagnosed by ultrasound examinations, which should be performed routinely on very small infants.

NERVE INJURIES

Most nerve injuries involve the face (facial palsy), or the brachial plexus and, usually, follow a forceps delivery, shoulder dystocia, or a difficult breech birth.

Facial palsy

Facial palsy is a lower motor neurone disorder with paresis or paralysis of the facial nerve and inability to close the eye on the affected side. The lesion usually resolves spontaneously within 2–3 weeks.

Brachial palsy

This is due to nerve damage, usually following difficulty in delivering the aftercoming head of a breech or in shoulder dystocia. In most cases, the nerve sheath is torn and the nerve is compressed by haemorrhage and oedema, but its integrity is preserved. *Erb's palsy* is due to compression of the fibres of C5 and C6. The infant's arm hangs limply by the baby's side. Treatment consists of placing the arm in abduction, with flexion of the elbow and extension of the wrist, and maintaining muscle tone by moving the arm

passively. Erb's palsy occurs in fewer than 1 in 2000 births. *Klumpke's paralysis* is rare and it occurs when nerves C7 and C8 are compressed. The infant has a paralysed arm, with wrist drop and flaccid paralysis of hand muscles. The prognosis is worse than that following Erb's palsy.

BONE AND MUSCLE INJURIES

These injuries may occur following a breech extraction. The clavicle, humerus or femur may be fractured. Injury to the sternomastoid muscle, due to a haematoma, may occur following a difficult delivery. It should be looked for after any difficult delivery as, unless treated by stretching the muscle, permanent shortening may result.

Congenital malformations

Congenital malformations affect between 1.5 and 3.5% of all infants. These defects are major in about 2% of all infants (*Fig. 27.4*). More than 60% of infants with congenital defects survive and benefit most by growing up in a family, if this is possible. When the diagnosis has been established, the doctor should talk with the parents, explaining the malformation and the prognosis calmly and sympathetically. Most parents go through a grieving period. They may express anger and guilt, questioning if anything

Fig. 27.4 Congenital defects (data from Australia, UK and Sweden)	
Major defects	**Per 1000 births**
Chromosomal (especially Down's syndrome)	1–3
CNS defects:	
a) Open neural tube defects	1–1.5
1. anencephaly	0.5
2. spina bifida	0.5
b) Hydrocephaly	0.3–0.6
CVS defects: Heart and great vessels	2–5
Gastrointestinal defects:	
a) Cleftlip, cleft palate	1–2
b) Alimentary tract (especially pyloric stenosis)	1–3
Urogenital defects	0.5–1
Skeletal defects:	
Talipes	1–3
Congenital dislocated hip	2–4
Polydactyly, etc	0.5–1
Multiple defects	0.5–1
Major defects total	**15–28**
Minor defects (skin blemishes, etc)	**2–15**

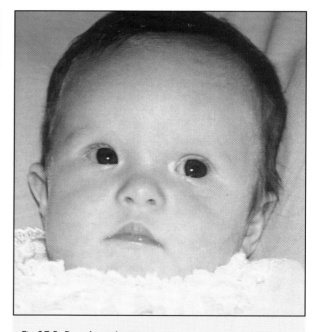

Fig. 27.5 Down's syndrome.

they did or did not do during the pregnancy caused the fetal malformation. Most appreciate counselling sessions.

The major malformations are now described.

DOWN'S SYNDROME

Down's syndrome is the most common genetic defect. The infant has slanting eyes with epicanthic folds, short hands, small fingers, and feet with abnormal skin creases. The head is short, the cheeks fat, the back of the neck short and fat, and the ears are squarish (see Fig. 27.5). Many children with Down's syndrome have some degree of mental handicap.

The incidence of Down's syndrome increases with the age of the mother (Fig. 27.6). As mentioned in Chapter 6,

page 39, Down's syndrome can now be diagnosed in early pregnancy and termination offered.

Sex-linked genetic disorders can be diagnosed in early pregnancy by chorionic villus sampling.

CENTRAL NERVOUS SYSTEM DEFECTS

Anencephaly (Fig. 27.7) and *spina bifida* (Fig. 27.8) can be diagnosed in pregnancy as described on page 40. *Hydrocephalus* can be diagnosed in the second half of pregnancy by ultrasound scanning, but may only be noticed when delivery is difficult.

CARDIOVASCULAR DEFECTS

Gross heart defects are usually demonstrated by cyanosis when the baby cries, and by marked cardiac thrills and murmurs. Care should be taken when a heart murmur is heard soon after birth as it may not be due to a congenital heart defect – the murmur may be transient. A reassessment should be made before discharge from hospital and a paediatric consultation obtained if abnormal signs persist.

GASTROINTESTINAL DEFECTS

Cleftlip and *cleft palate* are obvious. *Oesophageal atresia* should be considered in the babies of women who had polyhydramnios. A size-9 catheter should be passed through the mouth along the oesophagus and an ultrasound examination made. Oral feeding should not be started until the condition has been excluded or treated surgically. Duodenal stenosis or atresia should be suspected if persistent bile-stained vomiting occurs. Pyloric stenosis should be suspected if the infant, usually male, has projectile vomiting in the 3rd to 6th week of life. If the infant is relaxed, or feeding, the hypertrophied pyloric muscle may be palpable.

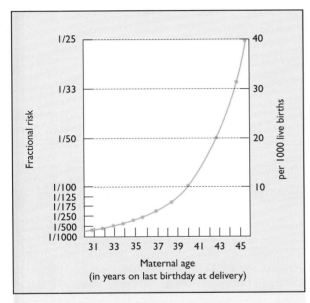

Fig. 27.6 The rate of Down's syndrome in live births in relation to maternal age.

Fig. 27.7 Anencephaly.

Fig. 27.8 Spina bifida.

UROGENITAL DEFECTS

Atresia of the kidneys is rare and fatal. In 2% of mature neonate boys, and 20% of preterm boys, one or both testes will have failed to have descended into the scrotum. By the infant's first birthday less than 1% have *undescended testes* (cryptorchidism). Surgical treatment is delayed until the child is 1.5–2.0 years old.

Circumcision

This is not required for medical reasons but some parents want it performed. Current advice is to delay circumcision until the infant is at least 10 days, and preferably 6 months, old. It should be performed under a local or a general anaesthetic.

SKELETAL DEFECTS

The most common skeletal disorders are *talipes calcaneus* (the foot is turned in and points down) and *talipes equinovarus* (the foot is turned out and points up). Usually no treatment other than gentle manipulation is needed.

Congenital dislocation of the hip is characterized by an anteverted femoral head and neck and a shallow acetabulum from which the femoral head may be displaced partially or completely. Between 1 and 3% of neonates show evidence of instability of the hip at birth but, in most cases, this resolves spontaneously within a week or two. In a few infants the defect persists. Examination of the newborn for congenital hip dislocation is described in *Figure 10.1*, page 93. If congenital dislocation of the hip is confirmed, treatment should be withheld until the infant is 5 months old, as 20% of babies treated earlier relapse or develop dysplasia or avascular necrosis of the femoral head.

SKIN

Defects involving the bladder (*ectopia vesicae*) and umbilicus (*exomphalos*) are obvious at birth. The former has a poor prognosis but the latter may be treated surgically. *Angiomata* (port wine stains and strawberry marks) occur. Most defects regress spontaneously or can be treated by laser when the infant is older. *Mongolian blue spots* are patches of slate blue discoloration over the sacrum or lower spine; these occur particularly in Asian infants. They have no clinical significance.

METABOLIC DISORDERS

Cystic fibrosis, affecting 1 baby in 2000; *congenital hypothyroidism*, affecting 1 baby in 6000; and *phenylketonuria*, affecting 1 baby per 10,000 can be detected by filter paper tests on blood samples taken on the 5th day of life. *Congenital adrenal hyperplasia* (1 in 10,000) can also be detected in the same way. The rare amino-acid disorders can be detected on a urine sample taken when an infant is 6 weeks old.

Risk of next baby being congenitally affected

A question of great concern to the parents of a congenitally affected baby is: 'What is the risk of our next baby being affected?' Available data are shown in *Figure 27.9*.

Maternal ingestion of drugs affecting the fetus

Pregnant women should avoid taking medications as far as possible, since many pharmaceutical agents cross the placenta and may affect the fetus adversely. If a drug is required, the doctor should read the product information document before prescribing it. In some countries, lists of drugs which should be avoided during pregnancy are obtainable from the health authorities.

Cerebral palsy

Cerebral palsy is a descriptive term for a collection of non-progressive neuromotor disorders which are not the result of cerebral malformations. The condition affects between 1.5 and 3.5% of all live born children. In most cases the cause of cerebral palsy is unknown, although low birth weight infants have a greater risk of developing it. If the infant weighs less than 1500g at birth the risk is increased 25-fold. Another factor may be the development of chorioamnionitis associated with prolonged rupture of the membranes or maternal infection. Birth trauma and hypoxia during labour (judged by a 5-minute Apgar score of 3 or less) are uncommon causes, accounting for less than 10% of all cases and, in many of these cases, the cerebral palsy may have been due to intrinsic fetal defects rather than to events occurring during childbirth.

Clinically, cerebral palsy may not be detected in the early neonatal period, although 25% of the victims have a seizure

Disorder	Incidence (per 100 births)	Risk (%) Normal parent having a second affected child	Risk (%) Affected parent having an affected child
Down's syndrome	0.2	1	33
Anencephaly	0.2	2	5
Spina bifida	0.3	4	5
Cleft palate	0.04	2	7
Cleft lip and palate	0.1	4	4
Congenital heart disease	0.6	2	2

Fig. 27.9 Risks of recurrence of some congenital defects

disorder at this time. The main clinical feature is a lack of motor control, usually presenting as spasticity, or, less commonly, as involuntary movements or muscle incoordination. Any muscle group may be affected, but quadriplegia and diplegia are seen most often. In 15% of affected people, choreo-athetoid, dystonic or ataxic movements predominate. If bulbar involvement occurs, the person will have difficulty in articulating. Over half of the people who have cerebral palsy have normal intelligence.

The stress on the parents and siblings is considerable, but much can be done to help them.

Neonatal infections

Any infant showing signs of infection should be isolated, together with the mother, until adequate treatment has controlled the infection. Infection may occur during pregnancy, as discussed in Chapter 18, Infections during pregnancy. During labour, infection may occur, particularly if the membranes have been ruptured for a long time; or from vaginal infection by group B streptococci (see page 140).

The common infections occurring after birth are:
* *Candida* spp. which infect the infant's mouth, white patches being formed.
* Staphylococcal infections which present as skin pustules, periumbilical infection, or blepharoconjunctivitis.
* *Chlamydia trachomatis* which may cause conjunctivitis, 1–3 weeks after birth, or pneumonia 3 weeks later.
* *Escherichia coli* infections causing gastroenteritis and urinary tract infection (which is difficult to diagnose).

Any ill infant with unexplained fever should have a urine specimen (obtained by suprapubic puncture) examined and, if the diagnosis remains unclear, a chest X-ray and a lumbar puncture should be made to exclude meningitis.

Treatment consists of giving the appropriate antibiotic depending on local bacterial sensitivities and experience. Care must be taken to prevent cross-infection by ensuring that the staff practice hygiene including hand washing.

CHAPTER 28

The low birth weight infant

The intra-uterine growth and birth weight of the fetus depends on its inherited growth potential and the effectiveness of the support to its growth provided by the utero-placental environment. The latter is affected, in a general sense, by the health of the mother and the presence, or absence, of maternal disease.

Provided the growth support exceeds the growth potential, fetal intra-uterine growth will continue; but when the fetal growth potential is limited, as in the case of many malformed fetuses, or maternal growth support diminishes, as in cases of multiple pregnancy and maternal diseases, a deviation from the normal growth curve occurs. The deviations usually arise after the 30th gestational week and are most marked after the 35th week of pregnancy (Fig. 28.1).

Fetal growth restriction is identified if the estimated weight of the infant is more than two standard deviations below the mean; a low birth weight baby is arbitrarily defined as weighing less than 2500g at birth. This definition presents some problems, as the mean birth weight of babies in many developing countries is less than for those in developed countries. For example, the mean birth weight of a baby born to a poor woman in Tamil Nadu, India, is about 2800g compared with a mean birth weight of 3400g in most developed countries. Defining low birth weight as less than 2500g in southern India would place over 15%

of healthy infants in the low birth weight category. The mean birth weight of babies born to mothers living in developed countries, at various gestational periods, is shown in *Figure 28.2*. The figure shows that the birth weight of 2500g is usually achieved at the end of the 35th week of pregnancy, and hospital statistics show that between 5 and 6% of the infants weigh less than 2500g at birth, in other words have a low birth weight.

Data are available from several developed countries which show the proportion of babies who are of low birth weight, their perinatal mortality and the survival of those babies born alive (*Figures 28.3 and 28.4*). These data obscure the fact that low birth weight babies comprise two populations: preterm (premature) babies and small for gestational age (SGA) babies.

Preterm babies have grown normally in the uterus but are born preterm, that is, by definition, before the 37th week of gestation.

SGA babies are also referred to as small-for-dates babies. These infants weigh less than their expected weight for a given gestational age, and comprise two groups. The growth potential of babies in the first group is low at all gestational ages and they are light-for-dates, but otherwise healthy. The growth of babies in the second group falters *in utero*, as detected by at least two measurements (usually by ultrasound scanning).

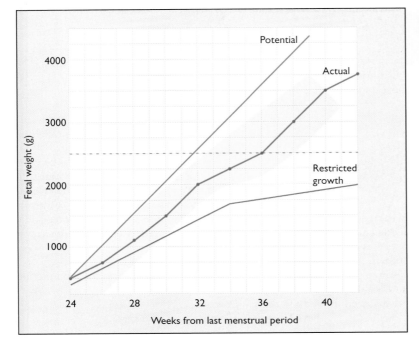

Fig. 28.1 Fetal weight versus gestation period (USA).

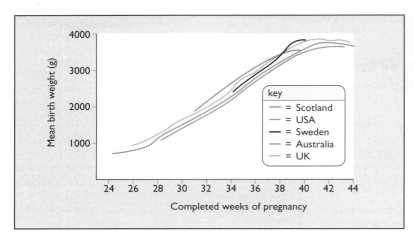

Fig. 28.2 The mean birth weight at various gestational ages in several developed nations. Note that the mean birth weight at the end of the 35th gestational week is approximately 2500g.

Gestation (weeks)	Total births	Fetal death rate (per 1000)	NND rate (per 1000)	PNM rate (per 1000)	Survivors (%)
<22	204	760	1000	1000	0
22–24	480	546	826	921	7.9
25–27	475	183	188	337	66.3
28–31	1304	103	37	136	86.4
32–36	8900	19.4	7.1	26.4	97.4
37–41	129014	1.8	1.2	3.1	99.7
>42	4181	1.9	1.7	3.6	99.6
Total	144558	7.3	4.0	11.3	98.9

Fig. 28.3 Perinatal mortality related to gestation (Queensland; Australia) 1994–96

These babies have suffered intra-uterine growth restriction and are at greater risk of dying, either in the uterus or during the neonatal period. The baby has a wasted appearance with little subcutaneous fat.

Combinations of the two main populations may occur: a preterm baby may also be small-for-dates.

Aetiological factors in low birth weight

The common aetiological factors are shown in *Figure 28.5*. It has to be said that in many cases no precise factor has been identified. The socio-economic factors are the most amenable to change with a possible reduction in the proportion of low birth weight babies born. However, trials of supplemental nutrients, the frequency of antenatal visits, or antenatal education have not significantly reduced the number of low birth weight infants born.

Management of the low birth weight infant

The birth weight and gestational age of the infant predict its morbidity and mortality to a large extent. A special category of high-risk babies are those whose birth weight is less than 1500g – the Very Low Birth Weight Baby.

The care of a low birth weight baby should be conducted by a neonatologist, with the resources available in an intensive neonatal-care unit. As mentioned in Chapter 20, Variations in the duration of pregnancy, a woman who goes into labour before the 35th week of pregnancy should, if possible, be transferred to a hospital with a level 3 nursery.

The objectives of management are:
• To provide an environment as close to the intra-uterine environment as possible.
• To prevent infection.
• To provide adequate nourishment.

Birthweight (g)	Total births	Fetal death rate (per 1000)	NND rate (per 1000)	PNM rate (per 1000)	Survivors (%)
<500	385	735	931	982	1.8
500–749	421	397	606	762	23.8
750–999	405	244	141	351	64.9
1000–1499	1013	92.8	44.4	137	86.3
1500–1999	2002	41.5	17.5	58.9	94.1
2000–2499	5526	13.2	7.05	20.4	98.0
2500–2999	21356	4.7	2.4	7.1	99.3
3000–3499	51849	1.5	1.2	2.7	99.7
3500–3999	44410	1.0	0.7	1.7	99.8
4000–4999	14642	1.1	0.8	1.8	99.8
>4500	2524	2.4	1.6	4.0	99.6
Total	144533	7.3	4.0	11.3	98.9

Fig. 28.4 Perinatal mortality related to birthweight (Queensland; Australia) 1994–96

- To detect and treat possible metabolic, and other, complications.

The best environment for a small baby is in a nursery maintained at a temperature of no less than 24°C or, if the infant is very small, in an incubator maintained at a temperature of 26–32°C and a humidity of 65–75%. Oxygen is provided via a head box or enters the incubator in a controlled manner.

Infection is controlled by careful attention to avoid overcrowding and medical attendants and others introducing infection into the nursery. Hand washing before handling a baby is the most important preventive measure.

Feeding is started about 6 hours after birth and breast milk is used as soon as possible. The baby is fed by gavage or spoon, and is put to the breast as soon as it suckles strongly. Vitamin supplements are given with, or after, feeding. Recommended daily doses are: vitamin D 400U; ascorbic acid 50mg; niacin 6mg; riboflavin 1mg; and vitamin A 5000U.

The following complications may occur:
- Hyaline membrane disease (see page 209).
- Cyanotic attacks, which may be due to inadequate ventilation of the lungs or cerebral damage.
- Jaundice (see page 93).
- Hypoglycaemia. This affects about 15% of low birth weight babies. For this reason regular checks of the infant's blood glucose are made until feeding has been established. If detected, glucose is given via intravenous infusion (6–9mg/kg per min).
- Hypocalcaemia may occur in very low birth weight babies, usually in the first 24 hours of life. If the plasma calcium level is less than 2mmol/L, calcium gluconate is given slowly intravenously.

- Intracranial haemorrhage. Periventricular haemorrhage (intraventricular or parenchymal haemorrhage) occurs mainly in babies weighing 1500g or less, about 20% thereof being affected. This complication is detected by real-time ultrasonography.

Retinopathy of prematurity

This disease of immature retinal vessels increases in incidence the lower the birth weight of the infant, affecting over 40% of infants weighing less than 1500g at birth. In most cases, the disease is mild, but 1 infant in 5 who has retinopathy is severely affected. Excessive doses and prolonged exposure to oxygen is thought to be the main cause, but other factors are probably involved. Continuous monitoring of oxygen supply has helped to reduce the incidence of the disease, but cases continue to occur. Treatment of established severe cases consists of using cryotherapy or laser, applied trans-sclerally.

Mortality and morbidity of low birth weight infants

Low birth weight infants contribute 70% of early neonatal deaths; the smaller the infant, the less is its chance of survival. With the development of special neonatal intensive care units, the mortality of these small babies has decreased. Few infants weighing 500g or less survive; 25% of infants weighing 501–750g survive, as do 65% of infants weighing 751–1000g. Babies weighing 1001–1500g have a 86% chance of surviving and those weighing 1501–2499g have a 94–98% survival rate.

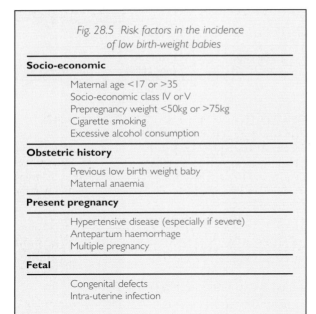

Fig. 28.5 *Risk factors in the incidence of low birth-weight babies*

Socio-economic

> Maternal age <17 or >35
> Socio-economic class IV or V
> Prepregnancy weight <50kg or >75kg
> Cigarette smoking
> Excessive alcohol consumption

Obstetric history

> Previous low birth weight baby
> Maternal anaemia

Present pregnancy

> Hypertensive disease (especially if severe)
> Antepartum haemorrhage
> Multiple pregnancy

Fetal

> Congenital defects
> Intra-uterine infection

at 5 years of age, of 95 surviving infants who were born at 24–26 weeks, gestational age showed that 15% were severely or moderately disabled. Five infants were blind with varying degrees of cerebral palsy, 5 had markedly low IQs, 6 had cerebral palsy and 2 were deaf. A further 23 (24%) had mild disability (17 a reduced IQ and 6 mild cerebral palsy).

An ultrasound scan of the infant's brain, if normal, is highly predictive of a normal neurological development. If the scan shows hypoxic ischaemic encephalopathy the chance of a good outcome for the baby is reduced. The encephalopathy can be graded from mild (no seizures) to severe (coma). Infants categorized as having mild encephalopathy have a good outcome. Those graded as having moderate encephalopathy have a 25% chance of severe handicap, whilst those with severe encephalopathy will die or have a severe neurological disability. These outcomes are irrespective of Apgar scores or acid–base status at delivery.

Even with this more accurate assessment, ethical problems remain. For example, the disability rate of survivors who weighed less than 700g at birth is over 50%. Should the parents have the choice to ask for continued resuscitation or be permitted to let their baby die? This raises an ethical question. Should the medical attendants persist with complex, expensive, traumatic procedures or, with the agreement of the parents, permit the infant to die peacefully?

The morbidity of the surviving infants has also decreased in recent years; the highest morbidity is among infants whose gestational age is less than 27 weeks and whose birth weight is 700g or less. An Australian study of outcome,

CHAPTER 29

Disorders of menstruation

Menstruation is normal if it occurs at intervals of 22–35 days (from day 1 of menstruation to the onset of the next menstrual period) as mentioned in Chapter 1, Gyniatric history and examination; if the duration of the bleeding is less than 7 days; and if the menstrual blood loss is less than 80ml. It was also noted that menstrual discharge consists of tissue fluid (20–40% of the total discharge), blood (50–80%) and fragments of the endometrium. However, to the woman menstrual discharge looks like blood and is so reported.

By convention, the notation of menstruation and its disturbances is written as, for example, 5/28. This indicates that the woman bled for 5 days and that menstruation occurred at an interval of 28 days. The quantity of menstrual loss is entered as slight, normal or heavy.

Disorders of menstruation occur, most commonly, at each extreme of the reproductive years, that is under the age of 19 and over the age of 39 years. The disorder may relate to the length of the menstrual cycle, or to the amount and duration of the menstrual loss. A woman may have both disturbances.

Definitions

CHANGES IN THE LENGTH OF THE MENSTRUAL CYCLE

Menstruation may occur at intervals longer than 35 days, when it is termed *oligomenorrhoea*; if menstruation does not occur for more than 70 days (in the absence of pregnancy) a diagnosis of *secondary amenorrhoea* is made. *Primary amenorrhoea* is diagnosed if menstruation has not commenced by the age of 16 years. Menstruation may also occur at intervals of less than 21 days, when it is given the term *epimenorrhoea* or *polymenorrhoea*.

CHANGES IN THE AMOUNT OF MENSTRUAL LOSS

The quantity of menstrual discharge may vary, without altering the cyclicity of menstruation. Scanty or light menstrual discharge is termed *hypomenorrhoea*; heavy 'bleeding' is termed *menorrhagia*. In menorrhagia there may be an excessive amount of blood lost, or the apparently heavy bleeding may be due to an increased loss of tissue fluid.

Menorrhagia may occur in association with an organic condition in the uterus, or may occur in the absence of any detectable uterine abnormality. In this case it is termed *dysfunctional uterine bleeding*.

DISTURBANCES IN CYCLICITY AND AMOUNT OF MENSTRUAL LOSS

In this disturbance the cyclicity of menstruation is lost, bleeding occurring at irregular intervals, the quantity of menstrual loss varying considerably. This pattern is termed *metrorrhagia*. Generally it indicates a local condition in the uterus.

Amenorrhoea and oligomenorrhoea

PRIMARY AMENORRHOEA

Primary amenorrhoea (affecting 5% of amenorrhoeic women) may be due to a genetic defect, such as gonadal dysgenesis, in which case the secondary sexual characteristics will not have developed. It may be due to a Müllerian duct abnormality, such as an absent uterus, vaginal agenesis, a transverse vaginal septum, or an imperforate hymen. In the last three causes, menstruation may occur but the menstrual discharge cannot escape from the genital tract. The condition is *cryptomenorrhoea* rather than amenorrhoea. Rarely is testicular feminization the cause.

In many cases, however, no abnormality is found and the young woman may be expected to menstruate in time. Some of these women have an eating disorder or exercise excessively. If the adolescent girl has not started menstruating by the age of 17, investigations should be made as described on page 318, and hormone treatment prescribed as appropriate.

SECONDARY AMENORRHOEA

The most common cause of secondary amenorrhoea is pregnancy but the condition may occur during the reproductive years from a variety of causes. In *Figures 29.1* and *29.2* the most common causes of amenorrhoea and their frequency are shown. Only these causes will be discussed in this chapter.

As noted in Chapter 1, Gyniatric history and examination, normal menstruation depends on a normal uterus and vagina, and on the reciprocal interaction between hormones released from the hypothalamus (gonadotrophic-releasing hormones), the pituitary [the gonadotrophins – follicle-stimulating hormone (FSH) and luteinizing hormone (LH)] and the ovaries (oestrogen and progesterone).

Fig. 29.1 The aetiology of secondary amenorrhoea.

Fig. 29.2 Causes of secondary amenorrhea

Cause	Incidence (%)
Weight loss	20–40
Polycystic ovaries	15–30
Pituitary insensitivity (post pill)	10–20
Hyperprolactinaemia	10–20
Primary ovarian failure	5–10
Asherman's syndrome	1–2
Hypothyroidism	1–2

Investigation of secondary amenorrhoea

Unless organic disease is suspected, or the woman is desperately seeking relief from infertility, most experts would not investigate amenorrhoea until it has lasted for 6–12 months, as most women start menstruating during this time.

When investigation is indicated, a careful history is essential, in which the doctor inquires about the woman's general health, and seeks to determine if she has an eating disorder or exercises excessively, or if any medical or psychiatric condition is present. A physical examination, including a vaginal examination, follows and a pelvic ultrasound examination may be made in certain cases. If these examinations reveal no definite diagnosis, the following tests are ordered.

- Hormone assays:
  FSH and *LH*. An FSH level above the normal range of the laboratory, confirmed by repeating the measurement, indicates primary ovarian failure.
  Prolactin (hPr). A raised hPr level on two or more occasions indicates hyperprolactinaemia.
  Thyroid-stimulating hormone (TSH) and serum T_4.
  Oestradiol 17-β. This may be measured or a 'progestogen stimulation test' made.
- *Progestogen stimulation test*. The test seeks to determine if the uterus responds to progestogen withdrawal. Progestogens will only provoke bleeding if there is sufficient circulating oestradiol (more than 150pmol/L). The test determines if the endometrium will respond and indirectly determines that the oestradiol is above a critical level. Medroxyprogesterone acetate 5mg is given daily for 5 days. If menstrual bleeding occurs within 7 days the test is positive, and clomiphene is likely to induce ovulation.
- *X-ray of the pituitary fossa or a CT scan* if the hPr level is raised, to exclude the presence of a pituitary tumour.

The purpose of the investigations is to exclude organic disease (for example, a prolactin-secreting microadenoma or hypothyroidism) and to treat anovulation as a cause of infertility. If organic disease is not detected and infertility is not a problem, amenorrhoea does not represent a danger to the woman, but because low oestrogen levels may lead to bone loss, after 6 months of amenorrhoea hormone replacement treatment (see page 321) should be advised.

The sequence of investigations is shown in *Figure 29.3*.

MORE COMMON CAUSES OF AMENORRHOEA
Weight loss

Women who have an eating disorder, particularly anorexia nervosa, cease to menstruate as do some women who are compulsive exercisers. The cause of the amenorrhoea is a failure of the hypothalamus to release sufficient gonadotrophic-releasing hormone (GnRH) to initiate the release of gonadotrophins and, in consequence, only a small quantity of oestrogen is secreted by the ovaries. If this persists for more than 6 months, bone loss may occur at a time when bone formation is reaching its peak. A consequence of this is a greater risk of osteoporosis in later life. Even during the recovery phase, menstruation may not occur for several months, which may aggravate the problem.

Hyperprolactinaemia and prolactin-secreting tumours

Prolactin secretion by the pituitary gland is inhibited, under normal conditions, by dopamine released from the hypothalamus. In certain circumstances, this control is diminished. Examples are, hypothyroidism and the administration of dopamine-depleting agents or dopamine-receptor blocking agents. A more common cause of hyperprolactinaemia is a potential, or actual, microadenoma of the pituitary gland. In these cases, the increased circulating levels of prolactin act directly on the hypothalamus to reduce the secretion of GnRH which, in turn, prevents the FSH and LH rises needed for follicle development and ovulation.

The woman develops oestrogen deficiency, with menstrual disturbances (usually amenorrhoea), a dry vagina and, often, a reduction of her libido. If the hyperprolactinaemia persists, osteopenia and, perhaps, osteoporosis will result. In 30% of women inappropriate milk secretion (galactorrhoea) occurs.

As hyperprolactinaemia accounts for 10–20% of cases of amenorrhoea, investigation is important. The diagnosis is made if a raised blood level of prolactin is found. If this

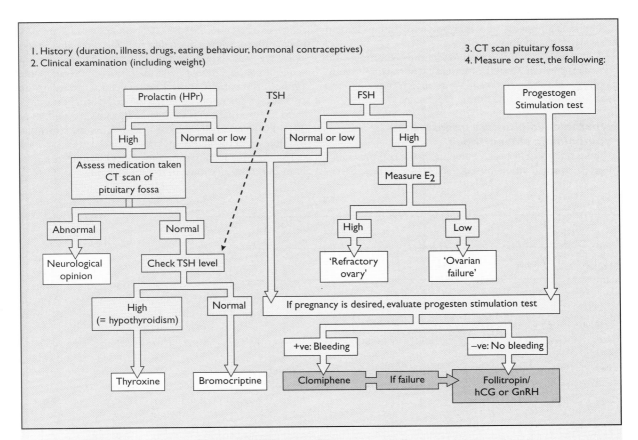

Fig. 29.3 *The investigation and treatment of secondary amenorrhoea.*

is noted during investigation, a high-resolution CT scan of the pituitary is made to detect a prolactin-secreting tumour, although in most cases none is found. A microadenoma (less than 10mm in diameter) is more common than a macroadenoma.

Treatment is needed if a macroadenoma is detected, or if the woman desires to become pregnant, but in all cases of hyperprolactinaemia careful follow-up is needed as some women with this condition, but no tumour, eventually develop one. Women who have functional hyperprolactinaemia require assessment at 1–3 year intervals, when the level of prolactin in a blood sample is measured and a CT scan made. Women who have a microadenoma need to be assessed annually, but treatment is not required unless they are infertile or have marked symptoms of low circulating levels of oestradiol. In both these groups, if amenorrhoea persists for more than 6 months, as is likely, hormone replacement treatment should be offered to prevent bone loss and the development of osteoporosis.

If a macroadenoma is detected, treatment consists of prescribing a dopamine agonist, such as bromocriptine or cabergoline, in a dose which reduces the prolactin levels to the normal range and maintains them in this range. The treatment causes the tumour to shrink in most women.

Surgery is only indicated if bromocriptine treatment fails. During treatment and after ceasing to take the drug, regular measurements of serum prolactin and an annual CT scan are mandatory.

A patient who has a macroadenoma should avoid becoming pregnant until the tumour has shrunk to lie completely within the pituitary fossa as shown by a CT scan, as the tumour may grow during pregnancy.

Hypothalamic–pituitary insensitivity: hypothalamic amenorrhoea

In about one-third of cases of amenorrhoea, hypothalamic-pituitary insensitivity is postulated. Many of these cases, coincidentally, follow the use of oral contraceptives, but eating disorders may also be involved, as may psychosomatic factors (for example, change of work, marital disharmony or separation). Severe depression or acute or chronic illness may be factors.

Treatment of hypothalamic amenorrhoea

If the amenorrhoea has persisted for 9–12 months and anovulation is the only or the main cause of the couple's infertility, treatment should be offered. Women whose body weight is low [Body Mass Index (BMI) less than 19] or who are compulsive exercisers should be persuaded to change their behaviour and try to obtain a body weight within the normal range for women (BMI 19.0–24.9) before starting drug treatment. The reasons are that these women are at greater risk of developing the ovarian hyperstimulation syndrome and, if they achieve a pregnancy, have a greater risk of delivering a preterm infant.

Clomiphene is an anti-oestrogen (which may sometimes act as a weak oestrogen). It acts by binding on to oestrogen receptors in target cells, thus preventing oestradiol binding to them. Transferred to the cell nucleus, it renders the cells relatively insensitive to the effects of endogenous oestradiol. This inhibits the negative feedback with the release of GnRH and, subsequently, FSH and LH. The regimen for clomiphene use is shown in *Figure 29.4*. Clomiphene will induce ovulation in over 80% of women who have hypothalmic amenorrhoea, particularly if the progestogen test is positive, and should be chosen first.

Should anovulation persist in spite of the clomiphene regimen, the patient should be referred to an infertility specialist, as laboratory control is needed if other drugs regimens are used. The regimens are follitropin (recombinant FSH: Puregon and Gonal-F) and human chorionic gonadotrophin (hCG, Pregnyl, Profasi).

The details of the treatments can be found in books about infertility as shown in the Bibliography.

Stage	Month	Dose
Fig. 29.4 Therapeutic regimen using clomiphene to induce ovulation		
1	1	Clomiphene 50mg daily for 5 days
2	2	Clomiphene 100mg daily for 5 days
3	3	Clomiphene 150mg daily for 5 days
4	4	Clomiphene 200mg daily for 5 days
5	6–8	No treatment
6	9	Clomiphene 100mg daily for 5 days + HCG 5000IU 7 days later
7	10	Clomiphene 150mg daily for 5 days + HCG 5000IU 7 days later

Using these treatments about 90% of women with amenorrhoea and 40% of women with oligomenorrhoea will ovulate, and 70% and 25% will conceive. A number of women continue to ovulate after the treatments have ceased and become pregnant.

Polycystic ovarian syndrome (PCO)

The ovary contains multiple (more than four) immature and atretic follicles (not cysts in spite of the name), which are aligned near the surface, often in a necklace-like formation (Fig. 29.5). Oligomenorrhoea or amenorrhoea usually occurs and may be associated with hirsutism, acne, infertility and, sometimes, obesity. The cause of PCO is not fully understood, but at least two hormones are involved. First, there is an increase in insulin resistance that leads to hyperinsulinaemia, which causes an increase in serum testosterone. Second, there is an increase in LH levels, which in turn may be due to hyperinsulinaemia.

A diagnostic problem has arisen with the increased use of transvaginal ultrasound to image pelvic organs. Using this technique, about 20% of normally menstruating women have been found to have more than 15 subcapsular follicles, measuring 2–10mm in diameter. In addition, three-quarters of women who have bulimia nervosa have been found to have either multiple small ovarian follicles or PCO. It is possible that chaotic eating, particularly of carbohydrates, leads to insulin resistance, which in turn indirectly causes PCO.

A key feature of PCO is that there is an increased level of LH. This may lead to hypertrophy of the theca interna with an increased secretion, by the ovaries, of androstenedione and, to a lesser extent, testosterone. The high level of LH may also prevent the proper maturation of oocytes when they complete the first meiotic division. This may account for the infertility of some women who have PCO.

Fig. 29.5 Polycystic ovary.

The diagnosis of PCO is made on the case history and confirmed by transvaginal ultrasound and the finding of a raised LH:FSH ratio.

Treatment depends on the presenting symptoms and on the wishes of the woman. If there are no symptoms no treatment is indicated. Hirsutism causing concern to the woman should be treated (see page 240). Life-style changes should be encouraged, and obese women persuaded to lose weight and all women to increase exercising.

In most cases the woman presents to the doctor complaining of infertility, usually because of anovulation. If this is found, the treatment is that described for hypothalamic-pituitary dysfunction. If medical treatment fails to lead to ovulation, some gynaecologists treat polycystic ovaries by laparoscopic diathermy or 'drilling' the cysts in an attempt to induce ovulation.

Women with PCO should be followed up as over 20% will be found to have, or will develop, impaired glucose tolerance or diabetes. They also have an increased risk of developing endometrial carcinoma if the anovulation persists for a number of years.

Uterine abnormalities

Surgical removal of the uterus, endometrial ablation or radiation results in amenorrhoea. Excessive curettage (particularly following an abortion or postpartum) may act in the same way as endometrial ablation, producing amenorrhoea by removing the basal endometrial layer and permitting synechiae to form (Asherman's syndrome). The diagnosis is made by hysteroscopy, transvaginal ultrasound scanning or from a hysterogram.

Primary gonadal (ovarian) failure

The cause of primary ovarian failure, in most cases, is unknown. In this condition the ovarian follicles disappear before the age of 40, and the woman reaches a premature menopause. In other women the follicles persist but the woman develops auto-antibodies which mask the gonadotrophin receptors in the ovaries with the result that the gonadotrophins can no longer bind to them. These women may have a premature menopause, but some months or years later, inexplicably, the woman ovulates and menstruates – the 'resistant ovarian syndrome'. Treatment consists of providing hormone replacement to control menopausal symptoms and to prevent bone loss and cardiovascular sequelae (see page 320). If the woman wishes to have a child, she may enter an assisted conception programme and receive a donor ovum.

Menorrhagia

Menorrhagia may be due to an organic cause but, in many instances, is dysfunctional; in other words menorrhagia is due to an alteration in the endocrine or local endometrial control of menstruation (see page 11). Ovulation has often occurred but not always. Organic causes include: uterine myomata, particularly if the myoma is intramural or submucous and distorts the endometrial cavity; diffuse adenomyosis; endometrial polyps and, rarely, chronic pelvic infection (pelvic inflammatory disease); a blood dyscrasia; and hypothyroidism. If the clinician thinks hypothyroidism is a possible diagnosis TSH and free T_4 levels should be measured. Treatment in these cases is directed to the cause.

INVESTIGATION

A careful history and a physical examination should be made and from this specific laboratory tests ordered. These include a full blood picture, including a coagulation screen if indicated, and possibly tests for thyroid function.

These tests may be sufficient to reach a diagnosis, but if the woman is over the age of 35 years it is usual to investigate further. The additional tests are hysteroscopy and endometrial biopsy, endometrial sampling, transvaginal ultrasound scanning and diagnostic curettage.

Hysteroscopy

Using a hysteroscope, the uterine cavity can be inspected and abnormalities, such as endometrial polyps or submucous myomata, can be detected and often removed. In addition, an endometrial sample can be taken for histological examination. Hysteroscopy is an office procedure which can be performed either with or without a local anaesthetic.

Hysteroscopy provides a clearer picture of the interior of the uterus and makes the diagnosis clearer than diagnostic curettage under anaesthesia, which it is replacing. In several large studies, hysteroscopy has shown that about 25% of women with menorrhagia or irregular menstruation have submucous myomata, usually projecting into the uterine cavity, and of that about 10% have endometrial polyps. Previously, these cases would have been identified as dysfunctional uterine bleeding. They can be treated at the time of hysteroscopic diagnosis by hysteroscopic resection.

Endometrial sampling (biopsy)

Endometrial sampling (biopsy) is made by introducing a narrow biopsy curette, through the uterine cervix, and obtaining a representative sample of the endometrium. The procedure can take place in the doctor's office.

Transvaginal ultrasound

This procedure has been suggested as a non-invasive method of imaging the uterine cavity. The presence of submucous myomata can be detected and the width of the endometrium measured. An endometrium more than 5mm in width in a postmenopausal woman indicates the need for a curettage to exclude endometrial pathology.

Diagnostic curettage

The procedure is invasive and is performed under general anaesthesia. It requires admission to hospital as a day case and is performed between bleeding episodes. The entire endometrium is curetted and sent for histological examination. It is being replaced by hysteroscopy and endometrial sampling.

DIAGNOSIS

If no organic cause for menorrhagia is found, a diagnosis of *dysfunctional uterine bleeding* is made. In these cases, the immediate cause of the menorrhagia is thought to be that there is reduced vasoconstriction and a lack of platelet aggregation, hence the haemostatic plugs occluding the endometrial blood vessels are less effective in achieving haemostasis. These changes may reflect increased prostacyclin and prostaglandin E_2 secretion by the endometrium. Dysfunctional uterine bleeding is more common under the age of 19 and after the age of 39 years.

Dysfunctional uterine bleeding

The importance of an accurate menstrual history cannot be overstated. If the patient is agreeable, and the bleeding is not too severe, or if she has not recorded a menstrual history herself, it is helpful if she records the duration of, the interval between, and the perceived amount of menstrual discharges for a 3-month period. The latter is difficult for a woman to measure and it is usually overestimated. Ideally, the actual blood loss should be determined (by collecting all pads and tampons and measuring the haemoglobin content by the alkaline haematin method) but this is not practicable except in a research programme. Certain clinical pointers help. These are: the occurrence of 'flooding'; saturation of tampons or pads or changing pads every 1/2 to 2 hours; the presence of large blood clots; and a prolonged duration of the menstrual period.

Although dysfunctional uterine bleeding is usually regular, the duration of the menstrual cycle may be increased with the result that the menorrhagia occurs less frequently. In this group of cases, which are usually found at the extremes of the reproductive period, oestrogen secretion may be less than normal and is not opposed by progesterone. In other words the bleeding is *anovulatory*. In other cases the unopposed oestrogen levels are high, resulting in an increased thickness of the endometrium and causing *cystic hyperplasia* (Fig. 29.6). The pathology of an endometrial sample may show simple (cystic) endometrial hyperplasia (Fig. 29.7); complex adenomatous hyperplasia (Fig. 29.8); simple hyperplasia with atypia or complex hyperplasia with atypia (Fig. 29.9). If the pathology shows atypical hyperplasia, (the treatment is that described on page 294), follow-up with further endometrial studies is mandatory (unless the woman chooses to have a hysterectomy) as between 10 and 25% of cases progress to endometrial carcinoma.

Fluctuations in the circulating levels of oestrogen tend to occur, resulting in a 'lack of support' for the endometrium leading to cyclical, profuse bleeding. In other cases, the heavy bleeding occurs at shorter intervals, the cycle length being reduced. This is referred to as *polymenorrhagia*. The treatment of these variants is the same as that of dysfunctional uterine bleeding.

TREATMENT OF DYSFUNCTIONAL UTERINE BLEEDING

Patients seen during a severe bleeding episode

In this situation treatment may be required urgently. Two methods are available: to perform a curettage and to administer hormones. The hormones usually chosen are combined equine oestrogens (CEE), 25mg given intravenously and repeated 6-hourly for 2–3 doses. CEE in this dosage may cause marked nausea in some women. Once CEE has stopped the bleeding, a progestogen must be given for 14 days to induce secretory change and then endometrial shedding. An alternative to CEE is to give 17-hydroxyprogesterone acetate 125–250mg intramuscularly, or oral norethisterone 20–30mg each day, in divided doses,

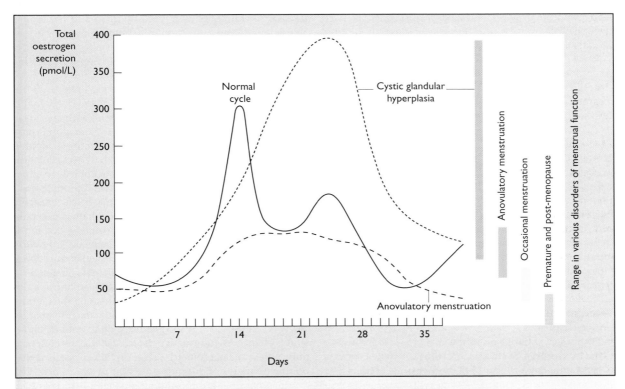

Fig. 29.6 Urinary oestrogen secretion in certain gynaecological conditions related to the menstrual cycle.

Fig. 29.7 Cystic endometrial hyperplasia.

Fig. 29.8 Complex adenomatous hyperplasia.

Fig. 29.9 Complex hyperplasia with atypia.

for 4 days. If a progestogen is used, a withdrawal bleed may be expected 3–6 days later. This can be avoided if norethisterone (5–10mg daily) is continued for 20 days.

Patients seen between bleeding episodes

In this situation several choices are available. They should be discussed with the woman as her wishes and concerns should be addressed before treatment is instituted. The choices fall into two main groups: hormonal treatment and surgical treatment.

Medical treatment

This consists of:

- *Progestogens*. Either norethisterone (5–15mg daily) or medroxyprogesterone acetate (10mg 2–3 times daily) is given from day 5 to day 25 of the menstrual cycle. A new progestogen, gestrinone 2.5mg twice weekly, is also being used. The treatment is continued for 4–6 menstrual cycles.
- *Non-steroidal anti-inflammatory drugs (NSAIDS)*. These drugs inhibit prostaglandin synthesis and reduce both the volume of blood loss (by 20%) and the associated dysmenorrhoea. A widely used example is mefenamic acid which is taken in a dose of 500mg 8 hourly if possible commencing 4 days before menstruation.
- *Oral contraceptives*. If the bleeding is not too severe, a monophasic, progestogen-dominant hormonal contraceptive may be used.
- *Danazol*. This hormone, in a dose of 200mg a day, may be used. If this dose does not control the bleeding it is increased to 400mg a day. At these doses side effects such as lassitude, weight gain, muscle pains and acne are uncommon, but may occur. Danazol is expensive, but is highly effective in courses of no more than 6 months.
- *A levonorgestrel intra-uterine device*. This device releases 20μg of levonorgestrel a day and is effective for 5 years. As well as regulating the menorrhagia it is an effective

contraceptive. The menorrhagia is cured within 3 months in 90% of women.
- *Antifibrinolytic agent tranexamic acid* reduces menstrual loss by 50%. The dose is 1g 6 hourly commencing on the first day of menstruation.

Surgical treatment
Curettage

Before the availability of hormones, or the newer surgical treatments, curettage was the only treatment of menorrhagia, apart from hysterectomy. Curettage controls heavy bleeding for a short time but there is usually a recurrence in 4–6 months. For this reason, it is being replaced by medical treatment or endometrial ablation.

Endometrial ablation

The concept of this procedure is that by ablating the basal layer of the endometrium, endometrial regeneration is prevented or reduced and the menorrhagia is cured. Endometrial ablation should only be performed by a gynaecologist experienced in the technique, or the results will be poor and the woman may be at risk of severe complications. Before endometrial ablation is carried out the cavity of the uterus is inspected with a hysteroscope. Many gynaecologists prescribe danazol 200mg 2 or 3 times a day for 4 weeks before the operation or a GnRH analogue (for example, depot leuprolide 7.5mg, 4 weeks before the procedure) to reduce endometrial thickness. Endometrial ablation may be performed using 'roller ball' electrocoagulation, loop resection or laser, after distending and flushing the uterine cavity with a glycine mixture. If laser is chosen, the uterine cavity is continuously flushed with a sodium chloride infusion system. An alternative is to use radiofrequency induced thermal endometrial ablation. In this method the uterine cavity is not distended with fluid.

The procedures are not without problems. In 1% of cases the uterine wall is perforated. Glycine and sodium chloride are absorbed into the vascular system and may cause fluid overload, pulmonary oedema and hyponatraemia.

These different methods produce similar results: 30–60% of women become amenorrhoeic, 35–60% become hypomenorrhoeic and the remaining 5–15% require a repeat of the procedure or a hysterectomy. Interviewed up to 2 years after the procedure, three-quarters of women express satisfaction, the remainder complaining of persistent menstruation, dysmenorrhoea or pelvic pain.

The benefits of endometrial ablation are that it is less invasive and painful than hysterectomy, the woman is in hospital for 1–2 days rather than 7–10 days and it is less expensive. The woman should be convalescent for 7–14 days.

Hysterectomy

Whilst there is no argument that hysterectomy is an appropriate operation in many cases of uterine myomata, adenomyosis, advanced endometriosis, uterine malignancy and in some cases of pelvic infection, its position in the treatment of dysfunctional uterine bleeding is not so clear. Although many women welcome hysterectomy for the relief of a distressing symptom, others believe that hysterectomy diminishes their femininity. The importance of this observation is that a woman must have the opportunity to discuss the choices for the treatment of menorrhagia, and be given time to reflect, if hysterectomy is recommended to her. There is rarely any need for an urgent hysterectomy and, once the operation has been recommended by a gynaecologist, it may be helpful for the woman to talk with her general practitioner about the benefits of and problems related to the operation. These matters are discussed further on page 233.

Metrorrhagia

In metrorrhagia, the bleeding is irregular in quantity, acyclical in character and often prolonged in duration. The condition is usually due to a pathological condition in the uterus or other internal genital organs. Its presence demands that the doctor investigate further. The investigations include either a hysteroscopy and endometrial biopsy or a diagnostic curettage. Treatment is directed to the underlying cause. Hysterectomy is often appropriate.

Other disturbances of menstruation

In some women the duration of the cycle is shortened to less than 21 days (*polymenorrhoea*). Most women have no concern about this but, if the change is annoying, the menstrual period can be regulated by prescribing an oral contraceptive.

Some women complain of *slight menstrual staining* occurring 2–3 days before or following the end of a normal menstrual period. Apart from being annoying, the condition has no sinister consequences, although some doctors believe that premenstrual staining is a sign of endometriosis. The woman should be reassured but, if she requests treatment, menstruation is usually regulated by prescribing oral contraceptives or norethisterone 2.5mg from days 20–25 of the menstrual cycle for a few months.

Another concern of some women is that the amount of menstrual discharge has decreased. The condition, known as *hypomenorrhoea*, occurs most commonly in women taking oral contraceptives. The woman should be reassured that it has no abnormal consequences.

CHAPTER 30

Psychosomatic and physical disorders of the menstrual cycle

In the proliferative phase of the menstrual cycle few problems occur. Some women experience pain in the lower abdomen which is unilateral and occurs at the time of ovulation. The pain is usually not severe and lasts for about 12 hours or less. The condition is called *mittelschmerz*. It indicates that ovulation has occurred, but investigations show no intra-abdominal pathology. If *mittelschmerz* is recurrent and distressing, relief can be obtained if the woman takes a hormonal contraceptive.

Mood and physical symptoms in the menstrual cycle

Most women, in the reproductive years, experience some psychological (negative mood) or physical symptoms in the luteal phase of the menstrual cycle. The symptoms vary in character and tend to become worse as menstruation approaches. They do not occur in every cycle and may vary in intensity in different cycles. A few women have severe mood and physical symptoms; a diagnosis of premenstrual syndrome is made in these cases.

Predominantly psychosomatic disorders

PREMENSTRUAL SYNDROME (LATE LUTEAL PHASE DYSPHORIC DISORDER, DSM-III-R)

In 5–15% of women, who are usually aged in their late 20s or early 30s (range 20–40 years), the negative mood and physical changes occurring in the luteal phase are of sufficient severity to affect day-to-day living and social and personal relationships, particularly with partners or children, most or all months. With the onset of menstruation, or during it, the symptoms disappear. During the postmenstrual period, for at least a week, the woman feels well, often euphoric. With, or soon after, ovulation the symptoms reappear. The condition is the *premenstrual syndrome* (PMS).

The symptoms vary in character and in severity in different menstrual cycles, but are always cyclic, a symptom-free interval occurring. The most common symptoms are shown in *Figure 30.1*. The mood changes tend to cluster together and can be grouped into one defined factor – general negative mood. The physical symptoms cluster into two groups: the first group, includes breast symptoms, abdominal fullness, increased appetite and food cravings;

the second group, of symptoms start during the 1–2 days before menstruation and include abdominal discomfort or pain, headache, backache, lassitude, decreased appetite and menstrual cramps. This second group may be identified as the *perimenstrual syndrome*.

Diagnosis of PMS

The diagnosis of PMS is made after evaluating the periodicity of the physical and mood symptoms, ascertaining that there is a symptom-free period after menstruation and ensuring that the symptoms cannot be explained by some other illness.

The suspected diagnosis should be confirmed by asking the woman to complete a daily record of symptoms over three menstrual cycles (*Fig. 30.2*). As well as establishing a firm diagnosis, the value of the daily record is that the woman develops an insight into her symptoms and is encouraged by the fact that the medical practitioner has an interest in her problems.

Aetiology of PMS

The aetiology of PMS is unknown. There may be a genetic component, but the current theory is that PMS is multifactorial. One underlying abnormality may be a fluctuation in the levels of oestradiol in the luteal phase, which may cause the symptoms directly or by decreasing brain serotonin activity. A problem in accepting this theory is that no consistent fluctuations have been detected with daily monitoring.

Management of PMS

The importance of obtaining an ongoing therapeutic relationship with the woman cannot be overestimated. Once this has been established, explanation and counselling will

Fig. 30.1 *Symptoms associated with PMS*	
Symptoms	
Mood (emotional)	**Physical**
Irritability	Abdominal bloating
Anxiety	Abdominal discomfort, tenderness or pain
Nervous tension	Breast swelling, tenderness or pain
Depression (feeling sad or blue)	Feeling of weight gain
Lethargy, exhaustion, mood swings, aggression, panic	Oedema
Confusion	Headache
Craving for sweet foods	Backache
	Nausea

be accepted. The woman's lifestyle should be explored and suggestions made to reduce 'stress'. The predominant symptoms should be identified from the completed charts and treatment directed to specific problems.

Several medications have been tried (*Fig. 30.3*) but, in spite of enthusiastic reports, none has proved better than placebo. If altered serotonin levels are relevant, the use of fluoxetine, a selective serotonin uptake inhibitor, may

Fig. 30.2 Menstrual history diary.

relieve the symptoms in some women. A recent pilot study shows that the drug may be effective.

The concept that PMS is associated with diurnal fluctuations of oestradiol is also being investigated. Three approaches for women who have severe, intractable PMS have been suggested. The first is to prescribe a hormonal contraceptive. The Pill (not a triphasic pill) has been prescribed for some years with varying rates of success in relieving PMS. More recently, transdermal oestrogen patches, or an oestrogen implant, have been prescribed. In these cases the woman has to be protected from the development of endometrial carcinoma from unopposed oestrogen and a progestogen is prescribed cyclically. During the period when the progestogen is taken, symptoms of PMS may recur. The third approach is radical. It is either to suppress ovarian activity with gonadotrophin-releasing hormone agonists or to perform a bilateral oophorectomy (and total hysterectomy).

Perimenstrual syndrome

Women with this syndrome complain of symptoms which occur within 2 days of the onset of menstruation, the earlier part of the menstrual cycle being symptom-free or they may exhibit symptoms of PMS.

The most common mood symptoms are lassitude and headache. The most common physical symptoms are abdominal discomfort and bloating, pelvic pressure and dysmenorrhoea. A few women may develop severe premenstrual migraine. The symptoms may vary in character and intensity in different menstrual cycles. They cease within 48 hours of the onset of menstruation.

Treatment, when requested, consists of prescribing one of the non-steroidal anti-inflammatory drugs.

IRRITABLE BOWEL SYNDROME

A number of PMS sufferers also have irritable bowel symptoms. The irritable bowel syndrome affects 15% of women aged 20–60, although only 1–2% seek medical help.

Normally, bursts of regular, powerful, propulsive contractions move the faeces along the bowel. Patients with irritable bowel syndrome have exaggerated patterns of bowel motility, the bursts of activity occurring at shorter or longer intervals. The cause of the bowel motility dysfunction is unknown, but as there is a strong psychosomatic element, the medical practitioner should determine whether the woman is depressed or anxious or has a sexual problem. The patient complains of abdominal pain (usually left-sided, which is relieved by defaecation), gaseous abdominal distention, an alteration in bowel habit and episodes of diarrhoea alternating with constipation. Investigations should be made to exclude organic disease, and the faeces should be examined for occult blood, giardiasis and other parasites.

Treatment

Treatment is unsatisfactory, unless a clear cause (for example giardiasis) has been detected. Explanation and reassurance that the woman does not have serious bowel disease or cancer is important and supportive psychotherapy may help. Patients should review their diet to ascertain whether any foods cause 'gas'. If the predominant symptom is pain and diarrhoea, loperidine or codeine phosphate may help. Support and explanation are required.

CHRONIC PELVIC PAIN

A few women complain of chronic pain in the lower abdomen and pelvis which fluctuates in intensity and tends to increase in the premenstruum. It may occur on either side of the abdomen and may be felt on different sides at different times. The woman may also complain of deep dyspareunia or a postcoital pelvic ache which may last for 24 hours. The woman may have a history of several episodes of 'pelvic inflammatory disease' which have been diagnosed on clinical findings rather than by laparoscopy and she may have had episodes of pelvic surgery.

The diagnosis is made after excluding organic causes of chronic pelvic pain such as adenomyosis, endometriosis and pelvic inflammatory disease, which are present in about one-third of cases. This indicates that laparoscopy is mandatory to make a diagnosis. The procedure should be made during menstruation to disclose endometriotic lesions deep in the cul-de-sac when the lesion is most likely to be seen. At laparoscopy, although the pelvis shows no evidence of disease, a venogram via the uterus may occasionally show varicosities in the broad ligament.

Fig. 30.3 Medications used to treat PMS	
Alprazolam	0.25mg three times a day
Bromocriptine	2.5mg twice daily (this may relieve breast symptoms but has no other benefit)
Diuretics	Including spirolactone
Dydrogesterone	10mg twice daily
Evening primrose oil	
Fluoxetine	20mg daily from day 3 of menstrual cycle
Mefenamic acid*	250mg four times a day (this may relieve the symptoms of PMS)
Oestradiol skin patches	100–200µg twice weekly
Oral monophasic contraceptives	
Progesterone	(vaginal suppositories) 200-800mg daily
Pyridoxine	(vitamin B$_6$) up to 300mg a day (a dose which may produce peripheral neuropathy)

*This drug is prescribed from 2 days before symptoms are expected until the onset of menstruation

Two studies in the USA showed that over half of the women who had chronic pelvic pain had been severely sexually abused (penetration or other contact with the patient's vagina or anus) before the age of 15 and 42% had also been physically abused. These issues are worth exploring.

In some cases chronic pelvic pain is associated with an ovarian remnant which was left behind after hysterectomy and bilateral oophorectomy.

Treatment

The investigations themselves may constitute a form of treatment as, in one study of 60 women in whom laparoscopy showed no pathology, 90% of the patients assessed 6 months later said that, since the laparoscopy, they had no pelvic pain or that there was much less pain.

The woman's psychological, marital and psychosexual problems need to be explored and supportive psychotherapy offered. If the woman asks for medications, medroxyprogesterone in a dose of 30mg a day may be prescribed. An alternative is to prescribe danazol 200mg three times daily for 2–3 months, although the side effects may deter the woman from taking this treatment.

Some gynaecologists prescribe antidepressants, particularly selective serotonin reuptake inhibitors (SSRIs), but the evaluation of this treatment has not been made rigorously.

Predominantly physical disorders

DYSMENORRHOEA

Dysmenorrhoea means painful menstruation. Two types are described: primary, or spasmodic dysmenorrhoea; and secondary dysmenorrhoea.

Primary dysmenorrhoea

This form usually starts 2–3 years after the menarche and is maximal between the ages of 15 and 25 years. It decreases with age and, usually, ceases after childbirth. The crampy pains start during the 24 hours before menstruation, and may last 24–36 hours, although they are only severe for the first 24 hours. The cramps are felt in the lower abdomen, but may radiate to the back or down the inner surface of the thighs. In severe cases vomiting or diarrhoea may accompany the cramps.

Spasmodic dysmenorrhoea is experienced by 60–75% of young women. In three-quarters of affected women the cramps are of minor or moderate severity, but in 25% they are severe and incapacitating.

The aetiology of spasmodic dysmenorrhoea has now been clarified. When progesterone is secreted following ovulation, the luteinized endometrium is able to synthesize prostaglandins. If the balance between prostacyclin (which causes vasodilatation and myometrial relaxation), prostaglandin $F_{2\alpha}$ (which causes vasoconstriction and myometrial contraction), and prostaglandin E_2 (which causes myometrial contraction and vasodilatation) is disturbed, causing $PGF_{2\alpha}$ to predominate, myometrial ischaemia (uterine angina) and uterine hypercontractility occur. In addition, vasopressin is involved in dysmenorrhoea. Vasopressin increases prostaglandin synthesis and may act on the uterine arteries directly.

Treatment

Treatment consists of either suppressing ovulation by prescribing an oral contraceptive or prescribing one of the prostaglandin synthetase inhibitors, such as mefenamic acid, ibuprofen, diclofenac sodium or naproxen. There appears to be little difference in their effectiveness.

- Oral contraceptives may be preferred by a woman who is sexually active as the Pill will protect her against an unwanted pregnancy as well as relieving the dysmenorrhoea.
- Non-steroidal anti-inflammatory drugs (NSAIDs) may be preferred by women who do not wish to use hormones and prefer to take medication for as short a time as possible. The chosen medication is taken at the first sign of pain and continued for up to 5 days.

Dysmenorrhoea is relieved in 95% of cases, whether oral contraceptives or NSAIDS are chosen. If the chosen treatment fails to relieve the dysmenorrhoea, an alternative can be tried.

Secondary dysmenorrhoea

Secondary, or acquired dysmenorrhoea is unusual before the age of 25 years and uncommon before the age of 30 years. In most cases the underlying cause is either endometriosis or pelvic inflammatory disease. Typically, the cramps start 2 or more days prior to menstruation, and the pain increases in severity, until late menstruation, when it peaks, taking 2 or more days to cease. The management is that of the primary condition.

Toxic shock syndrome

This syndrome, which is due to an endotoxin released by *Staphylococcus aureus*, may occur in women who use tampons for menstrual protection. The reported annual incidence is fewer than 1:25,000 tampon users. Toxic shock may also occur in men and in children following infected surgical wounds, furuncles or other skin infections. It is characterized by the acute onset of fever higher than 38.9°C, sore throat, headache, aching muscles, dizziness and, sometimes, watery diarrhoea. The woman may develop shock. A rash develops on the skin 3 days after the onset of the disease; later, dandruff-like desquamation of the skin occurs, which is followed a week later by epidermal sloughing of the skin from the hands and feet. Treatment consists of restoring blood volume and prescribing penicillinase-resistant antibiotics such as flucloxacillin. As the syndrome is associated, although rarely, with tampon use, tampons should be changed 4-hourly, and a pad used at night.

Psychosomatic problems after hysterectomy

In recent years, the frequency of hysterectomy has fallen as other methods of treatment for conditions previously treated by hysterectomy have been developed. The psychosomatic effects of the operation depend on the condition which led to the hysterectomy, and the woman's knowledge and attitude to hysterectomy. Some women recover quickly (after the first 24–48 hours when pain may be severe). Other women are mildly or moderately incapacitated for up to 3 months. One-third of women take 3 months to recover fully from the operation, and 20% take longer. Five to ten per cent of women feel well generally but have bowel or bladder symptoms, particularly genuine stress incontinence, which may persist for months.

Although most gynaecologists choose total hysterectomy so that cervical cancer will not develop, there is a small trend back to subtotal hysterectomy in selected cases. The reason for this are:

- The operation is less dangerous as the ureters are avoided.
- The sequelae of bowel and bladder symptoms occur less frequently.
- The woman's sexual response, sexual enjoyment and orgasm are less negatively affected.
- The risk of developing cervical cancer is very small if a woman has had regular cervical smears which have always been normal and she continues to have regular smears. If any cervical cell abnormality is detected it will be early and conisation or other local treatment can be offered.

Some women feel mutilated after hysterectomy and develop an anxiety state. This is more likely to occur if the woman believes that her body image, her femininity and her sexual attractiveness are reduced after the operation. The anxiety that her sexual attractiveness will be decreased follows misconceptions about hysterectomy. These include notions that:

- A woman will be unable to have or enjoy sexual intercourse because her vagina will be shorter.
- She will become obese.
- She will be severely depressed after the operation.
- She will become postmenopausal.

The patient should be reassured about the first two misconceptions before the operation takes place. The third misconception is untrue. There is no evidence that hysterectomy increases clinical depression, unless the woman had psychiatric morbidity prior to surgery. The fourth misconception is only likely to be true if she has her ovaries removed at the operation, or if the surgeon has damaged the ovarian blood supply. There exists data to the effect that up to 20% of women aged 40–45 experience ovarian failure within 3 years of hysterectomy. However, this and menopausal symptoms following bilateral oophorectomy at the time of hysterectomy can be eliminated if the woman is offered hormone replacement treatment (see page 321).

The question of bilateral oophorectomy of normal ovaries at the time of hysterectomy is contentious. Ovarian extirpation is not usually carried out in women aged under 45 but some gynaecologists perform it in older women. Their reasons for oophorectomy are first, that if the ovaries are left, 1 in 1000 women will develop ovarian cancer, and second, the ovaries have no function after the menopause. The woman should make her own decision, after discussion with her doctors and after she has had time to think it over and seek other advice if she wishes.

Hysterectomy is safe today, but it is not without mortality. A nationwide epidemiological study in Denmark in 1990, of hysterectomy for non-cancerous conditions, where no major 'co-surgery' took place, showed that the 30-day mortality rate, although only 16 per 10,000 cases, was four times as high as for a reference group. There is also some evidence that hysterectomy with oophorectomy under the age of 50 is associated with an increase in the risk of myocardial infarction later in life. This problem will be reduced if hormone replacement treatment is started following surgery. This finding suggests that if an alternative to hysterectomy is available (as it is in cases of dysfunctional uterine bleeding) this should be tried first.

To reduce the psychological and physical problems which may occur after hysterectomy, the attending doctors, whether specialist or GPs, have an obligation to talk with the woman and her partner. The reason for the operation should be explained, its extent described, alternative treatments discussed and problems which may arise mentioned. In most cases the woman should be given time to think about the discussion and to ask further questions, if she has any, before the operation is performed.

CHAPTER 31

Human sexuality and psychosexual problems

In the past three decades more people than ever before have been able to learn about human sexuality and the human sexual response. Discussion about human sexuality has become more open.

Sexual problems within a relationship are not uncommon and more women and men now feel able to seek advice about them. Often the first reference point is the person's general practitioner. General practitioners, like other people, have inhibitions about sexuality and a variety of values about sexual behaviour. These inhibitions and values are based on the person's religious beliefs, and upbringing and on values obtained from parents. Some medical practitioners are uncomfortable about discussing sexual problems with their patients; others are able to listen and give advice in a non-judgemental manner. If a medical practitioner is unable to do the latter he/she should refer the patient to a colleague and not impose his/her own sexual values on the patient. If the medical practitioner feels able to treat sexual dysfunctions, he/she should try to determine the patient's sexual values and try to solve the problem within that value system.

Sexual advice can only be given if the practitioner has some knowledge of sexuality and sexual behaviours.

Sexuality

Sexuality may be defined as the sum of a person's inherited characteristics, knowledge, experience, attitudes and behaviour as they relate to being a female or a male. It includes those ways of behaving which enrich the personality and increase love between people. Human sexuality is as much psychological as physical and involves feelings as well as physicality. It includes communication with the other person, not talking at him or her or remaining silent, but listening and interpreting. It also involves touching and exploring each other's bodies to learn the textures and surfaces, and the sight and smell of another person.

Sexuality includes the sexual drives, which is the sum of the desire to have sex and the ability to accomplish the act. Sexual drive varies considerably between different people. In some, a low drive is due to constitutional factors such as ill health or advanced age. In others, the low drive is due to a traumatic sexual experience in childhood or adolescence. Recently, more women are reporting that they have been sexually assaulted in childhood or early adolescence and this may be the basis of a fear of sex and a low sexual drive.

During adult life the intensity of the sexual drive is maximal in the years up to the age of 40 and tends to lessen after this time, but there are considerable variations. Problems arise if the sexual drive of two partners is markedly different.

Human sexual response

The physiology of the human sexual response was not described until 40 years ago, in the studies of Masters and Johnson. For descriptive purposes they divided the sexual response in women and men into five phases, although the distinction between each phase is often blurred and one phase tends to merge into the next provided the appropriate stimulation occurs.

The phases are:
* Sexual desire.
* Sexual arousal or excitement.
* Plateau.
* Orgasm.
* Resolution.

Sexual desire is stimulated by the thought, sight, touch or smell of another person. It may be suppressed or merge into the arousal phase.

In the *arousal phase*, a man's penis becomes erect and a woman's vagina becomes lubricated. In this phase, sexual enjoyment is increased if the couple pleasure each other sexually by cuddling, stroking and exploring each other's body with fingers, tongue, lips and thighs. Arousal is increased further if the erogenous zones of the body, a woman's clitoral area, breasts and vulva and a man's penis and scrotum, are stimulated. A woman's breasts become bigger due to engorgement with blood and her nipples become erect. Her clitoris increases in width and becomes more sensitive to touch and her labia and the lower part of her vagina become congested and softer and thicker. The subvaginal tissues become increasingly congested and fluid transudes between the vaginal cells to increase vaginal lubrication.

During the following *plateau phase*, the sexual pleasure is intensified and the partners desire to have penile–vaginal, penile–oral or penile–anal penetration. The thrusting movement of the penis in the vagina, or its oral stimulation, causes an *orgasm* in the man with the ejaculation of seminal fluid. In 90% of women, the thrusting of the man's penis in her vagina indirectly, or the digital or oral stimulation of her clitoral area directly, leads to orgasm. Fifty per cent of sexually active women reach orgasm when the clitoral area is stimulated by finger or tongue; 25% reach orgasm during penile thrusting in the vagina; 15% of women can achieve multiple orgasms and the remaining 10% are unable to achieve orgasm, although they may enjoy their partner's pleasure.

Orgasm provides an intense feeling of pleasure. During orgasm, the perineal muscles, the medial fibres of the levator ani and the sphincter ani muscles contract rhythmically and involuntarily, as do the muscles surrounding the vagina. Many other muscle groups, particularly those of the back, contract at the height of the orgasm and a deep feeling of ecstasy (in its original sense) and relaxation follows.

In the *resolution phase*, both sexual partners are relaxed. In the initial moments, the clitoris and the penis are exquisitely sensitive to touch, but this passes rapidly and the tissues of the lower genital tract, in both sexes, decongest; the penis becoming flaccid, the clitoris small and the woman's external genitals and vagina decongested.

The physiological basis of the observed changes during sexual response occurs in two parts. Both are mediated by psychic or physical sexual stimulation or, more usually, by both. Both parts can be inhibited by subconscious influences to a greater or lesser degree.

The phases of the sexual response up to orgasm are mediated by the parasympathetic nerves, which lead to vasodilatation and vasocongestion of the genital organs. In a man, this leads to an inflow of blood into the cavernous spaces of the penile cylinders and an inhibition of outflow from the cylinders. The result is an erection. In a woman, the changes lead to the development of congestive 'cushions' around the lower part of the vagina and to vaginal lubrication.

Failure of sexual arousal prevents these changes with resulting erectile failure in a man, and general sexual dysfunction in a woman.

The second, orgasmic phase is mediated by the sympathetic nerves, the stimulation of which leads to the clonic muscle contraction of the pelvic and other muscles. In a man, these contractions lead to ejaculation and, in both sexes, to the more general muscle contractions. The feeling of pleasure experienced by both sexes appears to have its origin in a 'sex centre' in the thalamic and limbic areas of the old cortex, which are closely related anatomically to the pleasure centres in the paleocortex. The messages which stimulate these centres are initiated from clitoral and vaginal stimulation in women and penile stimulation in men. Failure of the sympathetic element to proceed in an orderly fashion results in premature or restricted ejaculation in a man. Failure of the sensations invoked in the clitoris and vagina to be transmitted to the brain and interpreted as pleasurable is the reason for orgasm failing to occur in women.

Sexual dysfunctions

Most sexual dysfunctions arise from a poor relationship with the partner, ignorance about sexuality and sexual technique, a low sex drive, or performance anxiety. In addition, physical illness, the fear that sex will aggravate an existing illness, excessive alcohol use or clinical depression are factors.

As men and women age, changes occur in their sexual desire and sexual response. These are considered on page 321.

Women have three main sexual dysfunctions:
- Inhibited sexual desire.
- Failure to achieve orgasm.
- Dyspareunia (including vaginismus).

In *Figure 31.1*, the sexual dysfunctions which occur in men and women are listed.

INHIBITED SEXUAL DESIRE (HYPO-ACTIVE SEXUAL DESIRE DISORDER)

Women with this disorder do not have sexual fantasies and have no desire for sexual activity. Its prevalence in society is not known but may be as high as 10%. Allied to this disorder is a failure to become sexually aroused either by sexual fantasies or when sexually teased by the partner, and the woman may find the teasing distasteful. This may not mean that the woman will reject sexual advances by a partner, but that she will obtain little or no enjoyment from the contact.

Inhibited sexual desire, or inhibited sexual arousal, may have been present since puberty or may occur after some months or years of sexual activity. In the latter case, it may be the manifestation of a deteriorating relationship or a sign of depression. If both partners have inhibited sexual desire, problems are not perceived but, if one has inhibited sexual desire and the other has a normal or raised desire, the problem becomes manifest. The condition appears to affect more women than men.

FAILURE TO ACHIEVE ORGASM (ANORGASMIA)

Orgasm in females may be achieved during penile thrusting, but not usually simultaneously with the man's orgasm, or it may only be achieved if the woman's clitoral area is stimulated by finger or tongue. In both cases, orgasm is reached and the woman cannot be considered to be anorgasmic. However, some women (and men) believe that unless a woman reaches orgasm during penile thrusting, preferably simultaneously with the man, she is sexually dysfunctional.

APAREUNIA (VAGINISMUS) AND DYSPAREUNIA

In apareunia, the woman is unable to accept a penis penetrating her vagina. The condition may be due to vaginal atresia or to vulvovaginal infection. In some cases, the problem lies with the man, who is unable to acquire or sustain an erection, although this condition would be classified as erectile failure.

In most cases, the problem is psychosomatic, the woman involuntarily tightening the muscles which surround the vaginal introitus and the lower one-third of the vagina. This is termed *vaginismus* and, in severe cases, the woman is unable to accept an examiner's finger into her vagina, so marked is the muscle spasm. Vaginismus may be transient or permanent, and affects between 1 and 3% of women aged 15–50.

Although the woman is unable to have sexual intercourse, she may be able to enjoy masturbating her partner, but she avoids any contact with her own external genitals.

The cause of vaginismus lies in inadequate or faulty sex education, particularly in a belief that sex is 'dirty', or a fear based on ignorance that the penis may painfully damage the woman's body. Occasionally, vaginismus can be traced to a sexual assault during childhood, or to a painful, brutal initial experience of sexual intercourse.

Dyspareunia, or painful intercourse, is shown as recurrent and persistent pain during or after sexual intercourse. It usually has an organic component. Examples are vulvo-vaginal infections, a painful episiotomy scar, atrophic vulvovaginitis, endometriosis, pelvic inflammatory disease, and ovarian cysts or tumours. Organic disorders must be excluded before the condition is ascribed to psychosomatic factors. These are usually found in cases of prolonged dyspareunia. The aetiology of psychogenic dyspareunia is unclear, but lack of sexual knowledge, guilt about sexuality, or a childhood sexual assault have been postulated. The problem is aggravated when the woman fails to be aroused sexually and fails to lubricate.

GENERAL MANAGEMENT STRATEGIES

The objectives of treatment are to alter an existing destructive attitude to sexuality; to reduce or resolve any underlying interpersonal sexual conflict, anxiety or fear; and to help a couple create an environment in which sexuality is perceived as a mutually pleasurable experience. To achieve these objectives, the counsellor seeks to help the woman examine her attitudes to her sexuality and to discover what stimulates her sexually; to correct any false ideas or myths about sexuality; and to help her make her partner aware of her sexual feelings, needs, and desires, so that they can better express their needs to each other.

The management of sexual dysfunctions in women begins by the medical practitioner obtaining a comprehensive general and sexual history. The general history should pay particular attention to physical illness and psychiatric problems such as depression. The sexual history must be obtained with great sensitivity. During the history, the medical practitioner explores the current relationship and seeks to find out the woman's attitudes to her body, to menstruation and to her feelings about her sexuality.

This can be difficult and it may help to use the acronym LEPERS:
- Listen for hidden signals.
- Explore the patient's attitudes to her sexuality, sexual activities and responses.
- Provide information about the female and male body.
- Examine relationships.
- Reduce the patient's anxiety.
- Suggest strategies for helping the patient, such as giving permission and prescribing specific treatment, which may differ for different problems as discussed later.

The question of whether the partner should be involved depends on the sexual problem elucidated and, more particularly, on the patient's wishes.

Fig. 31.1 Sexual dysfunction		
	Clinical syndrome	
	Male	**Female**
Inhibited sexual desire	No arousal	No arousal
Fear of sexual (genital) activity	Primary erectile failure (impotence)	Vaginismus
Impairment of sexual arousal. Absence or inadequate vasocongestion* due to failure to respond to erotic stimulation because of anxiety, guilt, or fear of injury	Reduced libido and secondary erectile failure (impotence)	Reduced libido
Impairment or failure of orgasm. Extremely rapid, or absence of clonic rhythmic contractions of pelvic musculature due to inhibition of genital tactile or psychic erotic stimulation	Premature ejaculation Restricted ejaculation	Orgastic dysfunction
* In the male, penile erection; in the female, vaginal lubrication and perivaginal swelling		

MANAGEMENT OF SPECIFIC SEXUAL PROBLEMS

Although the general management of sexual problems is the same for all the sexual dysfunctions, the different categories of female sexual dysfunction require different strategies (*Fig. 31.2*).

Inhibited sexual desire

The most used approach is to involve both partners when possible. The partners attend together and are helped to communicate better with each other, through words and actions. If they are poorly informed, the therapist helps them learn the anatomy and physiology of sexual intercourse. The main part of treatment is for the couple to perform a series of graded 'tasks' at short intervals over a period of weeks. The tasks are undertaken at home in a relaxed atmosphere. In the first stage, lasting one week, the couple set aside at least 30 minutes each day for non-genital pleasuring. The man fondles, caresses and massages his partner at her direction, avoiding her breasts and genitals, and responding if she says that she does not like a particular area being touched. The couple then change roles.

At the end of the seven days, if the couple have made steady progress, they move to the second phase of genital

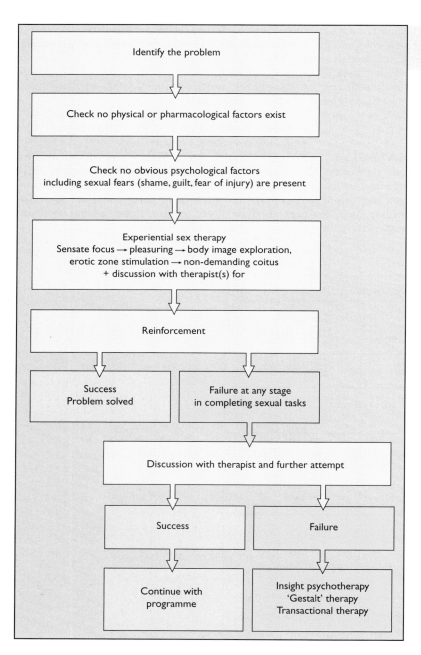

Fig. 31.2 Management of sexual problems.

pleasuring. In this phase the couple can touch, massage, kiss or lick each other's bodies and genitals. During the touching the active participant inquires: 'Do you like me touching you like this?', 'Does it feel good?' and 'How would you like me to do it?' After about 15 minutes the couple exchange roles.

The couple reach the third phase when they feel that they are confident that they have enjoyed the second phase. In the third phase, they proceed through the first two phases fairly quickly and then attempt sexual intercourse, preferably with the woman astride the man facing him so that she can introduce his penis into her vagina at her speed.

The couple see the therapist at intervals so that their progress can be reviewed and any problems discussed.

Anorgasmia

If a woman wishes to increase her ability to achieve orgasm, or has never achieved orgasm, several techniques are available. Of these masturbation has produced the most successes. Many young women have masturbated but have felt guilty about it and have not reached orgasm. Others have never masturbated. Learning to achieve orgasm by masturbation often cures anorgasmia, but the woman needs to supplement this with discussion and counselling with a trained practitioner. For masturbation to be effective in reaching orgasm, the woman has to give herself time, privacy and be able to fantasize, view or read erotic literature as she masturbates, either using her fingers or a vibrator.

Apareunia and dyspareunia

Any physical cause of these sexual dysfunctions must be identified, discussed with the woman and treated, if treatment is possible. If it is not, suggestions may be made about techniques with which the woman may better enjoy her sex. For example, if she has a chronic pelvic infection she may find a different position for sexual intercourse more pleasurable. If sexual intercourse is painful, whatever position the couple adopt, she may obtain sensual pleasure by body caressing and clitoral stimulation, whilst giving her partner pleasure by oral sex or by stimulating his sexual organs.

If the woman has vaginismus, the therapist reinforces the general strategies discussed earlier by stressing that she is not 'small made' and that she can learn to relax her perineal muscles. She may be asked to try to insert a lubricated finger in her vagina, and given instructions to continue with the exercise at home. If her relationship with her partner is good, she may ask him to insert his finger. Once one finger is accepted, she progresses to the insertion two and then three fingers or, if she prefers, a series of graded metal dilators. These steps require reinforcement and encouragement by the therapist who should be visited weekly. Once she has introduced three fingers with comfort and without muscle spasm occurring, she may be ready to sit above her partner and to

control his penis so that it touches the entrance to her vagina. In progressive steps, on different days, she inserts his penis into the entrance, then deeper into her vagina. When this is comfortable and accepted, she may move rhythmically with his penis deep in her vagina, and then permit him to thrust. Finally, having become confident that intercourse is painless, she will be able to have sexual intercourse with the man on top.

EVALUATION OF TREATMENT OUTCOMES

There is much confusion about treatment outcomes as many of the patients seen have been selected and the data collection uncontrolled. A literature survey suggests that 50–60% of women who have inhibited sexual desire or arousal are cured; 60–70% of women who have anorgasmia are cured; and over 75% of women who have vaginismus or psychosomatic dyspareunia enjoy normal sexual intercourse.

Other sexual problems

SEXUAL ABUSE

Sexual abuse includes incest and rape and, in the medical literature, the two terms are included in sexual abuse. It is defined as 'unlawful carnal knowledge of a woman without her consent by force, fear or fraud'. In over three-quarters of cases of rape, the offender is known to the woman. Evidence has been published that between 8 and 12% of women are abused during pregnancy, in addition to those who are 'battered' by their partner. Statistics about the prevalence of rape are difficult to obtain as fewer than one-third of rapes are reported, but about one woman in 200 has been raped or suffered attempted rape in a year.

A woman who has been raped needs to be treated with great care and consideration when she presents to a medical practitioner. In most cases, the woman attends a hospital or a 'rape crisis centre' where staff are trained to handle the woman's emotional and physical problems.

The woman should be listened to sympathetically and non-judgementally as she tells her story. She should then be examined. It is important to explain, during the examination, what is being done and why it is being done. The presence of scratches or bruises on the woman's arms or body should be looked for and the vulva examined for the presence of blood, bruising or seminal staining. A vaginal inspection is made and a vaginal smear taken to detect spermatozoa. The woman should be asked to return later, so that she can be tested to exclude gonorrhoea and so that serological tests can be made to exclude infection, particularly syphilis and HIV infection. If the rape took place at the time of ovulation, the woman should be given the choice of taking postcoital contraception, the 'morning after pill', or asked to return if she fails to menstruate.

It is important to record carefully all findings.

SEXUAL ABUSE IN CHILDHOOD AND ADOLESCENCE

A particular group of females require special consideration. These are children and young women under the age of 16 years. Data from several Western countries indicate that between 5 and 30% have been abused sexually, and repeatedly in half of them. Only the breasts or genitals were touched or fondled in half of the girls but, in 20%, the abuser made the girl practise fellatio, or was forced to have genital or anal intercourse. In over 40% of cases, the abuser was a family member.

Whilst most of the young women overcome their disgust and fear as they grow older; women who have been sexually abused in childhood or adolescence are three times as likely to seek psychiatric help as an adult and, if married, are three times as likely to be divorced. The reasons for seeking psychological and psychiatric help are many and common problems are depression, chronic pelvic pain, eating disorders and sexual problems. Women presenting to a doctor with what are perceived as psychosocial problems should be questioned sensitively about sexual abuse and help offered.

HIRSUTISM

The development of body hair is, to a large extent, genetic. Chinese people, for example, tend to have little body hair, whilst southern Europeans tend to have considerable amounts of body hair. Hirsutism is defined as a woman having increased, or excessive, body hair, particularly on her face, breasts or legs compared with other women of her ethnic group. Current fashion in most developed countries has decreed that, to be attractive, a woman should have no hair in her armpits, or on her body. Hirsutism is perceived as diminishing a woman's attractiveness and her femininity.

In most cases hirsutism is due to the benign androgen excess syndrome, which shows as raised levels of free testosterone and of the final degradation product, androstenedione glucuronide. Hirsutism is associated with polycystic ovarian syndrome in about half of the cases.

The diagnosis is reached after excluding other, uncommon, causes of hirsutism, such as Cushing's syndrome, congenital adrenal hyperplasia and virilism. These disorders account for only 1% of all cases of hirsutism. It is important to exclude virilism as this condition is usually due to virilizing ovarian or adrenal tumours. In affected women, as well as hirsutism, the clitoris is enlarged, the breasts are atrophic, the hairline recedes, the voice deepens and the muscle mass increases.

In the absence of virilism, few laboratory tests are needed. Blood should be taken to measure free testosterone, and androstenedione glucuronide. A transvaginal ultrasound test may be made, as some hirsute women also have polycystic ovaries.

Management of hirsutism

The management of benign androgen excess is broad. The medical practitioner should enquire about any psychosexual problems and explore the woman's concerns about her appearance. Information should be offered about cosmetic aids, such as bleaching, shaving (which contrary to popular belief does not accelerate hair growth), waxing, the use of depilatory creams and electrolysis.

Treatment

If the woman does not wish to use these methods, or they have been used and have not relieved her, several drugs are available to treat hirsutism:

- *Oral contraceptives*, particularly those containing one of the 'new generation' progestogens (such as Marvelon), often reduce the hirsutism. The oral contraceptive containing 35μg ethinyl oestradiol and 2mg cyproterone (Diane) is effective for mild cases.
- *Cyproterone acetate* in a dose of 100mg from day 5 to day 14 of the menstrual cycle, with ethinyl oestradiol (30μg from day 5 to day 25 of the cycle) to maintain a regular menstrual cycle. An alternative is to give cyproterone 300mg as a single intramuscular injection on day 5 of the menstrual cycle. Cyproterone is a competitive inhibitor of androgens at peripheral receptors and may reduce androgen synthesis. It takes about 3 months' use of cyproterone before any reduction of hirsutism is noted and the drug should be continued for 9 months to achieve the maximum effect. About 20% of women fail to respond, and a similar proportion develop side effects, if the larger-dose regimens are chosen. The side effects include lassitude, increase in body weight, loss of libido (10%) and breast discomfort. Fewer side effects occur if the oral contraceptive pill containing cyproterone is used.
- *Spironolactone*, given in a dose of 200mg a day in divided doses, reduces the amount of hirsutism over a 3-month period and, if continued, maintains the reduction. Spironolactone works in the same way as cyproterone. There is some concern that spironolactone, given for prolonged periods, may induce tumour formation. In the short term, it causes polymenorrhoea (a shorter menstrual cycle) in some women. If the woman becomes pregnant and the fetus is male, it may be feminized. For both these reasons, a woman taking spironolactone should also take an oral contraceptive.
- *Gonadotrophin-releasing hormone (GnRH)* agonists. If the above treatments fail to relieve the hirsutism, GnRH agonists given subcutaneously every 28 days with 'add back' oestrogen for a few days each month may be used instead.

CHAPTER 32

Conception control

The availability of safe modern contraceptives has enabled women to avoid having an unwanted pregnancy, and couples to space their children. Spacing children to intervals of 2 or more years, improves a woman's health.

Contraceptive choices now available permit the woman, or the couple, to choose the most appropriate contraceptive for their particular circumstances. Younger women usually prefer oral contraceptives or expect their male partners to use condoms, whilst the older woman is more inclined to choose the intra-uterine device or a permanent method of birth control such as tubal ligation or a vasectomy in her partner (*Fig. 32.1*).

Before choosing a particular contraceptive most people want to know its effectiveness in preventing pregnancy, its safety and the side effects associated with its use. A method of evaluating the effectiveness of the various contraceptive methods is the *Pearl Index*, which calculates the unintended pregnancy rate from the formula:

$$\frac{\text{The number of unintended pregnancies}}{\text{Total months of exposure to pregnancy}} \times 1200$$

The result is expressed as the *failure rate per 100 woman years (HWY)*.

In *Figure 32.2* the use of contraceptive methods worldwide is shown and, in *Figure 32.3*, the effectiveness of various available contraceptive methods in preventing pregnancy is shown.

Some women find it embarrassing to consult a medical practitioner about contraception and a sensitive doctor will do everything possible to diminish that embarrassment. The ability to listen to and to talk with the woman is of great importance.

The doctor should take a general history, a menstrual history and a sexual history in a non-judgemental way. With this information, the doctor will be better able to help the woman decide which method of contraception she would prefer.

A gynaecological examination should be made, although if the woman is teenaged and has not previously had a

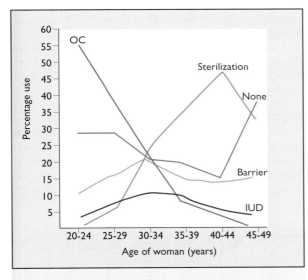

Fig. 32.1 *Methods of fertility control in Britain.*

Fig. 32.2 *Use of contraceptive methods by women worldwide*

- Sterilization. Used by 200 million women in 1994. Most popular in Asia (31% of all contraceptive users) and Latin America (25%).

- IUDs. Used by 112 million women, or about 25% of all contraceptive users. Most popular in Asia and Arab countries.

- The Pill. Used by around 70 million women, 50 million in developing countries, 25–30% of all contraceptive users in sub-Saharan Africa, Latin America and Europe, but only 8% in Asia.

- Injectables. More than 10 million women, 2.3 % of all contraceptive users (13% in sub-Saharan Africa).

- Implants. Used by 1.5 million women, the majority in developing countries (1.3 million in Indonesia).

- Condom. About 25 million condom users, although this may be a low estimate in view of AIDS prevention.

vaginal examination it can be deferred to a subsequent visit, when the woman may be less embarrassed. If she has not had a Pap smear taken in the previous year, the doctor should suggest that this is done, explaining how the smear is taken and the reason for it.

Fig. 32.3 Ranking of contraceptive methods by rate of effectiveness		Failure rates per 100HWY
Group A	**Most effective**	
	Tubal ligation/vasectomy	0.005–0.04
	Combined oral	0.005–0.30
	Sequential oral	0.20–0.56
Group B	**Highly effective**	
	IUD	0.5–3.5
	Continuous progestogen	1.5–2.3
	Diaphragm or condom and cream	
	All users	4.0–7.0
	Highly motivated	1.5–3.0
	Periodic abstinence	
	All users	10.0–30.0
	Highly motivated	2.5–5.0
Group C	**Less effective**	
	Coitus interruptus	30.0–40.0
	Vaginal foam or cream	30.0–40.0
Group D	**Least effective**	
	Postcoital douche	45.0
	Prolonged breastfeeding	45.0

Reversible methods of contraception used by the couple

PERIODIC ABSTINENCE

It is known that, if a woman has a menstrual cycle of normal duration, ovulation occurs 14±3 days before the start of her next menstruation. It is also known that pregnancy is most likely to occur if intercourse takes place in the 5 days before ovulation or on the day of ovulation. This interval is called the *fertile period*. This has led to the idea of *periodic abstinence* during the fertile period as a method of birth control.

The woman is taught to detect the presence of mucus at the vaginal entrance each morning (before any sexual arousal). Three types of mucus can be detected and, from this, the days on which sexual intercourse can take place can be calculated whilst avoiding, to some extent, the chance of an unwanted pregnancy occurring (*Fig. 32.4*). The compliance of the man is essential if pregnancy is to be avoided.

Because of the difficulties in assessing the mucus and the need for the man to cooperate fully, the pregnancy rate varies from 10 to 30 per HWY for all couples but, for motivated couples, it is 2.5–5.0 per HWY.

COITUS INTERRUPTUS

Withdrawal, or coitus interruptus, is the oldest form of birth control, apart from induced abortion. With the development of more modern contraceptives its frequency has declined, but it is still the favoured method among some sections of society. Its reliability for preventing pregnancy depends on

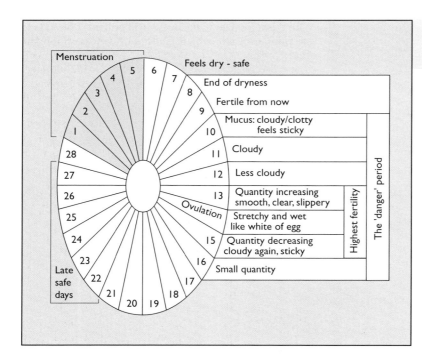

Fig. 32.4 Periodic abstinence: the mucus (ovulation) method.

the ability of the man to recognize the pre-ejaculatory phase and his agility in withdrawing his penis from the woman's vagina before ejaculation. Because of these constraints, the efficacy of coitus interruptus in preventing an unwanted pregnancy is rather low (see Figure 32.3).

Reversible methods of contraception used by men

CONDOM

Modern condoms, which are made of latex, prelubricated by adding silicone and supplied in hermetically sealed aluminium sachets, are cheap, efficient and hardly noticeable to either partner. Their advantages are that they can be obtained from a variety of outlets without a doctor's prescription and that they offer some protection against sexually transmitted diseases, including the human papilloma virus, chlamydia and the human immunodeficiency virus (HIV). The disadvantage of condoms is that many younger

Fig. 32.5 *Information for patients: how to use a condom. (a) Open the packet carefully, and do not unroll the condom before putting it on. (b) Semen can leak out soon after the penis becomes erect, prior to ejaculation. To prevent pregnancy or infection, the condom must be put on before any sexual contact takes place. (c) Ensure that the condom is the right way up. Squeeze the teat on the tip of the condom and hold it against the tip of the penis. (d) Unroll the condom all the way to the base of the penis. (e) After ejaculation, the penis should be withdrawn before the erection is totally lost. When withdrawing, hold onto the condom. (f) Do not allow the condom or penis to come into contact with the woman's genital area, and carefully dispose of the condom.*

men refuse to use them in the belief that they reduce sexual pleasure and may burst during use.

The pregnancy rate following condom use relates to usage, to the way the condom is put on the penis and how it is held on after penile detumescence. The doctor should explain how a condom should be used if consulted by a woman or her partner (*Fig. 32.5*).

Reversible methods of contraception used by women

Women have more choices of reversible or temporary contraception than men. Women may choose:
- *Barrier methods* – the vaginal diaphragm, the cervical cap, the vaginal sponge and the female condom.
- *Hormonal contraceptives* – the Pill, injectables and implants.
- *The intra-uterine device (IUD)*.

BARRIER METHODS
Vaginal diaphragm and the cervical cap
The vaginal diaphragm and the cervical cap consist of a thin plastic or latex dome attached to a circular flat, coiled or arching spring rim. The vaginal diaphragm is easier to use than the cervical cap as the diaphragm fits diagonally across the vagina. The correct size of the diaphragm is determined by a medical practitioner examining the woman vaginally, by inserting the index and middle fingers as far as they will go into the posterior vaginal fornix, and noting how far the index finger reaches behind the symphysis pubis. The diaphragm is made in sizes from 50mm to 100mm, in 5mm steps. After measuring the vagina, the doctor inserts a series of diaphragms or fitting rings until the most appropriate size is found.

Using a diaphragm, or a cervical cap, requires practise and, after teaching a woman how to use it (*Fig. 32.6*), many doctors ask the woman to learn the technique at home and return with the diaphragm, or cap, in her vagina for checking.

When the woman is confident about the technique, she inserts the diaphragm each day or at any convenient time before sexual intercourse is anticipated. It should not be removed for cleaning until at least 6 hours after the last ejaculation. Some women choose to smear a nonoxynol-9 spermicidal cream around the rim, but whether this adds to the effectiveness of the diaphragm in preventing pregnancy is uncertain. It is known to destroy the HIV, to some extent, which is a benefit.

If a woman chooses a cervical cap, she must have a healthy, short cervix. Fitting is carried out by a medical practitioner. The technique of insertion and removal is same as that of the vaginal diaphragm.

Vaginal sponges
These devices incorporate an active spermicide in a polyurethane mushroom-shaped sponge. The sponge is inserted before sexual intercourse and is not removed until 6 hours after the last ejaculation.

Female condom

This device is a tube of polyurethane plastic, about 15cm long and 7cm in diameter, that is closed at one end (*Fig. 32.7*). The lower, open end is surrounded by a soft ring, which holds it against the vulva. A problem is that the female condom may be pushed into the vagina during intercourse or slip out together with the penis.

HORMONAL CONTRACEPTIVES

Hormonal contraceptives contain oestrogen and a progestogen (combined oral contraceptives) or progestogen alone. Oestrogen suppresses follicle-stimulating hormone (FSH)

secretion and reduces luteinizing hormone (LH) secretion and, in this way, prevents ovulation. The progestogen further suppresses LH release, alters the quality of the cervical mucus, rendering it less penetrable to sperm, and produces endometrial changes culminating in glandular exhaustion. Importantly, the progestogen also permits a withdrawal bleed which is regular in onset, short in duration and light in amount.

Combined oral contraceptive (COC)

These formulations are chosen by most contraceptive users as they are effective in preventing pregnancy and are easy to take. Most types of currently available COCs contain less than 50μg of ethinyl oestradiol per dose (one type contains mestranol, which is rapidly converted into ethinyl oestradiol), and one of several progestogens. These COCs are called 'low-dose COCs'.

Most of the COCs prescribed are monophasic or triphasic. In the monophasic formulations, the amount of oestrogen and progestogen is constant in each tablet throughout the cycle. The triphasic formulation tablets contain varying doses of both oestrogen and progestogen. The total progestogen in a cycle is less and the total oestrogen is more than in the monophasic formulations. The two sequential (biphasic) formulations and a formulation containing

a Spermicidal cream applied around inside and on dome

b Diaphragm held ready for insertion

c A convenient position for insertion

d Correct placement

Anterior rim behind symphysis pubis

Dome uppermost

Posterior rim in posterior fornix

Finger checking that cervix is covered

e Removal by hooking out with a finger

Fig. 32.6 The use of vaginal diaphragm.

Fig. 32.7 The female condom.

cyproterone acetate have a limited use; they are prescribed for women who have acne or who are markedly hirsute.

The concept behind the development of the triphasic formulations was to reduce the effects of the Pill on lipid metabolism. Oestrogen increases high-density lipoprotein cholesterol (HDL-c) and reduces low-density lipoprotein (LDL-c); whilst the first generation progestogens decrease the level of HDL-c. Combined, as in the Pill, total cholesterol is not increased, but HDL-c is reduced slightly (compared with oestrogen alone), the decrease being related to the total dose of progestogen. The triphasic formulations reduce the total quantity of progestogen given in a cycle and, thus, reduce the decrease in the circulating levels of HDL-c.

Oral contraceptives containing the newer (second generation) progestogens, such as desogestrel and gestodene, do not reduce HDL-c and, thus, can be given in a monophasic preparation. They are replacing the older COCs.

Contra-indications to the prescription of COCs

The International Planned Parenthood Federation recommends that the following groups of women should not choose COCs if they have:

- A past or present history of venous or arterial thrombosis, ischaemic heart disease or severe hypertension.
- Familial hyperlipidaemia.
- Any condition favouring cerebral ischaemia, particularly severe focal migraine.
- Acute liver disease and some forms of chronic liver disease.
- Oestrogen-dependent cancer.
- Undiagnosed per vaginam bleeding.

Non-contraceptive benefits of COCs

As COCs are the most used form of contraception in the world, it is important to note the non-contraceptive benefits of the preparations:

- Most menstrual cycle disorders are reduced including menstrual blood loss, menorrhagia, dysmenorrhoea (by 80% or more) and the premenstrual syndrome. However, about 1% of COC users develop amenorrhoea.
- Pelvic infection (pelvic inflammatory disease) is reduced among women who have several sexual partners or whose partner has, or has had, several sexual partners.
- Benign breast disease and benign breast tumours are reduced by up to 50%.

- Breast carcinoma is not increased.
- Functional ovarian cysts are less common.
- Uterine myomata are less common, as is endometriosis.
- Endometrial and ovarian cancers are reduced.
- Rheumatoid arthritis appears to be reduced among COC users who have taken the medication for less than 5 years.

Clinical side effects of COCs

The two main areas of concern are circulatory disease and certain cancers. Other clinical conditions may also occur.

Circulatory disease

Thromboembolism is slightly more common among COC users, although the risk is small (from 4–6 to 10–15 per 100,000 women per year). The increase is due to an increase in fibrinogen concentration and of factors II, VII, IX, X and XII, and a decrease in antithrombin III. There is a concomitant increase in fibrinolysis but it does not equal the coagulation changes. The risk is increased in smokers and in obese women. If these two variables are excluded the relative risk of developing thromboembolism in a woman taking low-dose COCs is small. A worrying WHO report, in 1996, suggested that oral cotraceptives (OCs) containing third-generation progestogens (desogestrel and gestodene) may double the relative risk of a woman developing deep vein thrombosis or pulmonary embolus. A critique of the study suggests that the increased relative risk is due to bias in sampling, and subsequent reports have found no difference in the risk of DVT between second and third generation progestogens. Women should be informed that the absolute risk is very small (*Fig. 32.8*) and have their questions answered.

As major surgery adds to the risk of thromboembolism, women taking COCs should change to another form of contraception for 4 weeks before the surgery. Thrombotic stroke is increased 6-fold (compared with women using no, or other, forms of contraception) but is very uncommon in this age group.

The use of COCs leads to a small increase in the systolic blood pressure, which is reversible. *Hypertension* of greater magnitude occurs in about 2% of women and, particularly, in women who have a family history of hypertension, are overweight and over the age of 35 years. Women who have had pregnancy-induced hypertension are more likely to be affected. The cause is an increased sensitivity to the

Fig. 32.8 Risk of developing DVT or pulmonary embolus		Risk (per 100,000 women)
Healthy women who neither smoke nor take sex hormones		4–6
Women taking low-dose COCs with 2nd generation progestogens		10–15
Women taking COCs containing 3rd generation progestogens	??	20–30
Pregnant and parturient women		50–60

progestogen content of the Pill, but oestrogen may be involved, so a low-dose oestrogen Pill is to be preferred.

The use of low-dose COCs does not increase the risk of *myocardial infarction*, unless the woman is a smoker, overweight and over the age of 35, when a small increase in risk occurs. Among these women, stroke, mainly haemorrhagic stroke, is increased slightly (from 2 to 3 per 100,000 women per year).

Cancers

The use of COCs reduces the risk of developing ovarian cancer (by 40%) and endometrial cancer (by 50%). The prolonged use of COCs increases the risk of developing cervical cancer slightly, but this may be due to the sexual behaviour of the woman rather than to the use of COCs. The overall incidence of breast cancer does not increase except, perhaps, for a small subgroup of women presenting with breast cancer in their 30s, who have taken the Pill for at least 5 years before their first pregnancy.

Other clinical conditions occurring in women using COCs

Acne

The oestrogen content of the COCs tends to improve acne, whilst the progestogen tends to aggravate it. Monophasic COCs, especially these containing a second generation progestogen (eg Marvelon), sequential COCs or an OC containing cyproterone (eg Diane) should be chosen.

Break-through bleeding (BTB) and spotting

Many women starting to use hormonal contraception have episodes of break-through bleeding or spotting in the early months of use. In the first cycle 20% of women experience BTB; after 6 months less than 3% have the symptom. BTB is less likely if the woman takes the Pill *at the same time each day*. BTB causes considerable concern to many women, and doctors should advise women starting to use the Pill or 'switching' Pills, that BTB may occur. The doctor should explain that, in most cases, it settles within a few months and that it is not dangerous. If BTB continues for longer than 6 months, the woman should be prescribed a COC with a higher oestrogen content.

Chloasma

Hyperpigmentation of the skin may occur in susceptible women exposed to sunlight, but it is uncommon. The condition is thought to be due to oestrogen. Treatment consists of changing to a progesterone-only pill (POP) or using another form of contraception, avoiding direct sunlight, and if the woman is very concerned, applying 2% hydroquinone ointment. Even with these measures the chloasma takes up to 9 months to fade.

COCs and other drugs

Women who need to take antibiotics should take extra precautions during the time they take them, and for 7 days after, as absorption of the Pill is reduced and pregnancy may occur. Women who are prescribed carbamazepine, griseofulvin, phenytoin or rifampicin, should use a higher dose of COC preparation, as these antibiotics increase hepatic enzyme activity which, in turn, increases the metabolism of contraceptive steroids and reduces their efficacy.

Eye problems

A few women who use contact lenses may experience discomfort due to a change in the topography of the cornea.

Gall bladder disease

The development of gall bladder disease is accelerated among women taking a higher oestrogen dose COC (greater than 50μg).

Headaches and migraine

The prevalence of headaches among women taking COCs is variable and headaches may occur on days when no hormones are taken. If the headaches are severe and occur on days when the Pill is not taken (or when a non-active Pill is being taken in a 28-day pack), the frequency of headaches can be reduced by taking the Pill continuously for 3 months. The woman will not have a withdrawal bleed until the end of the 3-month cycle, but will have fewer headaches each year.

A few women develop migraine when taking COCs. If the migraine is focal or persists severely for 3 days or more, the woman should change to another form of contraception.

Mood changes, including depression

Some women who have premenstrual mood changes find that the symptoms decrease when taking a monophasic COC, particularly if it contains a second generation progestogen. Clinical depression is not increased among Pill users.

Nausea and vomiting

These symptoms may occur in the first few months of taking COCs as the body adjusts to the hormonal milieu.

Sexual desire

A few women report a decrease in libido when taking COCs; others report an increase.

Vaginal discharges

An increased amount of vaginal secretions is usual, but candidosis does not occur more frequently among women taking modern COCs.

Weight gain

Transient weight gain occurs in the premenstrual week in most women, and may be increased among women taking COCs; it is lost when menstruation starts. A few women gain weight after a few months' use of COCs. Whether this is due to the progestogen content of the COC or to an increased appetite is unclear.

Non-oestrogen hormonal contraceptives
Progesterone-only pill (POP) – the mini-Pill

This oral contraceptive is a good choice for women who have contra-indications for COCs or who are breastfeeding. It is an alternative for some diabetic women, women who have risk factors for cardiovascular disease, women who have hypertension related to COCs or are needing control by antihypertensives, and some migraine sufferers. The POP is associated with BTB and unpredictable menstruation in about one in four users. The failure rate (pregnancy rate) is shown in *Figure 32.3*.

Long-acting injectable progestogens

This formulation contains medroxyprogesterone acetate (DMPA) 150mg, injected 3-monthly, or norethisterone oenanthate (NET-OEN) 200mg, injected every 2 months. The advantage of the injectables is that they remove the need to take a Pill every day. Their disadvantage is that during the first 4–6 months of use, menstruation tends to be irregular. After this initial time period, amenorrhoea is usual and may lead to osteopenia.

Subdermal implants

Six silastic capsules, measuring 30mm × 2.5mm and each containing 36mg of levonorgestrel, are introduced subdermally into the anterior aspect of the forearm through a cannula, after making a 2mm incision through the skin. A recent development is to inject a single implant of desogestrel (Implanon), which is as effective in preventing pregnancy as the six silastic capsules. As with other progestogen formulations, such implants may provoke irregular episodes of uterine bleeding, which may be prolonged in the first year of use, in about 20% of women. The woman's fertility is not reduced once the implants have been removed.

Vaginal ring

This novel contraceptive, currently under study, has been developed in two forms:
- A ring containing an oestrogen and a progestogen mimicking the COCs.
- A ring containing levonorgestrel.

The ring fits in the upper vagina around the cervix. The advantage of the vaginal ring is that it is the only long-acting method under the woman's control. The woman removes the ring at will but generally replaces it at once after it has been washed. The disadvantage of the vaginal ring is that it may be associated with irregular bleeding in the first months of use and may be expelled from the vagina.

Prescribing hormonal contraceptives

The history is taken and the woman is examined as described in Chapter 1, Gyniatric history and examination. The choices of hormonal contraceptives available may be discussed with the woman, although often she has a good idea of the one she would prefer. She should be advised to read and to follow the instructions contained in the packet. Some doctors provide a pamphlet which reinforces these instructions.

The woman should be informed that these instructions include information on coping with forgotten pills to ensure maximum contraceptive effectiveness. If one OC pill is not taken at the regular time, it should be taken as soon as possible and the next pill taken at the regular time, even if this results in two tablets being taken on the same day. If two OC pills are missed, these two pills should be taken as soon as they are remembered, two pills should then be taken the following day and one pill each day until the pack is finished. Additional contraception, such as a condom, is needed for the next 7 days after two pills are missed.

POSTCOITAL CONTRACEPTION

If a woman has unprotected sexual intercourse at ovulation time she has two choices. The first is to wait and see if she misses a menstrual period and then have an immunological pregnancy test. If this is positive, she can then choose to continue with the pregnancy or to have an induced abortion (see page 111). The second choice is to use a form of postcoital contraception, provided she seeks help within 72 hours. Three methods are available:
- The woman may be prescribed a COC containing ethinyl oestradiol 50µg and levonorgestrel 250µg (the 'morning after' pill). Two of these tablets are taken together with an antiemetic, because of the side effects of nausea and vomiting. The dose is repeated after 12 hours.
- The woman is prescribed mifepristone (RU 486) in a dose of 600mg (at present), in countries where the drug is available. The advantage of mifepristone over the 'morning after' pill is that nausea and vomiting are less frequent.
- The woman may choose to have an IUD inserted within 5 days of the unprotected intercourse. This method is inadvisable if the woman is nulliparous.

Pregnancy is prevented in over 95% of cases, but the woman should return a week after the time of her expected period for a pregnancy test if she fails to menstruate.

INTRA-UTERINE DEVICE

Intra-uterine devices (IUDs) were used in humans in the last years of the 19th century, but had so many adverse side effects that their use was abandoned. The development of a polyethylene IUD in 1950, which had a memory for its shape, revived interest.

A satisfactory IUD should be easy to introduce, easy to remove, and have few side effects and a high degree of efficiency in preventing pregnancy. In the 1980s, a series of legal actions against IUD manufacturers led to the removal from the market of most IUDs, and, today, only three types remain. Two of the devices have fine copper wire surrounding the stem, which permits a smaller device to be used and reduces some of the side effects (*Fig. 32.9*). The third type of IUD contains levonorgestrel in its stem (*Fig. 32.10*). In the first 4 months of use, some women have unpredictable episodes of spotting or bleeding, and the woman may develop the unacceptable side effects of negative mood change, acne and sometimes, weight gain. After this time, the levonorgestrel IUD reduces the menstrual flow, controlling menorrhagia in women who have this menstrual disturbance; the device may cause amenorrhoea. This device may be chosen by women in their 40s who would otherwise consider tubal ligation.

Copper IUDs prevent pregnancy by incapacitating the sperms, making them dysfunctional for fertilization. The progestogen IUD releases 20µg of levonorgestrel a day and acts in the same manner as the progesterone-only Pill.

The 5-year cumulative pregnancy rate for the levonorgestrel IUD is 0.5–1.0%, whilst that of the copper-containing IUDs is between 2.0 and 5.5%.

Advantages of the IUD

The IUD requires only a single decision to have the device introduced into the uterus and, unless problems arise, will prevent pregnancy for 3–7 years (depending on the device). It is highly effective in preventing pregnancy (*see Fig. 32.3*).

Adverse effects of IUDs

During insertion

Perforation of the uterine wall occurs in about 1 per 1000 insertions and is directly proportional to the skill of the individual performing the insertion. Perforation may cause bleeding and pain, but is often silent. If perforation is suspected, the location of the IUD is determined using an ultrasound scan. If this indicates that the IUD has perforated the uterus and is wholly or partly in the abdominal pelvic cavity, it should be removed because the copper may cause a tissue reaction leading to intraperitoneal adhesions. The removal is effected by finding the IUD by using a laparoscope or by performing a laparotomy.

Expulsion

The uterus tends to expel 'foreign bodies' and the IUD is no exception; between 1 and 10 women, in every 100 who have an IUD inserted, expel the device. Expulsion may occur at any time after insertion, but usually occurs in the first 6–8 weeks, often during a menstrual period. Younger women and women who have never been pregnant are more likely to expel the device than other women.

Women using an IUD should be encouraged to check once each month that they can feel the string; to aid their memory it is suggested this is done immediately after each menstrual period.

Cramping and bleeding

Over a 2-year period these complications have been shown to occur with a frequency varying from 4 to 10% of women in the case of the copper-containing IUDs. The problem usually occurs in the first month after the insertion and diminishes as time passes. One half of the number of medical removals of an IUD is for this reason.

Pelvic inflammatory disease

Pelvic inflammatory disease (PID), or pelvic infection, is discussed in detail in Chapter 34, Infections of the genital tract. The background incidence of PID in the community is 1 per 100 women per year, aged 15–45 years. It has been claimed that the IUD increases the chance of developing PID. A recent meta-analysis has shown that this only applies if the infection occurs within the first month of the IUD insertion in women who have symptomless cervical

Fig. 32.9 Copper 375 multiload IUD.

Fig. 32.10 The levonorgestrel IUD.

infections due to *Chlamydia trachomatis*, *Neisseria gonorrhoeae* or, rarely, polymicrobial infection at the time of the IUD insertion.

These findings suggest that sexual activity rather than the IUD is the cause of PID, and that the introduction of an IUD through the infected cervix of a woman may increase slightly the chance that she will develop PID.

Tubal infertility

For a woman who has never been pregnant, the relative risk of developing tubal infertility (primary infertility) associated with the use of a copper IUD is 1.6. Women who have only one sexual partner have no increased risk of primary infertility.

Pregnancy and the IUD

Although the IUD is highly effective (greater than 98%) in protecting a woman against an unwanted pregnancy, occasionally a pregnancy occurs with the IUD in situ. The continued presence of the IUD increases the risk of miscarriage to 25% (compared with a 10% risk in a woman who has no IUD in situ), and thus, if the woman agrees, an attempt should be made to remove it from the uterine cavity. The procedure does not increase the miscarriage rate above that in the population. If the IUD cannot be removed and the woman chooses to continue with the pregnancy, a miscarriage occurring in the second quarter of pregnancy may be associated with infection (septic abortion), although the frequency of this complication is not known. Should infection occur, antibiotics should be given promptly and an attempt made to remove the IUD, if feasible. These problems should be discussed with the woman. Given the information she may choose to have an induced abortion.

Contra-indications to the use of an IUD

The IUD should not be inserted into a woman:

- Who has, or has had, several sexual partners or whose partner has, or has had, several sexual partners.
- With known or suspected pregnancy.
- With current or previous PID which has been accurately diagnosed.
- With a history of ectopic pregnancy.
- With abnormal genital tract bleeding which needs to be investigated.
- With congenital uterine abnormalities or myomata which distort the uterine cavity.

Insertion of the IUD

An IUD should only be inserted by a health-care practitioner who has received training in the insertion technique. The most appropriate time to insert an IUD is at midcycle, when the cervical canal is at its widest and the introduction of bacteria from the cervical canal is least likely.

Permanent methods of birth control

VASECTOMY

The vasectomy operation is simple to perform, effective and attended by little pain or inconvenience, particularly if the no-scalpel technique, developed in China, is used (*Fig. 32.11*). A few men develop scrotal swelling, bruising or a small haematoma, all of which settle quickly.

It is important that the medical practitioner discusses the procedure with the man and answers his questions. Many men equate vasectomy with castration; others are

Fig. 32.11 In a no-scalpel vasectomy, the vas (dotted line) is grasped by special ring forceps and the skin and the vas sheath are pierced by sharp-tipped dissecting forceps (a). The forceps then stretches an opening (b) and the vas is lifted out (c).

concerned that as sperm continues to be produced it will accumulate in the testes and swell them; others are anxious that after the vasectomy a man's desire and performance will diminish. None of these beliefs has any basis in fact. The man needs reassurance that vasectomy does not increase his risk of developing cardiovascular disease, prostatic disease, cancer, erectile failure or auto-immune disease.

He must be made aware that following vasectomy he is not immediately sterile, as the sperms in the epididymis proximal to the vasectomy are still potent. Until these sperm have been ejaculated, which takes on average 12 ejaculations, contraception must continue. The man should also be made aware that vasectomy should be considered a permanent method of birth control. Although the vasectomy can be reversed by microsurgery and patency obtained in 70% of cases, the pregnancy rate is less than 50%.

TUBAL LIGATION

In most cases tubal ligation, or more accurately tubal occlusive clipping, is performed through a laparoscope. A few women have the operation via a small suprapubic incision (minilaparotomy).

Although a failure rate of 2 per 1000 procedures at 5 years is often quoted, a study in the USA of 10,700 women who had had a tubal ligation showed a failure rate of more than 7 per 1000. The highest rate was 36 per 1000 procedures following clip sterilization and lowest, 7.5 per 1000 after unipolar procedures. The failure rate is three times lower if the operation is performed as an interval procedure, that is not immediately postpartum or after an abortion. A woman should be made aware of this before she decides to have the operation.

In the discussion before recommending the operation, the alternative methods of permanent birth control, including vasectomy, should be mentioned. Also, the stability of the current relationship should be explored.

Provided the woman has made an informed decision that she wants the operation and is aware that tubal ligation should be considered a permanent method of birth control, adverse reactions are few. As in the case of vasectomy, tubal patency can be restored by microsurgery and about 60% of women treated will conceive. In general, tubal ligation should not be made immediately after childbirth as 5% of women who have the operation at this time later regret their decision.

CHAPTER 33

Infertility

A couple who have had regular unprotected intercourse for a period of 12 months without a pregnancy occurring is considered to be infertile and may seek help from a medical practitioner. Infertility affects 10–15% of couples.

Factors in infertility

The factors which may be involved in the couple's infertility vary depending on local conditions, the population investigated and the referral procedures. Analyses reported by several clinics of large numbers of patients in the past two decades are given in *Figure 33.1*. In a quarter of cases, more than one of the factors is believed to be involved in the infertility.

Investigation of infertility

Of the many investigations suggested over the years, most have been found to be of little value and, today, there is relative agreement about what tests should be made to reach a diagnosis.

In most cases, the woman makes the first contact with a health professional. During this visit, the doctor should obtain information about the history of past illnesses and operations; the woman's menstrual history; and the couple's sexual behaviour, including frequency of sexual intercourse. Some women are concerned that they do not have an orgasm and that semen runs out of the vagina. The doctor should reassure the woman that neither of these affects the woman's fertility.

A general physical examination, including a pelvic examination, is made to exclude any current disease. The pelvic examination is made to detect any gross abnormalities of the genital tract, such as uterine myomata, ovarian tumours and endometriosis (see later). If a cervical smear (Pap smear) has not been made in the previous year this should be taken. Also, laboratory tests should be ordered and should include: a full blood examination, including tests for syphilis, rubella and HIV infection, and a urine analysis. If the woman has attended during the luteal phase of her menstrual cycle, blood may be taken to measure the progesterone level, to establish if she is ovulating.

Having completed these initial investigations the medical practitioner should outline the investigations which will be made, and their sequence. It is customary to start the investigations with a seminal analysis, as the man may have azoospermia or severe oligospermia. This finding would make further examinations of the woman unjustified initially.

SEMINAL ANALYSIS

Ideally, a man should accompany his partner at the first visit so that the investigation plan can be discussed with both people, a history can be obtained from the man and the man can also be examined. However, it is unusual for a man to attend with his partner. Because of this, and because a woman knows if penetration and ejaculation occur during sexual intercourse, the first step is to arrange for a semen analysis, and only if this is abnormal need the man be seen.

The seminal specimen can be obtained in two ways. The man can either attend the laboratory and masturbate there and so provide a fresh seminal specimen or he can masturbate at home (or have his partner masturbate him) and ejaculate into a clean, dry glass container. This is then taken to the laboratory within 1 hour, and the analysis made.

Standards for a normal seminal specimen have been developed by the World Health Organisation (WHO) and are shown in *Figure 33.2*. If the first seminal appraisal is abnormal, two further specimens should be evaluated before a prognosis is made.

Evaluation of the samples permits the specimens to be graded as:
- Normal.
- Oligospermia (a count of less than 20 million sperm per ml);
  - 1 with normally motile sperm
  - 2 with asthenospermia.
- Severe oligospermia (less than 5 million sperm in total specimen).
- Azoospermia.
- Asthenospermia with normal sperm count.

Fig. 33.1 Factors in infertility	
Factor	**Percentage of cases**
Male	
Defective sperm production, insemination difficulties	30–40
Female	
Ovulation factors	5–25
Tubal or uterine factors	15–25
Cervical/immunological factors	5–10
Unexplained after investigations	10–25

Fig. 33.2 Normal seminal analysis	
Volume	>2ml
Sperm concentration	>20 million per ml
Total sperm count	40 million
Motility 60 min after ejaculation	>50% with normal progression
Morphology	>30% with normal morphology

When the sperm count is less than 20 million per ml, abnormal morphology and motility is often found

Abnormal results indicate that the man should be examined and a history taken. The history may show that he is exposed to high heat, certain chemicals, or he is taking anticancer drugs. The examination of the man's genitals is important. The size of his testicles is evaluated and his scrotum is palpated, with the man standing, to detect if he has a varicocele, although the importance of this as a factor in infertility is disputed. If azoospermia or severe oligospermia is diagnosed, blood is drawn to measure the level of follicle-stimulating hormone (FSH). A raised level (3 times the normal upper limit) indicates testicular failure. If severe oligospermia is diagnosed, and the testicular volume and the FSH levels are normal, a testicular biopsy is sometimes made.

Absolute infertility is diagnosed if azoospermia and raised FSH levels are found. Severe infertility is diagnosed if severe oligospermia is found. Relative infertility is diagnosed if the sperm count is between 5 million and 20 million per ml. Treatment may be offered to men with relative infertility, although it has to be said that none has proved more effective than placebo.

The technique of micro-injection of a spermatozoon into the cytoplasm of the ovum is leading to pregnancies in cases of severe male infertility due to a very low sperm count. Sperm may also be retrieved from the epididymis in cases of blocked vasa defferentia, and the same technique applied.

INVESTIGATING THE WOMAN

The factors which may delay or prevent fertility in women are:

- Anovulation or infrequent ovulation.
- Tubal damage which prevents the passage of the sperm.
- Uterine factors such as intra-uterine adhesions (Asherman's syndrome).
- Cervical mucus 'hostility', which is an immunological defect in most cases.

These factors require to be investigated in the work-up of infertility.

Ovulation

The most effective way of determining if the woman is ovulating is to measure the serum progesterone level in the midluteal phase of the menstrual cycle. The older method of daily temperature charting is now obsolete. In past years, many gynaecologists performed a diagnostic curettage to obtain a specimen which could be examined to determine if endometrial luteinization had occurred, indicating ovulation. This invasive procedure is no longer justifiable except in countries where genital tuberculosis is common.

Time of ovulation

Knowledge of the time of ovulation is increasingly important in the treatment of some causes of infertility, because conception is most likely to occur on this day or on one of the 5 preceding days. The time of ovulation can be detected by measuring the plasma level of luteinizing hormone (LH) daily over this time period. The peak of LH release coincides with ovulation.

Anovulation is obvious if the woman is amenorrhoeic and may occur in women who have normal menstrual periods. The investigation of anovulation has been discussed in Chapter 29, Disorders of menstruation.

Defective luteal phase

A number of infertility specialists believe that some cases of infertility are due to the poor development of the luteal phase endometrium, with the result that the fertilized egg is unable to implant. Other specialists deny that the condition exists. Many treatments have been tried to treat the condition, but none has been evaluated scientifically or proved to be of value.

Tubal factors

The patency of the Fallopian tubes can be evaluated in three ways.

The first, hysterosalpingography, is performed by inserting a cannula, attached to a syringe, into the cervix and injecting a radio-opaque substance into the uterus under direct imaging. The passage of the dye is observed as it fills the uterine cavity and passes along the Fallopian tubes to spill into the peritoneal cavity. The advantages of hysterosalpingography are that it is a minor operation (the patient need not be admitted as a day-case) and that it will detect any intra-uterine abnormalities (Fig. 33.3).

A recent innovation is to use hysterosalpingo contrast sonography. Under transvaginal ultrasound scanning, a galactose solution is injected into the uterus and passes along the Fallopian tubes, which delineates them more accurately than hysterosalpingography using a radio-opaque substance.

The third method is to perform a laparoscopy and then to inject a water-soluble dye into the uterine cavity which is observed as it spills through the fimbrial ends of the Fallopian tubes. The advantage of laparoscopy is that, as well as ascertaining that the Fallopian tubes are patent, peritubal adhesions and endometrial deposits can be detected if they are present. Endometriosis is the only abnormality found in about 10% of infertile women and 40% of women who have endometriosis are involuntarily infertile, but the relationship between the two conditions is unclear. The topic is discussed further in Chapter 36, Endometriosis and adenomyosis.

Currently, the use of colour Doppler ultrasonography is being investigated, as is the use of tuboscopy.

Fig. 33.3 Hysterosalpingogram showing a normal uterus and tubes.

Cervical hostility

Although this term is usually used to indicate that the sperm fail to penetrate the cervical mucus at ovulation time, it is more likely that the failure is due to defective sperm function, probably immunological.

Many gynaecologists continue to believe in cervical hostility and test this by means of the *postcoital test*. The test has been in use for over 100 years and was originally carried out to detect sperm in the cervix. Today, the test is performed in the following way:
- The couple have intercourse on one of the two days before ovulation, or on the day of ovulation.
- After the man has ejaculated, the woman lies on her back for 20 minutes, and attends the doctor 8–12 hours later so that a sample of cervical mucus can be removed from her cervix (using a plastic tube attached to a syringe).
- The specimen is smeared on a slide and is examined to determine the degree of penetration of the mucus by actively moving sperm and their numbers per field.

A positive test (more than 20 actively moving sperm per field) indicates that there is unlikely to be an immunological problem causing the infertility; a negative test provides no useful information. Because of this, more specific sperm–mucus tests have been developed (*Fig. 33.4*). A second test is the Mixed Agglutinin Reaction (MAR). Human red cells are sensitised with IgG and mixed with sperm. If the spermatozoa are coated with antibody, the mixed agglutinates will be visable. However the value of these tests is unclear and the predictive value poor.

UNEXPLAINED INFERTILITY

After adequate investigation, about 15% of infertile couples will still not have had a cause for their infertility found. Unexplained infertility is frustrating both for the couple and the team of health professionals.

Fig. 33.4 Sperm–cervical mucus crossed hostility test				
Penetration of wife's cervical mucus with donor's sperm	+	−	+	−
Penetration of donor's cervical mucus with husband's sperm	+	+	−	−
Diagnosis	Specific immunological problem in couple	Cervical mucus of wife abnormal	Specific immunological problem in husband	Problem in husband and wife
Treatment	Donor insemination Intra-uterine insemination with husband's semen ?IVF	?Ethinyl oestradiol 0.01mg twice daily, days 10–14	Donor insemination or corticosteroids to husband	?

Treatment of infertility

INFERTILITY IN MEN

Azoospermia is an absolute barrier to conception, and it is unusual for a pregnancy to occur in a couple if the man has severe oligospermia. For these couples, donor semen insemination (DI) is a choice. Using DI monthly for 12 months, if necessary, will enable over 65% of women to become pregnant. If spermatozoa can be recovered a single spermatozoa can be micro-injected into the space under the zona pellucida or into the ovum (ICSI).

Improvement in the sperm count of men with non-severe oligospermia has been attempted using an oral form of testosterone (mestrolone) and more recently clomiphene prescribed for at least 12 weeks, but it is doubtful if any real improvement has occurred or that the pregnancy rate is higher than that obtained by chance.

An attractive alternative is to concentrate a seminal sample and fertilize several ova using the in-vitro fertilization (IVF) technique.

INFERTILITY IN WOMEN
Anovulation (usually associated with amenorrhoea)

The treatment is that discussed in the treatment of amenorrhoea on page 222. Inducing superovulation with ovulatory drugs can assist conception for men who have a low sperm count or women experiencing oligomenorrhoea.

Tubal damage

Two choices are available and the one chosen depends on the severity of the tubal damage and on the wishes of the patient. The first approach is to attempt to make the Fallopian tubes patent, using microsurgery. If only the fimbrial ends of the tubes are blocked, a salpingostomy or fimbriolysis is carried out. This results in a 40% chance of the woman conceiving in a 2-year period following the operation. Greater tubal damage necessitates a tubal anastomosis, with a success rate of no more than 20%, whilst reversal of a tubal ligation is followed by a pregnancy rate of 60%.

Given these relatively poor results (except in the case of reversal of a tubal ligation), the alternative approach, that of IVF, is recommended. The procedure is less invasive, the risk of ectopic gestation is lower and the chance of giving birth to a healthy baby is greater.

Cervical hostility (immunological infertility)

The oldest method of treatment is for the man to use condoms for 6 months in the hope that the antisperm antibodies will be eliminated. Other treatments are for the man to take low-dose corticosteroids (prednisone 20mg twice a day for the first 10 days of the woman's menstrual cycle) for 3 months; to use washed sperm introduced into the uterine cavity; or to use IVF or gamete intrafallopian transfer (GIFT) techniques. None of these treatments has been properly evaluated and it appears that as many pregnancies occur with treatment as when no treatment is given.

Unexplained infertility

Current opinion about the treatment of couples who have been diagnosed as having unexplained infertility is confused. If no treatment is given, beyond reassurance that no cause for the infertility has been found, over 40% of the women will become pregnant within 3 years. However, if the couple wish, or if the woman is over the age of 35 years, IVF or GIFT may be used soon after diagnosis, rather than delaying for 3 years.

NEW ASSISTED REPRODUCTIVE TECHNOLOGIES

These technologies, that is IVF and its variants (Fig. 33.5), have added a new dimension to the treatment of the infertile couple. In the past decade considerable advances have been made in reducing the pain involved, the invasiveness of the procedure and the cost. The procedure is as follows:

1. The woman is given ovulatory drugs, FSH, gonadotrophin-releasing hormone agonists and human chorionic gonadotrophin, to produce superovulation.
2. The eggs are retrieved from the ovaries by the transvaginal route under ultrasonic guidance.
3. The eggs are prepared for fertilization and only good ova are selected.
4. Sperm is added in vitro to the selected eggs.
5. Two (occasionally three) fertilized eggs are transferred into the uterus, or into the Fallopian tubes.

The GIFT technique involves similar procedures except fertilization does not taken place before transfer of the ova and sperm into the Fallopian tubes.

The success rate of a single IVF procedure, in terms of a live, healthy baby, is about 10%, whilst that of a single GIFT procedure is about 20%. If either procedure is repeated 5 times, the cumulative 'take-home baby' rate using IVF is 40% and that using GIFT about 50%.

SUCCESS RATE OF TREATMENT

Four couples in every 10 treated for infertility will have a 'take-home baby'. In most cases, the pregnancy occurs because of treatment but, in about 20%, it cannot be attributed to the treatment. The success rate for the treatment of various infertility factors is shown in Figure 33.6.

Psychosocial problems associated with infertility

The conception, and later the birth, of a healthy child is a significant life event. To most women, motherhood is the expression of her nurturing gender role and of her femininity and, to most men, the siring of a child is a visible demonstration of their masculinity and potency. For most couples, parenthood is an expression of their love for each other. However, to society infertility is still regarded as an illness.

The psychological impact of being infertile can be considerable and the necessary investigations psychologically disturbing, particularly to the woman who has more investigations performed than her partner. She may perceive these investigations as invasive and intimate, involving a loss of control over her body.

If a bar to fertility is detected in either partner or, if after investigation and treatment a pregnancy does not occur, the couple may be subjected to considerable psychological strain and may develop psychosexual problems.

The possibility of problems developing can be reduced in several ways, which involve the infertility specialist and the couple's general practitioner, who should have a key role as he knows the couple better. This implies that there must be good communication between specialist and doctor.

- As early as possible in the infertility 'work-up' the medical practitioner should provide the patients with a clear detail of the investigations proposed, the reasons for them, and the sequence in which they will be performed. As the patients may be so anxious that they may listen to but not hear what is being said, it is helpful to suggest that they read a book about infertility or are provided with pamphlets.
- The investigations should be kept to a minimum, and only those which produce reliable information should be made. Once information is obtained, the couple should be told the results and have the opportunity to ask questions.
- The attitude and behaviour of the doctor should be supportive, communicative and empathetic.

Fig. 33.5 Methods of assisted conception

Type	Assisted Insemination with Husband's sperm (AIH)	In-Vitro Fertilization (IVF)	Gamete Intrafallopian Transfer (GIFT)	Intracytoplasmic Sperm Injection (ICSI)	Zygote Intrafallopian Transfer (ZIFT), Tubal Embryo Stage Transfer (TEST)
Indications					
Male	Impotence Retrograde ejaculation Severe hypospadias	Oligospermia Presence of sperm antibodies	Moderate oligospermia	Severe oligospermia or azoospermia Vasectomy	Severe oligospermia
Female	Localized cervical or uterine problem	Endometriosis Damaged or absent Fallopian tubes	Endometriosis		
Male and/ or Female	Infrequent or absent sexual intercourse	Unexplained infertility		Failure of IVF	
Procedure	Sperm are transferred by catheter into uterus or Fallopian tube	Fertilized eggs are transferred into the uterus or Fallopian tube	Unfertilized eggs and sperm are transferred into one or both Fallopian tubes using laparoscopy or transvaginal ultrasound	Sperm is injected into the egg	Zygote or early embryo is transferred into the Fallopian tube using laparoscopy or transvaginal ultrasound the day after egg pickup
Pregnancy rate*	Up to 15% per cycle	10–25% per cycle; depends on maternal age	up to 30–40% per cycle	more than 50% per cycle	up to 30–40% per cycle

*'Take-home baby' rates are lower

Fig. 33.6 Pregnancy rates in infertility*		
	Proportion of all cases of infertility (%)	**Pregnancy rate** (%)**
Male:		
Azoospermia	7	65 (using DI)
Oligospermia	25	30
Female:		
Amenorrhoea	7	90
Other ovulatory	14	60
Tubal damage	16	20
Endometriosis (severe)	2	30
Uterine abnormalities	1	70
Male–female (immunological)	5	15
Unexplained	23	60

* 'Take-home baby' rates are about 7% lower
** Within 2 years of diagnosis with or without treatment

- If an absolute or severe barrier to conception is found, appropriate counselling should be offered. Inability to have a child represents a real loss, and mourning is an appropriate response. In counselling, the approach is to consider all the findings together as causing the couple's shared unhappiness, so that neither partner blames the other.

Couples who are in an IVF or a GIFT programme need special care, as in most cases these technologies are a 'last resort' in their attempt to have a child. The egg retrieval may be painful and the whole process psychologically traumatic, particularly if the woman perceives parenthood as a prerequisite for personal fulfilment. Most couples cope well but one-third of women experience anxiety or depression and one woman in 7 becomes severely distressed.

CHAPTER 34

Infections of the genital tract

Vulvovaginal infections

The skin of the vulva, in common with other parts of the skin which are liable to friction and chafing, may be infected by common skin pathogens. Boils may occur on the vulval skin, particularly when the standard of hygiene is low. Multiple vulval ulcers occur occasionally, particularly in debilitated women, and are due to staphylococcal infection. The ulcers are shallow with a grey, discharging base and surrounding oedema. The vulva is extremely tender. Treatment consists of prescribing antibiotics and applying 1% chlorhexidine cream if this can be done without causing much pain.

GENITAL HERPES

Herpetical infection of the vulva is becoming increasingly common. The virus, herpes simplex virus (HSV) exists in two forms, HSV1 and HSV2. HSV1 usually causes cold sores on the lips, but is the cause of genital herpes in 15% of cases. HSV2 causes genital herpes in 85% of cases. Serological testing shows that between 9 and 25% of adults have been infected at some time, but the infection was symptomatic in fewer than one-quarter of cases.

The first attack of genital herpes is the worst. It follows sexual contact with an infected person who, at the time, was recovering from an attack of genital herpes. The inner surfaces of the labia majora are most likely to be infected. After a short period of itching or burning, small crops of painful, reddish lumps appear which become blisters within 24 hours. The blisters ulcerate rapidly to form multiple shallow, painful ulcers (Fig. 34.1). The surrounding tissues become oedematous and secondary infection may occur, aggravating the oedema and pain, and, in some cases, making micturition painful and difficult. Over 5 days the ulcers crust over and heal slowly, the healing being complete in 7–12 days after the appearance of the blisters. During this time and for 7 days after healing, the virus is shed from the infected area. The virus also enters the myelin sheath of the sensory nerves supplying the affected area, and tracks to lie in the dorsal root ganglion. It may lie dormant for the rest of the person's life or may be reactivated and track back along the nerves to cause a new attack of herpes. Second and subsequent attacks are less severe but can cause considerable discomfort and affect relationships.

A single recurrence occurs in 30% of infected women, and between 2 and 5% have recurrent attacks, sometimes more than 6 times a year. As time passes the attacks become less frequent and may cease. In most cases, the cause of the recurrence is not known, but recurrences are more common in the luteal phase of the menstrual cycle, if the woman has other sexually transmitted infections, or if she is emotionally stressed.

Diagnosis

The appearance of the ulcers leads to a provisional diagnosis of genital herpes, which should be confirmed by pricking the blisters to obtain vesicular fluid or by rubbing the ulcers with a cotton tipped-bud (after applying 2% topical lignocaine a few minutes before) to obtain epithelial cells and sending the swab in a virus transport medium for culture.

Treatment

During an attack a woman should wear panties at all times as she may inadvertently scratch the infected area when sleeping and transfer the virus to her eyes. She should wash her hands after touching the infected area or applying medications. If the woman is unable to pass urine because of pain, a catheter may need to be inserted. Local applications of ice or anaesthetic jelly provide some relief.

Until recently, the only effective drug was acyclovir, but two new drugs – famciclovir and valaciclovir – are now available, increasing the therapeutic options. The antiviral drugs reduce the duration and severity of the initial and recurrent attacks, and shorten the time of viral shedding if given early in the attack. If a woman has five or more attacks each year or the outbreaks are particularly severe, long-lasting or interfere with the woman's psychosocial

Fig. 34.1 Genital herpes.

functioning, the drugs should be given as suppressive treatment for a period of about 12 months, or longer.

Women who have recurrent genital herpes are concerned more about the psychosocial sequelae of the disease, rather than the physical symptoms, and may need to be counselled.

GENITAL WARTS (CONDYLOMATA ACUMINATA)

Genital warts are caused by one or more types of the human papilloma virus (HPV), most commonly types 4 and 11, but sometimes types 16 and 18. The virus is usually transmitted sexually. Vulval infections are the most common, and the virus may spread to infect the vagina or the cervix; these areas may be infected initially.

Vulval warts usually present as cauliflower growths of varying sizes, but may be clinically undetectable. It has been estimated that 5–10% of sexually active adults are infected annually, and that 30% have evidence of previous infection (based on DNA hybridization).

The growths may occur on any part of the vulva and may involve the anal area (Fig. 34.2). In most cases the warts are symptomless but some women complain of vulval itching or burning. If the warts involve the vaginal entrance or the vagina, the woman may complain of dyspareunia.

The importance of HPV infection is that types 16 and 18 are involved, in some way, with the development of cervical carcinoma. The risk of this occurring from vulval warts is small (Relative Risk 1.5:0.9–2.5). This is discussed further in Chapter 38, Malignancies of the female genital tract.

Treatment

Genital warts, if not too exuberant, may be treated with podophyllotoxin (twice daily for 3 days, repeated if needed after 4 days) applied by the woman herself, after trimming away any vulval hair around the wart; or the medical practitioner may apply 20% podophyllin in benzoin tincture to the wart without touching the surrounding skin, to avoid skin burns and ulceration. The mixture is allowed to dry and the woman washes it off 4 hours later. This is repeated twice weekly, if necessary. Larger condylomata on the cervix may respond to the application of tricholoracetic acid. A new treatment, the application of imiquimod 5% cream 3 times weekly, has been developed.

Large warts, or warts which fail to respond to medical treatment, are treated by diathermy or by laser. The procedure is painful and anaesthesia is needed. Postoperatively, pain requires analgesics. A problem which has recently been reported is that neither diathermy nor laser may cure the woman, as the virus may have infected neighbouring normal cells and warts may recur. Because of the concern that HPV infection with types 16 and 18 may be involved with the development of cervical carcinoma, a woman who has vulval warts should have an annual Pap smear made.

SYPHILITIC VULVAL ULCER

Syphilis is caused by the invasion of the tissues by *Treponema pallidum* and is sexually transmitted. The initial lesion is a small papule which appears at the site of inoculation, usually 14–28 days after the person is infected. In women, the usual site of infection is one of the labia majora, but the cervix may be infected instead. The papule rapidly enlarges to form an oval lesion of variable size, the centre of which becomes eroded and granulomatous. The edges of the eroded area are sharp, and outside this a thickened, indurated zone occurs, hence the name for the lesion – hard chancre (*Fig. 34.3*). The chancre is painless and may be

Fig. 34.2 Genital warts.

Fig. 34.3 Primary lesion of syphilis – hard chancre.

ignored by the woman or considered a small sore of no consequence, but as it is teeming with *Treponema* it is highly infectious. The primary lesion disappears in 21 days or so.

Diagnosis

The diagnosis is confirmed by examining a swab taken from the ulcer, through a microscope under dark ground illumination. To obtain an accurate diagnosis the chancre is first cleaned with a swab, and then, if necessary, its edge and base is scarified using a scalpel so that exudate appears before the specimen is taken. Six weeks after the primary infection, serological tests for syphilis (VDRL or Rapid Plasma Reagin) become positive.

Treatment

Treatment consists of giving antibiotics, for example, procaine penicillin 1g daily for 10 days, a long-acting penicillin, benzathine penicillin 1.8g as a single dose or doxycycline 100mg twice daily for 14 days for penicillin sensitive individuals. Meticulous follow-up is essential.

INFECTION OF BARTHOLIN'S GLAND (BARTHOLINITIS)

The infection is usually due to *Escherichia coli* or *staphylococci* but may follow gonorrhoeal infection. In the acute stage, both the duct and gland are involved. If it is not treated the infection may subside or a Bartholin's abscess may form. Occasionally, the gland becomes chronically enlarged following an inflammatory conglutination of the duct epithelium, to form a Bartholin's cyst.

Diagnosis

In acute Bartholinitis, the woman complains of acute discomfort in the region of the gland, and a reddened, tender swelling appears beneath the posterior part of the labium majus.

Treatment

Treatment consists of prescribing analgesics and a broad-spectrum antibiotic. If an abscess has formed, marsupialization of the abscess should be performed. An elliptical piece of the vagina and abscess wall, just inside the hymen, is removed. The vaginal and abscess walls are sutured to maintain patency and a small drain is inserted.

VAGINAL DISCHARGES AND INFECTIONS

The vagina of a woman in the reproductive years is lined by a layer of stratified epithelium, 10–30 cells thick. As is described on page 329, the superficial cells of the vagina are shed constantly into the vaginal cavity and release glycogen, which is acted on by Doderlein's bacilli (lactobacilli) to produce lactic acid and hydrogen peroxide (natural defences against vaginal infection) and to maintain the vaginal pH between 3.5 and 4.5.

The vagina harbours large numbers of bacteria, which constitute its normal flora (*Fig. 34.4*). However, a significant number of women harbour potential pathogens in the vagina. These organisms are *Trichomonas*, *Candida* spp, and *Gardnerella* (*bacterial vaginosis*). They produce symptoms in only a few women.

The vagina is normally kept moist by transudation of fluid through the vaginal walls, which mixes with the exfoliated vaginal cells, aliphatic acids and the microorganisms mentioned earlier. The quantity of vaginal secretions varies through the menstrual cycle, peaking at ovulation time. The quantity is also increased by emotional stress. If an increased quantity of vaginal secretion is present, it may form a white coagulum, which may cause concern to the woman when she notices a whitish discharge that may cause itching. The discharge is termed leucorrhoea, which is defined as a non-infective, non-bloodstained physiological vaginal discharge.

LEUCORRHOEA

When a woman presents to a doctor with leucorrhoea, infection by pathogenic organisms must be excluded by obtaining a vaginal smear, which is examined or cultured.

Treatment

Treatment consists of reassuring the woman that the discharge is not pathogenic, that its fishy smell is undetectable to others, and exploring reasons for the woman's concern. A few women have recurrent vaginal discharges which show no pathogens on repeated laboratory investigations. These cases are difficult to treat. Many of these women have abnormal scores on psychometric tests, or have the somatizing syndrome, so the woman's life-style, including her sexuality, should be investigated rather than concentrating on the vaginal discharge. Some women repeatedly douche themselves for 'vaginal hygiene', a practice which may increase the chance of vaginal infection by reducing the number of vaginal lactobacilli.

If the woman wants medication, a vaginal acidifying jelly (Acijel) may be prescribed. Antibiotics should be avoided as they may aggravate the discharge rather than relieve it.

Organism	Percentage
Lactobacilli	80–90
Staphylococci, micrococci	50–70
Ureaplasma	40–50
Anaerobes	20–50
Streptococci	20–30
Gardnerella	10–30
E. coli	5–15
Candida spp.	5–15
Bacteroides	5–10
Trichomonas	3–7

Fig. 34.4 Normal vaginal flora

PATHOLOGICAL VAGINAL DISCHARGES

The three common irritating pathological vulvovaginal discharges are caused by:

- Trichomoniasis.
- Candidosis.
- Bacterial (amine) vaginosis.

In many cases they can be differentiated in the doctor's office or outpatient clinic by taking a sample of the discharge and looking at a smear under a microscope. Part of the swab is mixed with a drop of saline and part is mixed on a second slide with two drops of 10% potassium hydroxide (KOH). The saline preparation may reveal *trichomonal flagellates*, which can be observed moving and thrashing their tails (*Fig. 34.5*). This slide may also show vaginal epithelial cells with serrated borders, 'clue cells', which suggest that the woman has bacterial vaginosis (*Fig. 34.6*). Clue cells are more readily apparent on a Gram-stained slide. Bacterial vaginosis is also suggested by a strong fishy smell from the KOH preparation (the amine test). The KOH preparation is examined under a microscope, when hyphae of *Candida albicans* can be seen if this is the cause of the discharge (*Fig. 34.7*).

The alternative is to take the vaginal swab and place it in a culture medium, such as Transgrow, and send it to a laboratory for tests.

Trichomoniasis

The *Trichomonas vaginalis* parasite is a 20μm long flagellate. It is a little larger than a leucocyte (see *Fig. 34.5*). Once introduced into the vagina, it shelters at the bottom of the crypts of the velvet-like vaginal epithelium. As it is found in the vagina of symptomless women it appears only to become a pathogen in certain conditions, which raise the pH to 5.5 or more. The conditions are not known. It is readily sexually transmitted and infects the man's urethra, where it is also symptomless. The parasite may infect women who have not had sexual intercourse.

Clinical aspects

The main complaint is a moderate to profuse vaginal discharge which produces itching and irritation inside the vagina and around the vaginal introitus. In long-standing cases the discharge is greenish and frothy.

Treatment

The patient is given a single oral dose of tinidazole 3g or metronidazole 2g. Alternatively, oral metronidazole is prescribed in a dose of 200mg three times a day for 7 days. The woman's sexual partner should be invited to take the same treatment. These regimens cure 90% of infected women. A vaginal swab is taken 7 days after completing treatment and, if the flagellates are still present, a second course of treatment is given. All patients are asked to have a further vaginal swab made 2 months after the completion of treatment but few do. Side effects of treatment are minimal: a few women feel nauseated and alcohol should be avoided whilst taking the tablets as it may lead to headaches and flushing.

Candidosis

Candida spp. infect the vaginal epithelial cells, particularly if in the fungal-germinating stage, when they develop spores and long threads (hyphae) (see *Fig. 34.7*). Inside the vaginal epithelial cells they may lie dormant until environmental conditions encourage germination. *Candida* spp. may also infect the vulval skin, the anogenital region, the mouth and the intestinal tract. If the vaginal acidity falls, candidial growth is encouraged, as occurs in diabetic women and women taking antibiotics or corticosteroids.

Clinical aspects

The woman complains of severe vulvovaginal irritation which is associated with a vaginal discharge. In some cases, her sexual partner may complain of itching of his glans and foreskin.

Fig. 34.5 *Trichomonas vaginalis.*

Fig. 34.6 *'Clue cells', seen in Bacterial vaginitis.*

Typically the discharge is thick, 'cheesy' and adheres to the vaginal wall in plaques, but often these findings are not present.

Diagnosis
Diabetes mellitus should be excluded, and a vaginal swab should be taken and processed as mentioned earlier.

Treatment
One of the imidazole group of drugs (clotrimazole, econazole, isoconazole or miconazole) is prescribed as a vaginal tablet, either as a single dose or daily for 3 days. If vaginal treatment fails or oral treatment is preferred, a single dose of fluconazole or ketoconazole may be prescribed.

Alternatively, local treatment with an imidazole given every 2–4 weeks may control the infection. Vulval irritation may be intense and an imidazole cream may be applied at intervals. A course of treatment cures 85% of patients.

The woman should also be advised to wipe her vulva from the front to the rear to avoid possible faecal contamination.

Recurrent candidosis
Between 5 and 15% of women with vaginal candidosis have recurrent attacks, sometimes four times a year. Most are relapses of the initial infection, possibly because of a reduced local host defence against *Candida* spp. Recurrent attacks can cause a considerable disruption to the woman's personal and sexual life, and she may resort to alternative medicine.

Ha.

Treatment
It is difficult to treat this condition. In women who have frequent recurrences, prophylactic ketoconazole 100mg by mouth daily for 6 months or fluconazole 150mg weekly, may offer protection. Some women complain of nausea.

Fig. 34.7 Candida albicans.

Ketoconazole causes liver damage in 1 in 15,000 users, and the woman should have liver function tests at the start of treatment and again after 3 months. The woman is usually told not to wear nylon pantyhose or tight jeans, but the value of this has not been established.

Bacterial vaginosis
This vaginal infection is common, affecting 10–20% of women. In bacterial vaginosis, the numbers of vaginal organisms are increased considerably but only 6% of the lactobacilli produce hydrogen peroxidase compared with the normal 60%. This leads to a rise in the vaginal pH and an increase in the growth of *Gardnerella vaginalis* and vaginal anaerobes. As mentioned on page 149, bacterial vaginosis may increase the chance of preterm birth and the risk of cervical dysplasia.

Half of infections are symptomless, in others the woman complains of a thin, greyish discharge which has a strong, fishy smell. The clinical diagnosis is difficult but a vaginal smear which shows clue cells is diagnostic (see *Fig. 34.6*).

Treatment consists of prescribing metronidazole 2g orally as a single dose. An alternative is clindamycin given orally, or as a vaginal cream, 5g daily for 7 days. If these regimens do not clear the infection, metronidazole should be given 400mg three times a day for 7 days. In pregnancy, metronidazole 400mg twice daily for 2 days seems to clear the infection.

Infections of the internal genital organs

The fact that the genital tract, apart from the lowest third, derives from the Müllerian duct and has anastomosing systems of arteries, veins and lymphatics, means that infections of individual organs are less frequent than sequential ascending infection of the genital tract.

Ascending vaginal infection is controlled, to some extent, by the following mechanisms. First, the vaginal walls lie in apposition and the vaginal secretions are acidic, which inhibits bacterial growth; second, the cervical mucus forms a meshwork, except at the time of ovulation, which limits upward spread; and, third, the endometrium is shed each month during menstruation. However, if the cervix is infected directly, the above mechanisms are less effective.

Most cervical infections occur in sexually active women and usually follow a sexually transmitted organism acquired from an infected man who has gonorrhoea or nongonococcal genital infection (in most cases *Chlamydia trachomatis*). In a few cases, microbial agents which are normal vaginal inhabitants may spread upwards and cause infection of the internal genital organs. These polymicrobial infections are usually found in long-standing cases of pelvic infection and may be secondary contaminants.

As it may be difficult, clinically, to determine which organ is infected, and as more than one organ is usually infected, the condition is generally diagnosed as acute pelvic infection or *pelvic inflammatory disease (PID)*. It is currently thought that chlamydial infection causes 50–65% of all cases of PID and gonorrhoea 15–30%; in the remaining cases the aetiology is unclear, but may be polymicrobial. The women in this last group tend to be older and to have had PID for a longer time.

Infection of the internal genital organs may also occur following an abortion or after childbirth. In these cases the infective agents (which are usually staphylococci, streptococci, *E. coli* or anaerobes) enter the tissues through cervical lacerations, or more frequently, through the placental bed. Infections following pregnancy or childbirth are discussed in Chapter 24, Disorders of the puerperium.

In a few cases, pelvic infections occur either from haematogenous spread, as in tuberculosis, or from pelvic peritonitis.

NON-GONOCOCCAL AND GONOCOCCAL GENITAL INFECTIONS

As mentioned, most cases of PID follow sexual intercourse with a man who has gonorrhoea or non-gonococcal urethritis. In many cases, the man has no symptoms and may be unaware that he is infected. The microorganisms invade the columnar cells lining the crypts of the cervical canal. They may be eliminated by the body's immune system, spread rapidly to cause an acute infection, or remain quiescent in the columnar cells, with the potential

to spread to other pelvic organs. Spread occurs via the lymphatics, the veins or, possibly, by 'riding on the back of spermatozoa'. In a few instances, the infection is carried into the uterus during the insertion of an intra-uterine device (see page 247).

The endometrium is first infected, causing endometritis. From here the infection may spread to the myometrium causing myometritis, or through the uterine cavity to the Fallopian tubes causing acute or subacute salpingitis. In some cases the ovaries and the pelvic peritoneum may be involved (*Fig. 34.8*).

The two principal infecting agents are *C. trachomatis* and *Neisseria gonorrhoeae*. They require further discussion.

Chlamydial infection

Infection with *C. trachomatis* is usually symptomless, but a few women (less than 20%) may complain of a mucopurulent discharge from the cervix, or of dysuria. Community studies have shown that between 15 and 30% of healthy women have circulating antichlamydial antibodies, indicating previous subclinical infection and that between 4 and 12% of women have symptomless infection of their cervical cells (as have men who have symptomless infection of the urethral cells). Symptomatic infection affects between 1 and 3% of sexually active women, aged 15–50 years (and rather more men) each year. With the availability of polymerase chain reaction (PCR) and ligase chain

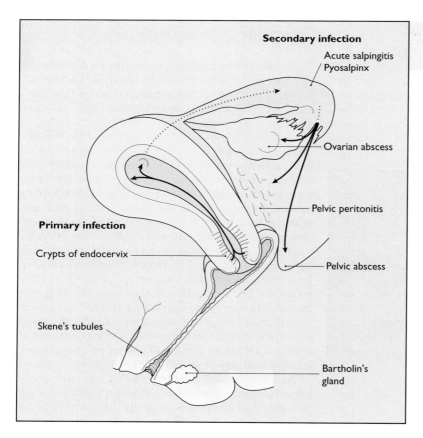

Fig. 34.8 Route of spread of non-gonococcal and gonococcal infection.

Secondary infection

Acute salpingitis / Pyosalpinx

Ovarian abscess

Pelvic peritonitis

Primary infection

Crypts of endocervix

Pelvic abscess

Skene's tubules

Bartholin's gland

reaction testing on urine, greater diagnostic accuracy has been obtained. A higher incidence occurs in women under the age of 25 years who have a history of a sexually transmitted disease and who have had several sexual partners, or whose sexual partners have had several partners.

Gonococcal genital infection

Gonococcal genital infection may be symptomless or may produce early symptoms of dysuria, urinary frequency and a purulent discharge *per vaginam*. The discharge originates from infected endocervical cells and from Bartholin's gland, but not from the vaginal mucosa as the gonococcus is unable to penetrate vaginal stratified epithelium. The severity of the initial infection varies and, in 50–80% of infected women, symptoms are so mild that they are ignored. Spread, if it occurs, is upwards to the endometrium and Fallopian tubes, or downwards to infect Bartholin's gland.

CLINICAL PRESENTATIONS OF PID

Cervical infection has been discussed and endometritis is usually symptomless except when it follows a bacterial infection after abortion or childbirth.

Salpingitis may be symptomless or symptomatic. In acute symptomatic cases, the growth of organisms of the cells lining the oviduct produces the acute phase of primary infection. A large amount of mucus is secreted, together with a fibrinous exudate which produces agglutination of the mucosal folds of the endosalpinx. The Fallopian tubes become inflamed and oedematous, producing recognizable symptoms. These are:

- Severe bilateral lower abdominal tenderness and pain.
- Abdominal muscle spasm.
- Fever (higher than 38.0°C), often with rigors.
- Leucocytosis.

On examination, the lower abdomen is tender and, on pelvic examination, bimanual palpation of the lateral vaginal fornices is excruciatingly painful.

In particularly virulent infections, pus may collect in the Fallopian tube, producing a pyosalpinx, or the infection may spread to the ovaries.

Low-grade infections will either be symptomless or associated with non-specific lower abdominal pain.

Diagnosis

The diagnosis may be established clinically, but confirmation by laparoscopy is required in most cases as the symptoms are non-specific and may occur in tubal pregnancy, accompany a complication of an ovarian cyst, or have a psychosomatic basis. Recently, it has been suggested that an endometrial sample (using a Vabra or similar biopsy curette) sent to a laboratory to detect plasma cells and transvaginal pelvic ultrasound scanning are as accurate as laparoscopy and less invasive. The transvaginal ultrasound looks for:

- Multiple ovarian cysts.
- Thickened fluid-filled Fallopian tubes.
- Free fluid in the pelvis.

Laboratory tests should be made: urethral and cervical swabs should be taken and sent in appropriate transport media for examination. Screening for chlamydia is made by an immunofluorescence test or an enzyme linked immunosorbent assay (ELISA) test using a monoclonal antibody.

Treatment

In most cases treatment should be started before the exact infective agent has been identified. In severely ill patients, antibiotics should be started intravenously. In less severe cases intramuscular or oral antibiotics should be given. Because of the frequent association of chlamydia and gonococcal infection, and the increasing prevalence of penicillin-resistant N. gonococci, the Center for Disease Control in the USA recommends that the current treatment of doxycycline and metronidazole should be replaced with a single dose of probenecid 1g and ceftriaxone 250mg intramuscularly (one dose), or cefixime 400–800mg orally, followed by doxycycline 100mg orally twice daily for 14–21 days. Other authorities recommend clindamycin 450mg four times a day for 10 days or ciprofloxacin 750mg twice daily for 12 days.

In severe infections, including tubo-ovarian abscess, intravenous treatment should be started with cefoxitin 2g four times daily plus doxycycline 100mg twice daily. This regimen is continued for 4 days and is followed by doxycycline 100mg twice daily for a further 10 days.

A recent study has shown that azithromycin has a major role in combating bacterial sexually transmitted diseases, particularly chlamydia infections, and may be superior to other treatments. As the recommended antibiotic treatment is changing constantly, it is important that the doctor keeps up to date and adopts the latest recommendations for treatment.

Surgery is indicated if the drug treatment fails in the presence of obvious abscesses which do not respond to antibiotic treatment. The surgery should be as conservative as possible, draining being preferred. A 'total clearance' of the genital organs is rarely indicated.

Prevention

Both chlamydia and gonorrhoea are sexually transmitted. Prevention is, therefore, best obtained if people are prepared to use 'safer sex', that is, limiting the number of sexual partners and insisting on the use of a condom if the couple choose vaginal or anal penetration and either partner cannot be relied on to disclose his or her previous sexual behaviour. This advice is idealistic, and usually is ignored. An alternative is to suggest that a person who has several sexual partners or whose partner has several sexual partners is screened for chlamydia and gonorrhoea every 6 months or so.

Long-term effects of PID

A first chlamydial genital infection, unless treated, causes damage to the Fallopian tubes in 10% of cases. If a second infection occurs the proportion of women who develop tubal damage increases to 25% and, after a third infection, to over 50%. Gonococcal infection, unless treated, is associated with an even higher chance of tubal damage. As many infections, particularly chlamydial infections, are symptomless, it is not surprising that evidence of previous tubal infection is often first detected during investigations for infertility. If a previously infected woman, who has had tubal damage, does succeed in getting pregnant, she has 5–7 times the risk of having an ectopic pregnancy compared with a woman who has not had PID.

SUBACUTE SALPINGITIS

This is often symptomless, but the woman may feel unwell. A vaginal examination may show a tubal mass. This is found in half the number of women infected with gonorrhoea, but in only a quarter of those infected with chlamydia.

CHRONIC GENITAL INFECTION (CHRONIC PID)

Chronic genital infection is a long-term sequel of acute or subacute infection and may follow post-abortion or puerperal infection. It may present as a pyosalpinx, a hydrosalpinx or a chronic tubo-ovarian abscess (*Fig. 34.9*). In other cases, the infection involves the connective tissues of the pelvis, causing chronic pelvic cellulitis.

Pyosalpinx

Pyosalpinx, or 'chronic pus tube', forms as a result of blockage of the lumen of the oviduct at the fimbrial end and at one or more points along the Fallopian tube. This occurs in the acute phase of the infection, and exudate

accumulates distending the oviduct to a greater or lesser degree (*Fig. 34.10*). The distension of the oviduct flattens the endosalpinx and the wall of the oviduct is thickened by the inflammatory process. Since the inflammatory process extends through the wall of the oviduct, adhesions to surrounding structures are usual occurrences. The ovary may be involved to form a chronic tubo-ovarian abscess.

There may be no symptoms, or vague pelvic pain may occur which is intermittent or constant. It is often worse in the premenstrual phase of the menstrual cycle and some women complain of deep dyspareunia. These symptoms are not specific for chronic pelvic infection and may be due to psychosomatic conditions. The symptoms may vary in severity, possibly because of an exacerbation of the infective process. This may occur months or years after the first infection. Laparoscopy may be needed to establish the diagnosis. In some cases the woman becomes acutely ill.

Treatment of chronic pyosalpinx which is causing symptoms is surgical. The extent of the surgery depends on the severity of the condition and, in general, requires bilateral salpingectomy and often oophorectomy, although some ovarian tissue may be saved. Hysterectomy is also usually performed in case residual infection is present.

Hydrosalpinx

Hydrosalpinx is the end result of burnt-out pyogenic salpingitis, which was of low virulence but highly irritating, producing large quantities of clear exudate within the closed portion of the oviduct. The distended oviduct has a thin

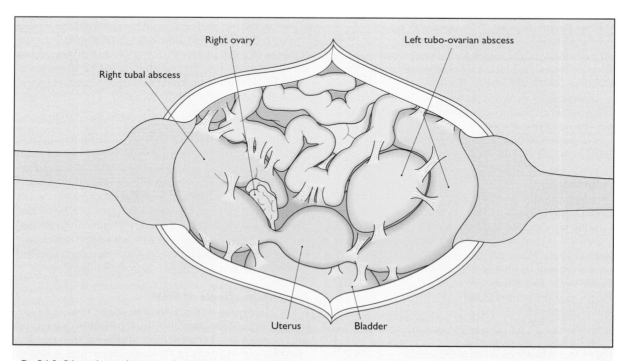

Fig. 34.9 *Bilateral pyosalpingitis – the appearance at operation.*

wall, which is translucent and usually retort-shaped (*Fig. 34.11*). Adhesions to contiguous structures may be present.

Hydrosalpinx may be symptomless but if symptoms are present they are many and variable. They include general ill-health, lassitude, disturbances of menstruation and chronic aching in the lower abdomen, which is worse premenstrually. Abdominal examination often shows no abnormality. Vaginal examination may reveal generalized tenderness or a smooth cystic enlargement. Because of these non-specific complaints, laparoscopy is often required to make a diagnosis, Treatment is surgical. The extent of the surgery is determined by the condition of the other Fallopian tube and the woman's desire to have children.

Chronic pelvic cellulitis

Chronic pelvic cellulitis is less common today but still occurs. It is usually the sequel of acute pelvic cellulitis and results in thickening and fibrosis of the connective tissues of the parametrium, with the result that the position of the uterus is distorted and it is relatively or absolutely immobilized (*Fig. 34.12*). The symptoms of chronic pain cellulitis are variable. The most common complaint is a chronic deep pelvic ache, often localized to one side, and backache. Deep dyspareunia is frequent and may be so severe as to prevent sexual intercourse. Vaginal examination shows a tender uterus drawn to one side and relatively fixed in position.

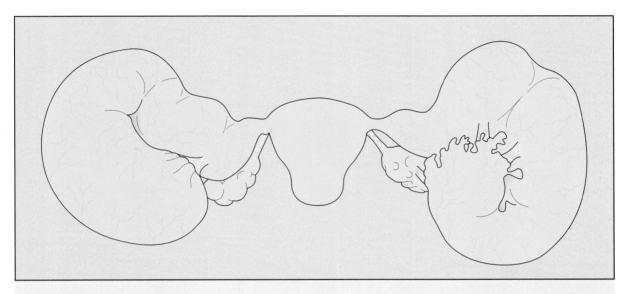

Fig. 34.10 Bilateral chronic salpingitis.

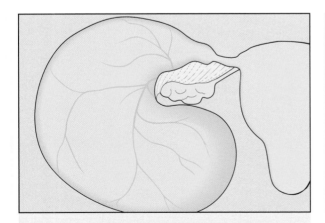

Fig 34.11 Hydrosalpinx. Note the retort-shaped distension of the oviduct.

Fig 34.12 Chronic pelvic cellulitis.

Treatment is unsatisfactory; some patients respond to pelvic short-wave diathermy, while hysterectomy is another option. Unfortunately, in spite of treatment, in many women the pain persists.

TUBERCULOUS INFECTION OF THE GENITAL TRACT

In the developed countries, genital tract tuberculosis is very uncommon, accounting for less than 0.5% of all pelvic infections. In the developing countries, the incidence is much higher. The disease is spread in the postprimary haematogenous phase of tuberculosis. If this happens to coincide with puberty, when increased growth both of the internal genital organs and of the supply of blood thereto occurs, infection may also occur. The disease may be limited to the oviducts, but spread to the endometrium is common. Symptoms are minimal, and the condition is detected when investigations for infertility are made. Treatment is that for pulmonary tuberculosis, surgery only being used when there are large adnexal masses and after medical treatment has been tried.

CHAPTER 35

Atrophic and dystrophic conditions

In the years after the menopause, the internal genital organs become smaller and atrophic. The changes occur because the amount of circulating oestrogen falls to a very low level.

Internal genital organs

By the age of 75 years, the uterus, the Fallopian tubes and the ovaries have shrunk considerably (*Fig. 35.1*). In the uterus, the endometrium has become atrophic and the muscle fibres of the myometrium have been replaced, progressively, by fibrous tissue. The cervix has atrophied and the cervical canal may become obliterated. If the woman develops uterine infection, the pus might not escape, leading to a *pyometra*. This may also occur if the woman develops an endometrial or cervical carcinoma. The woman may complain of lower abdominal pain and an examination shows that the uterus is larger than expected for her age. The diagnosis is confirmed by ultrasound scanning which shows that the uterine cavity is enlarged and filled with fluid. If carcinoma is detected it is treated appropriately; if it is not present, the cervix is dilated and a drain inserted for a few days.

VAGINA

The changes in the vagina depend on levels of oestrogen, which continues to be synthesized in peripheral tissues, but in most women the vaginal epithelium becomes atrophic. The superficial cells diminish in number, and intermediate and parabasal cells predominate. These changes show clinically as vaginal discomfort and burning, and painful intercourse.

THE PELVIC FLOOR

Deprived of oestrogen, the blood supply to the muscles of the pelvic floor diminishes. The pelvic floor muscles lose their tone and the connective tissue loses its elasticity, with

25 Years   Nulipara   55 Years   Multipara   75 Years

Fig. 35.1 *Reduction in the size of the uterus in old age.*

the result that relaxation of the pelvic floor tissues damaged during childbirth is likely to occur with varying degrees of prolapse (see Chapter 39, Uterovaginal displacements, damage and prolapse).

THE VULVA

As a woman's age increases, the labia majora lose their fat and elastic tissue content and become smaller, and the vaginal introitus is exposed. In very old women, only a narrow cleft indicates the presence of the vaginal introitus.

The vulval epithelium becomes thin, with loss of elastic and collagen fibres. These changes may lead to vulval irritation, although this may occur at earlier ages.

Itchy vulva (pruritus vulvae)

One woman in 10 who attends a medical practitioner for genital tract disorders, will say, among other complaints, that she has an itchy vulva. The reason may be infection, general skin or medical disease, or emotional problems. Emotional problems are thought to cause vulval itch in some women because both the skin covering the vulva, and its underlying capillaries, are unstable. Thus sexual or marital problems, anxiety and depression may manifest somatically as vulval itch.

Whatever the cause, the itch, mediated by a release of histamines, leads to scratching, which aggravates the itch. Over a period of months, the itch–scratch cycle may initiate a variety of histological changes in the vulval skin – non-neoplastic epithelial disorders of the skin and mucosa.

NON-NEOPLASTIC EPITHELIAL DISORDERS (SPECIFIC VULVAL DYSTROPHIES)

Two forms are described: lichen sclerosis (atrophic dystrophy) and squamous cell hyperplasia (hypertrophic dystrophy). Mixed forms of these two patterns may be found and it is worth noting that, if the itching has persisted for less than 6 months, the skin biopsy may show a normal vulval skin (Fig. 35.2).

Lichen sclerosis

The skin may be reddish, or of normal colour, and atrophic white, shiny plaques are seen. A skin biopsy shows that the horny layer is unchanged or hyperkeratinized with thinning of the epidermis and the disappearance of the rete pegs. The dermis is oedematous with some degree of hyalization and collections of round cells are seen (Fig. 35.3).

Squamous cell hyperplasia (hypertrophic dysplasia)

The skin is usually reddened with exaggerated skin-folds. In certain areas, lichenified white patches may be seen. A biopsy specimen will show a thickened epithelium, with elongated papillae, which retain their normal shape. The dermis is oedematous and contains numbers of plasma cells (Fig. 35.4)

Fig. 35.2 Histology of normal vulval skin.

Fig. 35.3 Lichen sclerosis (atrophic pattern).

Fig. 35.4 Squamous cell hyperplasia (hypertrophic patterns).

Vulval intra-epithelial neoplasia (VIN)

In a few instances, squamous cell hyperplasia or the mixed form may progress to VIN. For this reason, patients treated for squamous cell hyperplasia must be followed up at regular intervals. Like cervical intra-epithelial neoplasia (CIN), VIN is classified histologically in three grades, from VIN1 (mild dysplasia) (Fig. 35.5) to VIN3 (severe dysplasia and carcinoma in situ).

AETIOLOGY

Studies of women who have pruritus show that this disease has a varied aetiology.

General skin diseases

The conditions listed in Figure 35.6 are the usual skin diseases which may manifest as pruritus vulvae. Fungal infections may also cause vulval itch, although the itch is generally intercrural.

Fig 35.5 Dysplasia.

Fig. 35.6 The itchy vulva: aetiology	
	Percentage of cases
General skin diseases (psoriasis, leucoderma, lichen planus, intertrigo, scabies)	5
General diseases (diabetes,? deficiency diseases)	5
Allergic dermatitis	5
Vaginal discharges Trichomoniasis Candidosis	50
Psychosomatic conditions	35

General diseases

The most common general disease causing pruritus vulvae is diabetes mellitus. In diabetes, as well as being itchy, the vulva is swollen and dark-red in colour.

Allergic dermatitis

Sensitivity to soap (usually perfumed), some detergents used to wash pantihose, and other contact allergens may cause vulval itch.

Vaginal infections

The most common causes of vulval itch, particularly in younger women, are vaginal infections, particularly candidosis and trichomoniasis. As candidal infection of the vulval skin is common, vulval skin scrapings should be taken in cases where general diseases and allergic causes have been eliminated. It may also be helpful to inspect the vulval skin through a magnifying glass or a colposcope.

Human papilloma virus (HPV) infection is no longer thought to be a cause of pruritus vulvae.

Psychosocial causes

Pruritus vulvae is of organic aetiology in more than two-thirds of women with the disease. It is thought that psychosocial causes account for the remainder of cases.

INVESTIGATION OF PRURITUS VULVAE

Because psychosocial factors are involved in many cases, the history of the condition is crucial and questions should be asked about the period before the itchy vulva became distressing. The patient's general health should be assessed and questions asked about her general and sexual relationships (including, when appropriate, sexual abuse in childhood). Any concerns raised should be explored. The history will determine if the main area of itch is vulval, anal or intercrural. If it is one of the last two, the cause is probably threadworms, tinea or intertrigo. The woman should be asked about any allergic conditions including contact dermatitis and drug sensitivity. The duration of the pruritus should be determined. If it is longer than 12 months, multiple skin biopsies (Fig. 35.7) using a dermatome should be considered, irrespective of the age of the woman or the appearance of the vulva.

General skin condition should be assessed by examining the patient in a good light, and inspecting all body surfaces including the interdigital folds of the feet and hands.

General medical causes should be considered, particularly glycosuria. The urine should also be checked for protein. In elderly women, a 2-hour postprandial or fasting blood sugar test should be ordered.

The vagina should be inspected and swabs taken, on more than one occasion, to exclude candidosis and trichomoniasis. A skin scraping for vulval candida infection should be taken if the pruritus has persisted for more than 6 months.

Fig. 35.7 Sites from which a biopsy should be made.

Candidal infection of the vulval skin may cause cyclic, episodic itching or burning and, occasionally, postcoital vulvovaginal irritation. The syndrome is termed *cyclical vulvo-vestibulitis*.

TREATMENT

Any aetiological factor detected should be treated. Medical treatment is the appropriate course in cases of lichen sclerosis and squamous cell hyperplasia, unless a skin biopsy shows VIN3, when surgical or laser treatment is indicated. Surgery by simple vulvectomy has been largely abandoned because pruritus recurs in more than 50% of cases. The patient must be made aware that to obtain a cure, medical treatment must be continued over a long period. During this time, attempts should be made to discover any psychological upsets which might have precipitated the pruritus.

Perfumed sprays should not be applied to the vulva: in fact, it is preferable to apply nothing but water. Douching, if used, should cease and nylon knickers and pantihose should be avoided.

Topical corticosteroids are prescribed. Initially, a high-potency topical steroid cream, such as diprosone OV or clobetasone (Dermovate), is applied twice daily for 2–3 weeks and then daily for 1 month. After this, a less potent topical corticosteroid, such as hydrocortisone or Trimovate, is prescribed.

If the itch is severe, a sedative should be prescribed to help the woman sleep at night. Elderly women may obtain relief if hormone replacement treatment (see page 321) is tried. The patient requires a good deal of support and reassurance over the period of treatment but should be made aware that, in time, the itch ceases in about 90% of patients.

If the biopsies show severe dysplasia (vulval intra-epithelial dysplasia) or carcinoma *in situ*, vulvectomy is the correct treatment (see Chapter 38, Malignancies of the female genital tract).

Vulval atrophy in younger women

Vulval atrophy may occur in a few younger women. It can cause considerable distress not only because it is uncomfortable but because it prevents sexual intercourse, or makes it painful. The woman should be investigated for the presence of impaired glucose tolerance, and allergic conditions sought. Treatment is not very effective. The woman should be advised not to wear pantihose, as these garments prevent ventilation and increase vulval moisture.

Most medications are ineffective, but some success has been obtained using a 2% testosterone propionate ointment or a 2% dihydrotestosterone cream.

Chronic vulval burning or pain (vulvodynia)

A few women complain of chronic burning, stinging, irritation, rawness and, sometimes, pain in the vulvo-vestibular area. There is little or no itching. The condition is called *vulvodynia*. In a subset of vulvodynia, the woman complains of severe vulval pain during attempted penile entry or when one or more areas of the vulva is touched with a cotton wool swab. The area of tenderness may be reddened.

Treatment is unsatisfactory. Low-dose antidepressants and psychotherapy may be tried. If these treatments fail to relieve the symptoms, some gynaecologists offer laser excision of the area, including the Bartholin glands. If a skin biopsy is taken it shows non-specific chronic inflammation. The diagnosis is by exclusion. The aetiology is not known.

CHAPTER 36

Endometriosis and adenomyosis

Endometriosis

Endometriosis denotes the presence of functioning endometrial tissue in an abnormal location, in other words outside the uterus. The locations and the approximate chance of the lesion affecting the organ or structure is shown in *Figure 36.1*.

The incidence of endometriosis is difficult to determine, as in many instances it is only discovered at laparoscopy when the patient presents with infertility or obscure abdominal pain. A probable estimate is that between 1 and 7% of women in their reproductive years have endometriosis. Endometriosis is found more commonly among women who are infertile or who delay childbearing until after the age of 30 years.

AETIOLOGY

How the endometrium reaches the ectopic locations is not entirely understood. It probably results from the retrograde passage along the Fallopian tubes of endometrial tissue during menstruation. It is now believed that, in most women, retrograde menstruation occurs, but the development of other than temporary endometrial nodules (blisters) only occurs in some women. The retrograde menstruation explains why most endometrial lesions occur on the ovaries or in the cul-de-sac (pouch of Douglas). Lymphatic or haematogenous spread may be the reason for the rare deposits of endometriosis in distant sites, for example, the umbilicus.

Once viable endometriotic tissue has reached and adhered to the ectopic location, it still has to be explained why it survives and grows in that location, instead of being eliminated by macrophages. A current theory is that there may be a defect in cell-mediated immunity which permits the endometrial tissue to survive. In order to grow in these ectopic sites, the endometrial tissue has to respond to cyclical oestrogen and, to a lesser extent, progesterone. If a constant oestrogen milieu occurs, as in pregnancy, the lesions tend to be attacked by macrophages and become fibrotic.

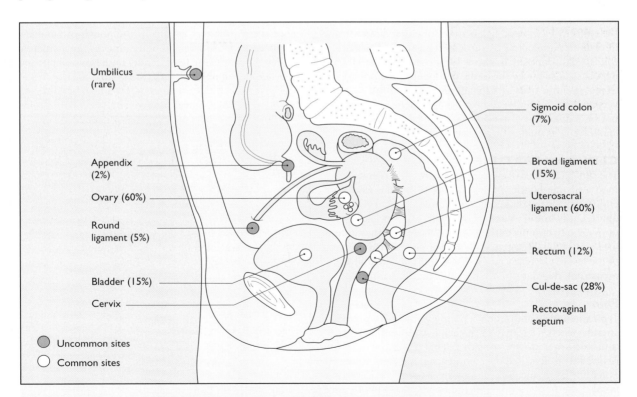

Fig. 36.1 *Common and uncommon sites of extra-uterine endometriosis. The figures given in parentheses indicate the approximate chance of the lesion affecting the organ or structure.*

PATHOLOGY

Whatever the location, the ectopic endometrium, surrounded by stroma, implants and forms a miniature cyst, which responds to the cyclic secretion of oestrogen and progesterone, just as the uterine endometrium does. During menstruation, bleeding in the cyst occurs. The blood, endometrial tissue and tissue fluid are trapped in the cyst. Over the next cycle, the tissue fluid and the blood plasma are absorbed, leaving dark, thickened blood. The cycle recurs each month and slowly the cyst enlarges, containing increased amounts of tarry, chocolate-coloured inspissated blood. The maximal size of the cyst depends on its location. Small cysts may remain small or be attacked by macrophages and become small fibrotic lesions. Ovarian cysts (endometriomata) tend to be larger than other cysts, but do not usually become larger than a medium-sized orange. As the cyst grows, internal pressure may destroy the active endometrial lining, making the cyst non-functional.

Rupture or leakage of material from even small cysts is not uncommon. The released inspissated blood is very irritating with the result that multiple adhesions surround the cysts. The ectopic endometrium and stromal cells also tend to infiltrate adjacent tissues, leading to more pelvic adhesions and fixation (Fig. 36.2). If an ovarian cyst is found which looks like an endometrioma, but there are no adhesions, the diagnosis is unlikely to be endometriosis.

As mentioned, the ovary is most often involved and ovarian endometriosis may present as small superficial implants (red or black spots) or a larger endometrial cyst. Lesions on the surface of the broad ligament occur either directly from implanting endometrial tissue or as a secondary spread from the ovarian deposit. In these locations the endometrial deposits cause puckering of the peritoneum and adhesions to the posterior surface of the uterus, often fixing it in retroversion. Lesions in the cul-de-sac are of interest as they may not be palpable or visualized by a laparoscope unless the laparoscopy is made during menstruation.

CLINICAL FEATURES

The clinical features of endometriosis are often non-specific. In at least one-quarter of the number of women who have endometriosis the disease is symptomless and, in a further quarter, it is found in association with other pelvic conditions. The symptoms may be bizarre because of the varying locations of the disease, and do not correlate with the extent of the lesions in many cases. The symptoms include pain, menstrual irregularities, dyspareunia and infertility.

Pain

Typically, lower abdominal crampy pain starts premenstrually, reaches its peak in the last few days of menstruation and then slowly subsides. This symptom is often referred to as acquired dysmenorrhoea. If the endometrial cysts are large and adhesions are present, or if lesions involve the peritoneum over the bowel, the woman may complain of constant lower abdominal or pelvic pain, which varies in intensity.

Menstrual disturbances

In 60% of women menstrual irregularities occur. The woman may complain of premenstrual staining or spotting, heavy menstrual periods (menorrhagia), or more frequent periods, which may be heavy.

Dyspareunia

If the endometriotic lesions involve the cul-de-sac, particularly if the uterus is retroverted and fixed by adhesions, the woman may complain of dyspareunia on deep penile penetration. If the peritoneum over the bowel is involved, she may have pain on defaecation.

Infertility

Although endometriosis is associated with infertility, whether it is a cause of infertility is disputed, unless the lesions are severe and distort the anatomy. Usually endometriosis is not suspected until a laparoscopy, made during the course of infertility investigations, reveals the disease. Mild endometriosis associated with infertility is treated with hormones by some specialists and not by others. In 1992, a group of European experts concluded that there were no reliable data to support treating mild endometriosis with drugs.

CLINICAL EXAMINATION

Abdominal and pelvic examination may show no abnormality if the lesions are small. It has been suggested that the pelvic examination should be made during menstruation, or soon after, to detect lesions in the pouch of Douglas, which may not be apparent at other times of the menstrual cycle. Larger cysts cause fixed, tender nodular swellings and may be easily palpable.

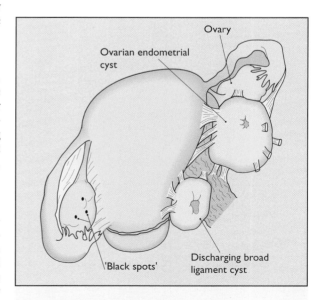

Fig. 36.2 Extra-uterine endometriosis.

DIAGNOSIS

It is often difficult, clinically, to distinguish endometriosis from pelvic inflammatory disease or an ovarian cyst. Because of this, it is prudent to examine the pelvis through a laparoscope if endometriosis is suspected. At laparoscopy, the extent of the disease should be determined as this will influence the treatment (Fig. 36.3).

MANAGEMENT OF ENDOMETRIOSIS

The management of endometriosis depends on the extent of the disease as determined by laparoscopy (see Fig. 36.3), on the symptoms, and on the desire of the woman to retain her fecundity. Figure 36.4 is an algorithm showing management of this disease, details of which will now be discussed.

Hormonal treatment

Currently, four regimens of hormonal treatment are advocated. The treatments suppress or reduce oestrogen synthesis and release. In consequence, menstruation ceases and this inhibits further growth of the lesions, permits the body defences to absorb the contents of the lesions and leads to their fibrosis. The hormonal treatments are:
- Danazol.
- Gonadotrophin-releasing hormone (GnRH) agonists.
- Gestrinone.
- Medroxyprogesterone acetate.

Danazol

Danazol, an isoxazol derivative of 17-α-ethinyl testosterone, reduces the number of GnRH receptors in the pituitary gland and causes a reduction in the level of sex hormone-binding globulin (SHBG). The fall in SHBG causes an increase in free testosterone and a fall in unbound oestradiol. Danazol may also act directly on the ovary to reduce steroid synthesis.

Danazol is given in a dose of 200mg two to four times a day for 3–12 months, depending on the extent of the lesions and on the response. The symptoms are usually relieved in 2–6 weeks in three-quarters of women treated. The effect of danazol on the endometriotic lesions is discussed later. Adverse effects include:
- Amenorrhoea in 60% of women and oligomenorrhoea in the remainder.
- Increase in weight, often more than 3kg.
- Oily skin or acne in 20% of women.
- Deepening voice in 10% of women.

GnRH agonists

GnRH agonists render the pituitary gonadotrophs insensitive to stimulation by endogenous GnRH, with resulting suppression of ovarian steroid secretion. The drug is given in a dose of 200μg intranasally twice daily for 3–6 months or as a long-acting injection monthly. The effect on the endometriosis is similar to that of danazol. Adverse effects include:
- Nearly all women experience hot flushes, which may be severe.
- Amenorrhoea develops in 70% of women.
- Reversible bone loss of 2–4% over a 6-month period occurs in 3% of women. However, fewer patients complain of side effects compared with danazol.

Stage	Characteristics	Diagnosis	Treatment
I, II	**Minimal, Mild** Small surface nodules with no scarring or peritubal adhesions.	Only by laparoscope in investigation of infertility.	At most, electrocautery or CO_2 laser to lesions. Do not give hormones.
III	**Moderate** Small scattered surface lesions with scarring; ovarian endometriomata, <2.5cm, few periovarian or peritubal adhesions; nodules in the cul-de-sac or uterosacral ligaments.	Often symptoms but confirmation by laparoscopy needed.	Electrocautery or CO_2 laser to lesions. Hormones. Conservative surgery if hormones fail to relieve symptoms.
IV	**Severe** Ovarian endometriomata >2.5cm; marked adhesions of ovary or tubes, cul-de-sac obliteration.	Symptoms and signs. Laparotomy confirms.	Conservative surgery. Hormones. Hysterectomy and salpingo-oophorectomy.
V	**Very severe** Stage III plus involvement of bowel, bladder, ureter, etc.	Laparotomy. Barium enema. IVP.	Surgery. Hormones, if surgery incomplete.

Fig. 36.3 The management of endometriosis

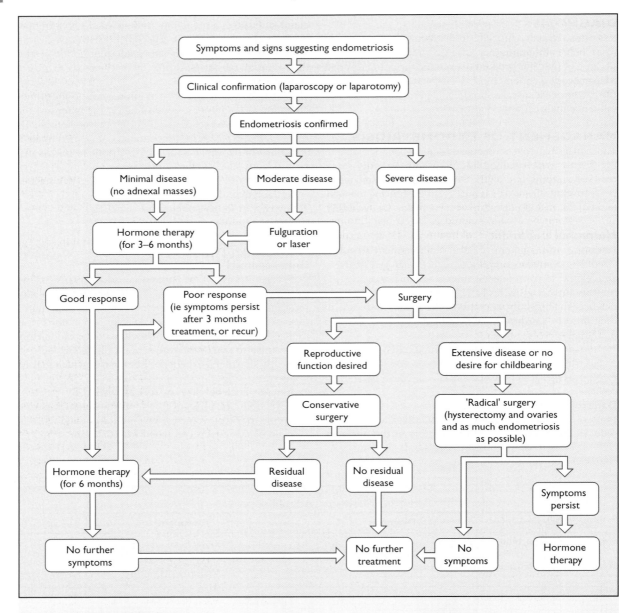

Fig. 36.4 Management of endometriosis.

Gestrinone
This is a 'new generation' progestogen and it is prescribed in a dose of 2.5mg twice weekly and, in early studies, seems as effective as danazol.

Medroxyprogesterone acetate
This progestogen has been used for the past 20 years; 30mg is given daily and the dose increased if the symptoms are not relieved, or it may be given intramuscularly

(150mg every 3 months). The side effects of nausea, weight gain, oily hair, acne and mood disturbances are common.

Longer-term adverse effects of the medications
The four regimens of treatment if continued for more than 6 months lead to bone loss, which is increased if GnRH agonists are used. Some women develop severe hot flushes and other symptoms of oestrogen deficiency. These

women, and women who require a longer course of GnRH agonists, can be treated with hormone replacement therapy (HRT) (see page 321), preferably using tibolone, the so-called 'add back' treatment.

Outcome

The effect of each of these hormonal treatments is similar in terms of relief of pain and reduction in the severity of the endometriosis judged by a second-look laparoscopy made after treatment has ceased and the woman has had at least one menstrual period. The results are: in 30% of the women complete regression of the disease will have occurred; in 60% partial regression will have occurred; and in 10% the extent of the disease is unchanged, although the symptoms have been relieved or cured. The findings suggest that further courses of treatment may be needed. It also appears that once hormonal treatment ceases, endometriosis recurs in about 50% of women over a 5-year period.

It should be noted that the greater the stage of the disease at diagnosis, the greater is the chance of recurrence.

It could be argued that surgery gives better results, though this is only true if an oophorectomy is performed in addition to other surgery. If the ovaries are conserved endometriosis may recur.

Surgery

Small lesions detected with laparoscopy can be treated by electrocautery or laser under laparoscopic vision. Larger lesions, particularly those involving the ovaries, require more extensive surgery. The procedure depends on the patient's age, her desire for children and the difficulty of the operation. There is evidence that, in extensive endometriosis, a 3-month course of hormone treatment may make the surgery easier. If the woman desires a pregnancy (provided no other bars to conception are present), the aim should be to conserve as much ovarian tissue as possible, by dissecting out or marsupializing the endometrial cysts. In women who have no desire for a further pregnancy, total hysterectomy and oophorectomy may be appropriate treatment, provided that the woman is informed about the procedure and has had the opportunity to think about it and discuss it with the surgeon. In some cases, hysterectomy will not relieve the symptoms as the endometrial nodules are extra-uterine and often deep in the pouch of Douglas. These deposits are difficult to access.

PSCHOLOGICAL ASPECTS OF ENDOMETRIOSIS

The knowledge that she has endometriosis can cause considerable distress to a woman. In part, this is because of the poor correlation between the size and number of the lesions and the symptomatology and, in part, it is due to the publicity that endometriosis receives in the popular press.

The woman's doctor should explain what endometriosis is and what it is not. The differentiation between endometriosis and the premenstrual syndrome needs to be discussed because some of the symptoms are similar. The relationship between endometriosis and infertility also needs to be discussed and treatment strategies outlined. The woman should be made aware of the choices of hormonal treatment and surgery (or a combination of each), and of their relative merits in her case. The fact that endometriosis may recur following either treatment needs to be brought to her attention. However, the doctor should offer qualified optimism about the outcome, and should stress the importance of adequate follow-up.

Adenomyosis

Adenomyosis denotes the presence of functioning endometrial tissue which has penetrated the myometrium by direct spread from the uterine lining.

PATHOLOGY

The cells which infiltrate the muscle derive mainly from the basal layer of the endometrium. As this layer is relatively insensitive to hormonal stimulation, the adenomyotic nodules tend to be small, containing little blood, but they provoke a marked stromal reaction. The lesion also appears to stimulate myometrial proliferation, causing the tumour to enlarge slowly (*Fig. 36.5*). Clinically, adenomyosis may be indistinguishable from a myoma, and both may coexist. As the growth of the clinical adenomyoma takes time, clinical adenomyosis tends to occur later in the reproductive years, often in parous women after a long period of secondary infertility.

CLINICAL FEATURES

One-third of patients are asymptomatic. In the remaining women, the main symptoms are:
- Progressively increasing pain, often associated with menstruation. In this case the pain increases throughout menstruation, reaching its peak towards the latter stages.
- Menstrual irregularities, such as premenstrual staining and spotting, increased flow or more frequent periods.

MANAGEMENT OF ADENOMYOSIS

At pelvic examination the uterus is found to be enlarged and tender, and there may be discrete adenomyomata which are indistinguishable from myomata. If the woman has no symptoms and the adenomyoma is not large, no treatment is needed. If the woman has symptoms, hysterectomy is the preferred treatment as adenomyosis does not respond well to hormone treatment.

Fig. 36.5 The microscopic appearance of adenomyosis. (a) The adenomyotic nodule is lying deep in the myometrium, and both glands and stroma are present.

(b) Another specimen at higher magnification showing the glands and the stroma, which is quite dense.

CHAPTER 37

Benign tumours, cysts and malformations of the genital tract

Benign tumours or cysts may form in any part of the genital tract. Benign tumours occur most often in the uterus (myomata) and most benign cysts occur in the ovaries. Malformations tend to involve the uterus and the vagina.

Malformations of the genital tract

The Müllerian ducts develop in a female fetus from the paramesonephric ducts, growing caudally on each side.

By the 35th day after fertilization, the lower part of the ducts change direction and grow towards the midline where they meet and fuse with each other and then grow caudally once again. By the 65th day, they have completed the fusion and their medial walls have gradually disappeared to form a single hollow tube (*Fig. 37.1*). The most caudal portion, which will become the vagina, becomes solid and fuses with an ingrowth of endodermal cells from the cloaca. By the 20th gestational week, the

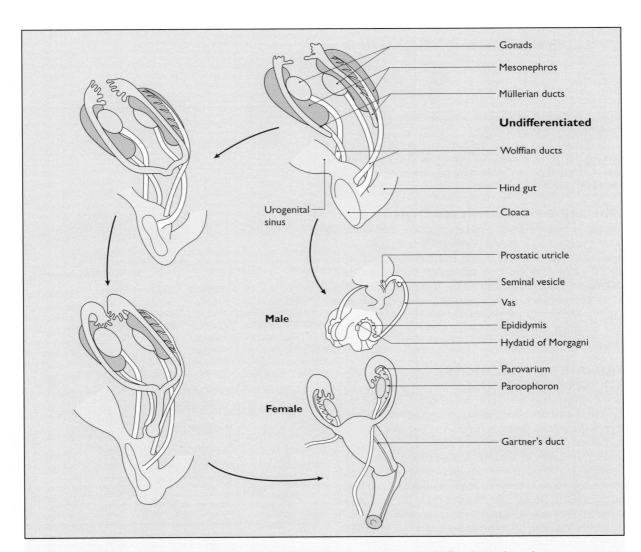

Fig. 37.1 Development of the genital organs, from the Müllerian duct in the female and the Wolffian duct in the male.

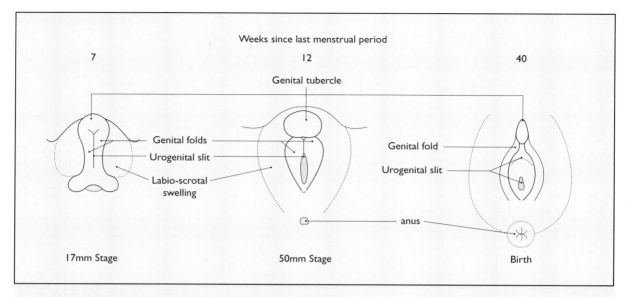

Fig. 37.2 Differentiation of the female external genitalia (not to scale).

solid growth has recanalized and the external genitalia have formed (*Fig. 37.2*).

Malformations of the genital tract occur when the process described above does not occur. The error may be one of failure of the recanalization process or may be a failure of the two Müllerian ducts to fuse.

FAILURE OF RECANALIZATION

The most common defect is an imperforate hymen or transverse septum, which should be detectable during the examination of the neonate. If it is not detected until after puberty, menstrual discharge may collect in the vagina and, in long-term cases, may distend the uterus and tubes (*Fig. 37.3*). Treatment is to make a cruciate incision in the hymen septum and permit the inspissated fluid to escape slowly. Less common defects produce complete or partial vaginal atresia.

FAILURE OF THE DUCTS TO FORM OR TO FUSE

One or other duct may fail to form, and only one Fallopian tube and a distorted unicornate uterus may be found. If both ducts fail to form the woman will be amenorrhoeic.

Failure of the two Müllerian ducts to fuse leads to one of several malformations (*Fig. 37.4*). Most of these malformations do not reduce the woman's fertility, but should pregnancy occur, late abortion, premature labour or intra-uterine fetal death are four times as likely to occur. A sub-septate uterus may lead to recurrent abortion, and can be treated by excising the septum by surgery or laser. If the woman has a bicornuate uterus and becomes pregnant, the fetus may present as a transverse lie in late pregnancy.

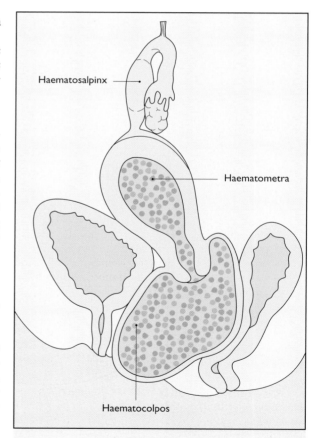

Fig. 37.3 Haematocolpos due to imperforate hymen septum.

Subseptate uterus   Arcuate uterus

Bicornuate uterus

Double uterus   Septate vagina

Fig. 37.4 Common genital tract malformations.

Vulval tumours

Since the tissues of the vulva are covered by skin, tumours arising in the vulval tissues are similar to those occurring in any part of the integument. A few women develop vulval varicosities, which may cause discomfort and are more marked in pregnancy.

Vaginal tumours

Vaginal cysts are uncommon but occasionally one develops in the lateral wall of the upper vagina. It is a cyst of a remnant of the degenerate Wolffian duct and is referred to as a *Gartner's duct cyst*. A cystic swelling may occur in the anterior wall of the vagina, directly below the urethra: this is a *urethral diverticulum*. If it becomes infected, the woman complains of dysuria and frequency of urination. Occasionally, a *myoma* may develop beneath the vaginal epithelium.

Cervical tumours

The most common cervical tumour is a cervical polyp, which occurs as the result of localized hyperplasia of the epithelium and stroma covering a ridge between two clefts in the cervical canal. The columnar epithelium covering the polyp may undergo squamous metaplasia, or ulcerate. The main symptoms are intermittent or post coital bleeding though many cervical polyps are symptomless. The diagnosis is made on inspection of the cervix. The polyp can be removed by twisting the pedicle and the tissue should be sent for histopathology. Other tumours which may be detected occasionally are genital papillomata and myomata or fibromyomata.

Uterine tumours

ENDOMETRIAL POLYPS

Endometrial polyps may occur in association with endometrial hyperplasia and may be a cause of abnormal uterine bleeding. They are detected by curettage provided a polyp forceps is also introduced into the uterus (*Fig. 37.5*), or by hysteroscopy.

UTERINE MYOMATA (FIBROMYOMATA, FIBROIDS)

These are the most common tumours of the genital tract. A myoma is composed of smooth muscle bundles interspersed with strands of connective tissue, surrounded by a thin capsule. The tumour may arise in any part of the Müllerian duct, but occurs most often in the myometrium, where several tumours may develop simultaneously. The tumour may vary from the size of a pea to a football.

Myomata occur in about 5% of women during the reproductive years. The tumours grow slowly and may only be detectable clinically in the fourth decade of life, when the incidence increases to about 20%. They are more common in nulliparous women or women who have had only one child.

Their aetiology is unclear. They may arise from normal muscle cells, from immature muscle cells in the myometrium or from embryonal cells in the walls of uterine blood vessels. Whatever their origin, the tumours begin as tiny multiple seedlings which are scattered through the myometrium. The seedlings grow very slowly but progressively (over years rather than months), under the influence of circulating oestrogens, and unless detected and treated as most are today, may form a tumour weighing 10kg or more. At first, the tumour is intramural, but as it grows it may develop in several directions. This is shown in *Figure 37.6*. After the menopause, as oestrogen is no longer secreted in any great quantity, myomata tend to atrophy.

Pathology

If the tumour is cut, it pouts above the surrounding myometrium as its capsule contracts. Whitish-grey in colour, it is composed of whorled intertwining bundles of

Fig. 37.5 The use of polyp forceps to secure and remove endometrial polyps.

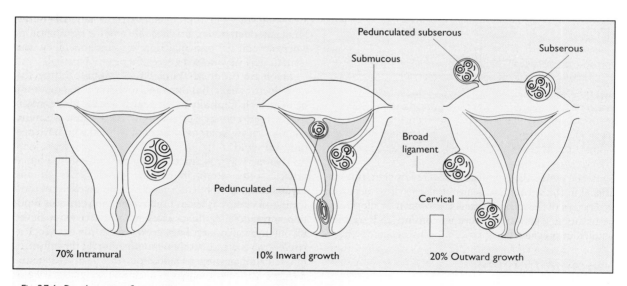

Fig. 37.6 Development of myomata.

muscles, in a matrix of connective tissue (*Fig. 37.7*). At its periphery, the muscle fibres are arranged in concentric layers, and the normal muscle fibres surrounding the tumour are similarly oriented. Between the tumour and the normal myometrium, a thin layer of areolar tissue forms a pseudocapsule, through which the blood vessels enter the myoma.

On microscopy, groups of spindle-shaped muscle cells, with elongated nuclei, are separated into bundles by connective tissue (*Fig. 37.8*). As the entire blood supply of the

Fig. 37.7 Gross appearance of a myoma.

Fig. 37.8 The microscopic appearance of a myoma. The bundles of spindle-shaped muscle cells run in several directions and tend to form a whorl-like pattern.

myoma is derived from the few vessels entering from the pseudocapsule, the growth of the tumour means that it often outstrips its blood supply. This leads to degeneration, particularly in the central portion of the myoma. Initially, *hyaline degeneration* occurs, which may become *cystic*, or *calcification* may occur over time – the 'womb stones' of 19th-century gynaecologists. In pregnancy, a rare complication (red degeneration) may occur. This follows extravasation of blood through the tumour, giving it a raw beef appearance. In fewer than 0.1% of tumours, sarcomatous change occurs.

Symptomatology

The symptoms depend on the size and the position of the myoma. Most small myomata, and some larger ones, are symptomless and are only detected during a routine examination. If the myoma is submucous, it may be associated with menorrhagia. If the heavy bleeding persists the woman may become anaemic and, as the uterus contracts, it may cause crampy pains. Submucous myomata which become pedunculated may cause a persistent bloody discharge from the uterus.

Irrespective of their position in the uterus, large myomata may cause pressure symptoms in the pelvis, dysuria and frequency, and constipation or backache if the enlarged uterus presses on the rectum. A cervical myoma may cause pelvic pain and make sexual intercourse impossible.

Diagnosis

Abdominal and vaginal examination may show a 'knobbly' uterus, or a smooth enlargement of the uterus. On moving the cervix, the whole firm mass moves. In some cases the diagnosis is obvious, in others the smooth enlargement may be due to a pregnancy or to an ovarian mass. A pelvic ultrasound examination will establish the diagnosis.

Management

Four choices exist:

- To continue to observe the myoma.
- To perform a myomectomy.
- To perform a hysterectomy.
- To offer the woman gonadotrophin-releasing hormone analogue (GnRHa).

Observation

Symptomless myomata, less than the size of a 14-week pregnancy, may be observed. Other types of myomata:

- Distort the uterine cavity and are considered a factor in the couple's infertility.
- Are situated in the lower part of the uterus or the cervix, which would complicate childbirth.
- Grow rapidly, which might suggest sarcomatous change.

If the myoma is associated with menstrual disturbances, the woman has the choice to have a hysteroscopy or a careful diagnostic curettage to exclude intra-uterine pathology, or to have surgical treatment.

Myomectomy

If the woman is wishes to preserve her reproductive function, myomectomy may be chosen. The operation removes all detected myomata and reconstitutes the uterus. The woman must accept that, if problems arise during myomectomy, the surgeon may have to proceed to hysterectomy. Following myomectomy, 40% of women who have the opportunity to conceive will do so. Against this is the fact that in 5% of women, the myomata recur and a similar number of women continue to have menorrhagia, which necessitates the use of hormones (see page 226), hysteroscopic resection or hysterectomy.

Hysterectomy

Total hysterectomy is the treatment of choice in older women, women who have no wish for a further pregnancy and women who have menorrhagia or marked pressure symptoms. A patient should not be rushed into making a decision to have a hysterectomy. She should be given time to think and to ask questions about the procedure. The gynaecologist should also make sure that misconceptions about the operation are addressed. This was discussed on page 233.

GnRH analogue

Given by injection at intervals, the drug will suppress oestrogen secretion and, consequently, the myomata will atrophy. The greatest effect is in the first month when, on average, a 27% reduction in size occurs. After 3 months little further reduction in the size of the myoma is apparent. In 10% of cases the treatment is ineffective and, after ceasing the treatment, the myomata will grow again. GnRH analogue has a small place in the treatment of selected cases of symptomatic myomata prior to myomectomy, or if the woman is nearing the menopause. However, this drug produces a hypo-oestrogenic state, and bone loss may increase and predispose the woman to osteoporosis.

MYOHYPERPLASIA

Occasionally, vaginal examination shows an enlarged uterus which does not contain myomata as determined by ultra-sound. The condition is termed myohyperplasia (*Fig. 37.9*) and it is thought that it may be caused by psychosomatic factors, but no clearly identified problem has been detected. The uterus rarely exceeds the size of a 10-week pregnancy and the endometrium may be hypertrophic or normal. Myohyperplasia is often symptomless, but may be associated with menorrhagia. Treatment for menorrhagia is discussed on page 226.

MYOMAS AND PREGNANCY

The prevalence of myomas complicating pregnancy is 1 in 200, but the majority of myomata are small and cause no problems. The complications which may occur depend on the number, the size and the position of the myomata in the uterus.

Effect of pregnancy on the myomata

The increased vascularity of the uterus together with the increased circulating levels of oestrogen often lead to an increase in the size and a softening of the myoma. If the growth of the myoma increases too fast, it may outstrip its blood supply, causing degenerative changes in the tumour. The most serious outcome is necrobiosis (red degeneration). The patient may complain of pain and low-grade fever, usually in the second quarter of pregnancy. Palpation reveals that the myoma is very tender and the treatment entails giving analgesics. The pain resolves within a few days and the pregnancy continues.

Effect of the myoma on the pregnancy

This depends on the size and position of the tumour. If it distorts the uterine cavity, the risk of spontaneous abortion is doubled and there is an increased chance that labour will start prematurely. Large tumours in the myometrium may also distort the uterine cavity causing malposition or malpresentation of the fetus. Tumours in the lower part of the uterus may obstruct the birth canal, preventing vaginal delivery. Large tumours may cause pressure symptoms on the bladder or the rectum. Postdelivery, they can interfere with uterine muscle contraction leading to postpartum haemorrhage.

Diagnosis

If the patient presents early in pregnancy, the myoma may be felt on vaginal examination. A single fundal myoma may cause diagnostic difficulty but this can be resolved by an ultrasound examination.

Management

In most cases, no treatment is needed during pregnancy. Myomectomy is inadvisable as the operation is attended by marked bleeding, and haemostasis can be difficult. In late pregnancy, the position of the myoma in relation to the fetal-presenting part and the pelvic cavity will affect the decision on the method of delivery. The patient and her partner should be involved in the discussion and the reason for the final decision explained.

As the tumour is usually in the upper segment of the uterus, vaginal delivery is possible for most patients. A few women with low-lying myomata which obstruct the birth canal require caesarean section. Myomectomy should not be performed during this operation because of the dangers of haemorrhage and infection.

Fallopian tube tumours

Benign tumours and cysts of the Fallopian tubes and the broad ligament are rare. Occasionally, cysts are found in remnants of the Wolffian duct at surgery (hydatid of

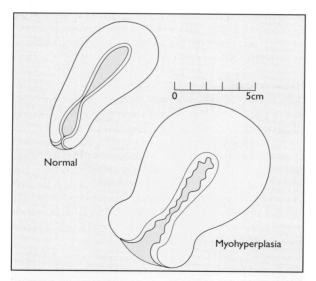

Fig. 37.9 Myohyperplasia.

Morgagni). Parovarian cysts are often large and may be thought to be ovarian until exposed at surgery.

Benign ovarian cysts and tumours

The ovary consists of:
* Coelomic epithelium.
* Oocytes, derived from primitive germ cells.
* Mesenchymal elements which form the medulla.

These tissues are particularly dynamic, being affected by hormonal stimuli from puberty to the menopause. This may be the reason why so many benign cysts and tumours arise in the ovary.

CLASSIFICATION OF BENIGN OVARIAN CYSTS AND TUMOURS

There is no entirely satisfactory classification of ovarian cysts and tumours. This is because of the complexity of ovarian new growths and because the distinction between some of them can only be made after histological examination. In *Figure 37.10*, a classification is presented and the proportions of benign cysts and tumours encountered is shown.

Functional cysts

A *follicle cyst* is an enlargement of an unruptured Graffian follicle which has continued to secrete fluid. The cyst is usually unilateral and less than 5cm in diameter. The cells may secrete oestrogen or be relatively quiescent and, because of this, the symptoms vary. The woman's menstrual cycle may be lengthened and menorrhagia may occur, or it may be of normal length or shorter.

Multiple follicle cysts may occur following the use of clomiphene or gonadotrophins for inducing ovulation.

Corpus luteum cysts occur when, instead of degenerating when implantation of the embryo fails to occur, the corpus luteum survives and grows. *Theca lutein cysts* occur in gestational trophoblastic disease (see page 146).

If the clinical findings are insufficient to reach a diagnosis, a transvaginal ultrasound examination will help to diagnose an ovarian cyst. However, small cystic enlargements should not be reported as ovarian cysts without qualification. For example, just before ovulation, follicles may measure 20mm (± 10mm). A simple cyst measuring less than 30mm on ultrasound scanning is better described as a follicle, to avoid unnecessary investigations and, perhaps, surgery.

Treatment

The cyst should be observed for 2–3 months, during which time it will probably disappear. Should it still persist and be unilocular, showing no solid areas on ultrasound, it may be aspirated under ultrasonic or laparoscopic guidance. If needle aspiration shows blood-stained fluid a laparotomy is needed. Multilocular persistent cysts require surgical removal.

Benign ovarian neoplasms

Mucinous cystadenoma and serous cystadenoma account for 40% of benign ovarian cysts and tumours. Both derive from the multipotential coelomic epithelium, which forms the Müllerian duct and can imitate tubal, uterine or cervical epithelium.

Mucinous cystadenoma

The cysts occur most frequently between the ages of 35 and 55 years. They can grow to a considerable size, and are multilocular (*Fig. 37.11*). They are usually unilateral and rarely become malignant. The cyst is lined with tall columnar cells, each of which has a basal nucleus and cystoplasmic mucin (*Fig. 37.12*). Mucin is constantly secreted into the cyst with the result that its wall becomes tense. Often a portion of the wall bulges outwards and a depression may form at the neck of the bulge, which may become occluded, forming a daughter

Tumour (benign)	Cell origin	Type	Proportional incidence %
Functional cysts (follicle, corpus luteum)	Normal follicle	Cystic	24
Serous cystadenoma	Coelomic epithelium	Cystic	20
Mucinous cystadenoma	Coelomic epithelium	Cystic	20
Teratoma (dermoid cyst)	Oogonia	Cystic	15
Endometrioma	Ectopic endometrium	Cystic	10
Fibroma (inc, Brenner's tumour)	Mesenchyme	Solid	5

Fig 37.10 A classification of benign ovarian cysts and tumours

Fig. 37.11 Benign mucinous cystadenoma.

Fig. 37.12 Microscopic appearance of mucinous cystadenoma – note the cells lining the tumour resemble those of the endocervix (× 256).

cyst (*Fig. 37.13*). Occasionally the cyst may rupture, releasing mucinous cells, which may become attached to the peritoneum and omentum, leading to an intraperitoneal accumulation of mucin (*pseudomyxoma peritonei*).

Serous cystadenoma

These cysts are also more frequently detected in women aged 35–55 years. They are lined with cuboidal epithelium, resembling that of the oviduct (*Fig. 37.14*). The cells secrete thin, watery fluid, but the quantity secreted is not great. In consequence, the tension inside the cyst is low and the epithelial cells proliferate to form intracystic papillomata. In some cases, the cells penetrate the cyst wall to form external papillary projections. Serous cystadenoma are uni- or multilocular and are bilateral in 30% of cases (*Fig. 37.15*). They only grow to a moderate size, with malignant changes occurring in one-third of cases, usually when the woman is in her 50s.

Endometriomata

These ovarian tumours (chocolate cysts) are usually associated with other evidence of endometriosis. They rarely become malignant. Endometriosis is discussed on page 272.

Benign teratoma (dermoid cyst)

Deriving from germ cells, benign teratomata are relatively common. The cyst contains epithelial, mesodermal and endothelial elements. Thus the dermoid may contain hair, teeth and pultaceous material from sebaceous glands. The tumour is bilateral in 10% of cases. It may occur at any age, but mostly is detected when the woman is aged between 20 and 40 years. The nature of the tumour is confirmed by ultrasound examination or radiology.

Connective tissue neoplasms

Fibromata constitute 5% of benign ovarian neoplasms. The tumour may consist entirely of connective tissue or may be found in association with serous cystadenoma, or with the rare Brenner tumour. Fibromata are usually small, and are bilateral in 10% of cases. Rarely, the fibroma is associated with hydrothorax and ascites (Meigs' syndrome).

DIAGNOSIS OF OVARIAN TUMOURS

Benign ovarian cysts and tumours grow silently and are often undetected for some years. They do not cause pain, but if large may cause discomfort. They rarely affect menstrual function. Periodic abdominal and vaginal examinations will detect benign tumours. A painless cystic or solid mass in the cul-de-sac, or in the position of an ovary, or distending the abdomen, which is cystic to firm on palpation suggests an ovarian tumour. The diagnosis can be confirmed by an abdominal or transvaginal ultrasound scan, which differentiates the tumour from pregnancy, obesity, pseudocyesis, a full bladder or cystic degeneration of a myoma (Fig. 37.16).

MANAGEMENT OF BENIGN OVARIAN TUMOURS

The treatment of mucinous cystadenoma is surgical, the extent of the operation depending on the age of the patient. In younger women ovarian cystectomy is possible, the ovary being reconstructed after the tumour has been shelled out. A similar approach can be used in cases of serous cystadenoma, but in women over the age of 40 years, bilateral salpingo-oophorectomy and total hysterectomy is preferred, because of the possibility of malignant change. Endometriomata, benign teratomata and fibromata can often be shelled out of the normal ovarian tissue and the ovary reconstructed.

OVARIAN TUMOURS AND PREGNANCY

One pregnancy in 1500 is complicated by a clinically detectable ovarian tumour, measuring more than 50mm in diameter. If an ultrasound examination of the pelvis is made routinely, ovarian tumours are detected in 1 in 200 pregnancies. Most of them are cysts, usually an enlarged corpus luteum which resolves spontaneously. Neoplastic tumours are less common in pregnancy. Most are serous cystadenomas, a few are mucinous cystadenomas and these two account for 65% of all neoplasias complicating pregnancy. Teratomata account for 25% and the remaining 10% is made up of a wide variety of ovarian tumours.

Fig. 37.13 Formation of daughter cysts in the wall of a mucinous cystadenoma.

Fig. 37.14 Microscopic appearance of a serous cystadenoma. Note that the cells lining the tumour resemble those of the endosalpinx (× 256).

Fig. 37.15 Gross appearance of a serous cystadenoma.

Effect of the pregnancy of the tumour

The size of the tumour may not change during the pregnancy, but the growing uterus may displace it so that it becomes more obvious. Rarely, torsion of the ovary containing the tumour may occur and, even more rarely, the tumour may rupture.

Effect of the tumour on the pregnancy

The only problem is that the tumour may become incarcerated in the cul-de-sac and obstruct the birth canal (Fig. 37.17).

Diagnosis

In early pregnancy, a vaginal examination may reveal two masses, the pregnant uterus and the ovarian tumour. If any doubt exists, a pelvic ultrasound examination will clarify the diagnosis.

Treatment

Treatment depends on the size and consistency of the tumour and its appearance on ultrasound examination. Ovarian tumours less than 80mm in diameter and echo-free, can be observed, repeat scans being made to see if the tumour increases in size. If treatment is decided upon, the cyst may be aspirated or an ovarian cystectomy performed. A multilocular cyst or a tumour greater than 80mm in size which is thick-walled or semi-solid, requires surgical removal, after the 12th gestational week. A tumour detected after the 30th gestational week may be difficult to remove surgically and premature labour may follow. The decision to operate can only be made after careful consideration and involvement of the patient and her partner. If the tumour obstructs the birth canal and cannot be moved digitally, the patient should be delivered by caesarean section and an ovarian cystectomy performed.

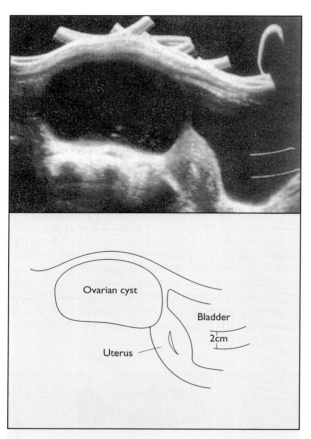

Fig. 37.16 Ovarian cyst (ultrasound-sagittal scan). Line drawing showing the identification of relevant points.

Fig. 37.17 Ovarian cyst obstructing labour.

CHAPTER 38

Malignancies of the female genital tract

Only four cancers can be either prevented or diagnosed at a stage when treatment is curative in most cases. Skin cancer can be prevented by avoiding excessive exposure to the sun; lung cancer can largely be prevented by avoiding smoking tobacco. The other two cancers – cancer of the uterine cervix and breast cancer – can be detected, in most cases, at a stage when treatment is curative.

In this chapter, cancers of the genital tract will be discussed, the most common being mentioned first. Rare cancers such as vaginal cancer and cancer of the Fallopian tubes will not be discussed.

Cervical precancer and cancer

The cervical epithelium undergoes changes through the menstrual cycle and is readily accessible for examination. The epithelium covering the ectocervix is stratified and identical with that of the vagina (*Fig. 38.1*). It is separated from the underlying stroma by an apparent basement membrane. Superior to this is a layer of basal cells from which the other cell layers differentiate. Above the basal layer are five or six layers of parabasal cells. Above them are intermediate and superficial cell layers. The intermediate cell layer consists of large cells, each with reticulated nuclei and vacuoles of glycogen in the cytoplasm. The superficial cell layer varies in thickness, depending on the oestradiol:progesterone ratio present. The superficial cells are flattened and have small nuclei, the cytoplasm containing glycogen (*Fig. 38.2*). A small amount of keratin is produced in some of the cells, which becomes 'cornified'. During the reproductive years, the superficial cells are constantly shed or exfoliated into the vagina, and differentiation of cells from the basal layer also proceeds constantly.

The characteristics of the superficial cells can be studied by taking a smear from the cervix and staining it with Papanicolaou's stain. In some women, the nuclei become abnormally shaped or dyskaryotic, which may indicate a precancerous change; this can be detected by cervical smears.

EPIDEMIOLOGY OF CERVICAL CANCER

Cervical cancer occurs, almost exclusively, among women who are or have been sexually active, but the cause of cervical cancer is not known. There is increasing evidence that infection by certain strains of the human papilloma virus (HPV) is a factor. Studies have shown that between 10 and 30% of sexually active women have acquired HPV infection of the genital tract (including the vulva) by the age of 30 years. The proportion of women infected is higher if the woman or her partner have had several sexual partners. In most cases, the infection is symptomless and persists (see page 258). However, an unknown proportion of women have a transient infection, the body eliminating the virus. The initial infection may be vulval or vaginal, from which the virus spreads to the uterine cervix; the cervix may, however, be infected directly.

The genesis of HPV infection is complex as the presence of cervical cell infection by the virus does not mean that it is always transmitted by sexual intercourse, nor that it necessarily leads to cervical cancer. If cervical cancer does develop it may manifest itself soon or many years after the HPV infection.

Fig. 38.1 Normal squamous epithelium which covers the vaginal portion of the cervix.

Fig. 38.2 Normal exfoliated cervical cells.

This suggests that, if cervical carcinoma develops, it must be due to the added affect of a co-agent. One theory is that HPV sensitizes the cells and, acting with another agent (such as tobacco smoke), may reduce the effectiveness of the woman's immune system to deal with the virus, permitting the development of the abnormal cells. The reason for postulating that certain strains of HPV, notably strains 16 and 18, are involved in the development of cervical cancer, is that over 80% of women who have cervical carcinoma have evidence of HPV infection. If hybrid capture using polymerase chain reaction (PCR) testing is carried out, a higher detection rate is achieved.

CERVICAL EXFOLIATIVE CYTOLOGY

The development of cervical carcinoma is preceded by the appearance of abnormal (dyskaryotic) cervical cells. These cells can be detected by examining an exfoliative cervical smear, stained using the papanicolaou stain (the Pap test), microscopically. As this is a screening test, false negatives may occur, estimated at 5–15%. The proportion of false-negative smears will be reduced if strict criteria are adopted for taking and for examining the smear.

Recently, a new technique has been suggested to clarify smears showing atypical squamous cells of uncertain significance (ASCUS) and to reduce the false-negative rate. The test involves taking cervical cells with a Cervex sampler brush and rinsing the brush into a vial of fixative. The cells are not obscured by blood or mucus and are all fixed properly. In the laboratory, a monolayer of cells is made which is easier to interpret. If the result is inconclusive, the remaining cells in the vial can be used to make a hybrid capture test, which will detect the presence of oncogenic HPVs. A further advantage of this test is that it is likely to reduce the number of colposcopies which gynaecologists make when an inconclusive Pap smear abnormality is found. In the future, the test may also be used to detect other sexually transmitted diseases, such as chlamydia and gonorrhoea.

To reduce the incidence of cervical cancer it is recommended that all sexually active women should have Pap smears made regularly. The first smear should be made soon after the woman starts sexual intercourse and should be repeated after 1 year, as abnormal cells may be missed in a single smear. If no abnormality is found on either smear, regular smears at 2-year intervals should be made, at least until the woman reaches the age of 65 years.

In women aged 30 years and over, the doctor or nurse taking the smear should also examine the woman's breasts, teach her breast self-examination and after the age of 40 years measure her blood pressure.

Technique of taking a cervical smear

A tray is provided on which a bivalve vaginal speculum, some slides, a spray-on fixative plastic, a modified Ayre spatula and an endocervical brush are placed. Before performing a vaginal examination, the warmed speculum is inserted to expose the cervix. The cytobrush is inserted into the cervical canal and rotated. The sample is smeared onto the slide. The ectocervix is sampled with the Ayre spatulum by rotating it through 360° twice and the sample is smeared on to a slide (*Fig. 38.3*).

The smears are sent to a reliable, quality assured cytological laboratory for examination.

Reporting on smears

Cytologists have agreed that nuclear abnormalities should form the basis of a cytological diagnosis. They have agreed to report smears as follows:

- *Unsatisfactory*. A diagnosis cannot be made because there are too few cells, there are no endocervical cells or the slide has been processed incorrectly. The smear should be repeated 4 weeks later.
- *Inflammatory or inconclusive*. The nuclei are distorted by the effects of vaginal infections, such as trichomoniasis and gardnerella. The referring doctor is asked to treat the infection appropriately and then to repeat the smear.
- *Normal*. Repeat the smear in 1–3 years.
- *Mild dyskaryosis* (predictive of CIN 1). The slide may show HPV infection with no dyskaryosis, HPV infection and dyskaryosis, or dyskaryosis without HPV infection.
- *Moderate dyskaryosis* (predictive of CIN 2).
- *Severe dyskaryosis* (predictive of CIN 3) (*Fig. 38.4*).

The Bethesda Classification

An alternative classification is used in the USA (the Bethesda Classification). Smears showing abnormal cells are placed in three categories. These are:

- *Atypical squamous cells of uncertain significance (ASCUS).*
- *Low-grade squamous intra-epithelial lesions (SIL)*, which includes HPV infection as shown by koilocytosis (a halo around the nucleus of some cells) and mild dyskaryosis.
- *High-grade SIL* which includes moderate dyskaryosis (predictive of CIN 2), severe dyskaryosis (predictive of CIN 3) and carcinoma *in situ*.

Telling the patient

The result of the smear should be reported to the woman by phone or by letter. This applies to all smears not just abnormal ones. If an abnormal smear is reported, the need to counsel and explain is imperative.

To many women, the finding of a dyskaryotic smear suggests the presence of cancer. If HPV is found, many women question their own and their partner's previous sexual behaviour. Either finding can lead to guilt, misery and anxiety. Doctors should be aware of this and should talk with the woman, explaining the meaning of the result of the smear and that HPV is not always sexually transmitted. The woman should also be told, in clear non-jargon language, what procedures may be needed. In one reported study, the term 'pre-cancer' was perceived as threatening and the authors suggested that a better term would be 'early warning cells'.

Fig. 38.3 Methods of obtaining cells from the cervix for cytological examination: using (1) special wooden spatula, (2) an Ayre spatula, and (3) a Cervex sampler

Fig. 38.4 Exfoliated cervical cells showing severe dyskaryosis.

MANAGEMENT OF ABNORMAL CERVICAL SMEARS

Approaches to the management of abnormal cervical smears are summarized in *Figure 38.5*.

HPV infection with no evidence of dyskaryosis

Smears should be taken at 6-monthly intervals until the smear is negative for HPV, then annually for 2 years. If there is no evidence of HPV at this time, the patient should return to having a smear every 2 years. If dyskaryosis appears in any smear, treat as recommended below.

Mild dyskaryosis (predictive of CIN 1) with or without HPV

The treatment for this condition is controversial and no consensus has been reached. The reason is that there is no agreement what proportion of cases of mild dyskaryosis progress to, or on biopsy are in, a more severe form. One group of gynaecologists believe that the risk is high and that, in many cases, an immediate biopsy will show moderate or severe dysplasia. They recommend that patients are referred for immediate colposcopy and cervical biopsy.

The other group believe that no immediate action need be taken for 6 months when a second smear is made (some delaying for a third smear at 12 months). They believe that colposcopy and biopsy need be performed only if either or both of the smears show moderate or severe dyskaryosis.

The development of hybrid capture of oncogenic HPV (see page 258) may help resolve the problem.

At present the concept of immediate referral is gaining ground, in spite of the strain it will place on colposcopy services. With increasing women being referred for colposcopy, delays of up to 2 months may occur. Levels of anxiety and distress between being referred for colposcopy because of an abnormal smear and the procedure itself may be considerable. This can be reduced if the doctor or clinic nurse takes time to explain the implications of an abnormal smear and, in detail, the colposcopy procedure. The woman should also be told that she may talk with one of the clinic staff if she becomes anxious or has not understood what they have said.

Moderate and severe dyskaryosis (predictive of in CIN 1 or CIN 2)

These degrees of dyskaryosis require referral for colposcopy and cervical biopsy.

COLPOSCOPY

Dyskaryosis is a cytological diagnosis and observer error is not uncommon. For this reason, a colposcope is often used to verify abnormal findings. A colposcope is a system of lenses which magnifies the cervix 5–20 times and enables a trained observer to translate changes in colour tone, opacity, surface configuration, vascular pattern and intercapillary distance into a diagnosis (Figs. 38.6–38.9).

Abnormal epithelium is white in colour after application of aqueous acetic acid solution (acido-white epithelium), white keratotic patches may be seen and the blood vessels may appear as punctate dots or as a mosaic arrangement (Figs. 38.6–38.9). Bizarre branching vessels usually denote invasive cancer. A trained observer can differentiate between the minor and major cervical precancer lesions and carcinoma with a

Lesion	Low-grade squamous intra-epithelial		High-grade squamous intra-epithelial	
Normal	HPV infection	Mild dyskaryosis	Moderate dyskaryosis	Severe dyskaryosis
If first Pap smear repeat within 1 year. Otherwise every 2 years.	Repeat Pap smear every 6 months, 3 times. If HPV persists, refer for colposcopy.	Either repeat Pap smear 3 times every 6 months and if persists refer, or refer at once for colposcopy.	Refer for colposcopy and biopsy.	Refer for colposcopy and biopsy.

Fig. 38.5 Management of an abnormal Pap smear

Fig. 38.6 Normal cervix. Opening the bivalve speculum exposes the endocervical canal allowing examination of the full transformation zone.

Fig. 38.7 CIN 1. The abnormal epithelium is visible on both the anterior and posterior margins of the cervix having turned white after application of acetic acid.

reasonable degree of accuracy. The predicted diagnosis is confirmed by punch biopsies which are examined histologically.

HISTOLOGY

Mild dysplasia is characterized by nuclear abnormalities in the basal third of the epithelium; the upper layers are not affected. In *moderate dysplasia* some dyskaryotic nuclei are found in the upper layers of the epithelium and abnormal nuclei are more common (*Fig. 38.10*). In *severe dysplasia* the abnormal nuclei occupy all the epithelial layers, and there is a high nuclear:cytoplasmic ratio (*Fig. 38.11*). Severe dysplasia may be difficult to differentiate from carcinoma *in situ*. In carcinoma *in situ* there is no differentiation as the surface layers are reached; the nuclei vary in size and stain deeply, the cells are crowded and the cytoplasm is scanty (*Fig. 38.12*).

Cervical intra-epithelial neoplasia (CIN)

In some cases there is uncertainty about the exact histological diagnosis and whether the identified lesion will regress, persist or progress. This has led to a classification which includes all grades of dysplasia, the CIN classification (*Fig. 38.13*).

Fig. 38.8 *The appearance of the cervix following diathermic ablation of the dysplastic epithelium. The abnormal transformation zone has been replaced by mature squamous epithelium.*

Fig. 38.9 *Invasive cancer of the cervix. The cervix bleeds readily on contact.*

Fig. 38.10 *Dysplasia (moderate) (CIN 2).*

Fig. 38.11 *Dysplasia (severe) (CIN 3).*

Fig. 38.12 *Cervical biopsy from the patient whose cervical smear is shown in Figure 38.4. Carcinoma in situ was found. (a) (× 40) There appears to be invasion of the tissues but in reality the cells have only crept into endocervical crypts. (b) (× 160) The lack of stratification and pleomorphism of the cells is seen at higher magnification.*

NATURAL HISTORY OF CIN

The current belief about the natural history of CIN is shown in *Figure 38.14*.

MANAGEMENT OF CIN

The management of CIN depends on the age of the woman, her desire to reproduce and on the location and extent of the lesion.

Current recommendations for treatment are described below.

CIN grade I

There is a lack of agreement about the management if colposcopically controlled biopsy shows mild dysplasia (CIN 1). Some gynaecologists recommend careful observation as the majority of lesions will resolve spontaneously, but increasingly specialists are recommending that the lesion be obliterated using one of the methods outlined in the management of CIN 2 and 3.

CIN grades 2 and 3

These major grade lesions require either local destructive treatment or excision of the suspect area. Local destructive treatment includes laser, cryosurgery and electrocoagulation diathermy. Each of these methods has its ardent advocates. The selection of patients is important and the whole lesion must be visible and invasive cancer must have been excluded. All treatments can be given under local anaesthesia (2ml

lignocaine 2% in normal saline) or general anaesthesia depending on the patient's and the gynaecologist's preference. Laser protagonists claim that the accuracy of the method and the absence of cervical scarring makes it the preferred method, although they admit the equipment is expensive and requires regular maintenance.

Proponents of other modalities claim that their results are as good as those following laser therapy (over 90% of women have normal smears and normal colposcopic findings after 5 years of follow-up), and that the techniques are simpler, quicker and cheaper.

Each of these treatments may be followed by blood-stained or clear discharge for 1–3 weeks. About 5% of women have vaginal bleeding and the patient may complain of pain or severe discomfort. Sexual intercourse and the use of tampons should be avoided for 4 weeks to allow complete healing. The treatments do not affect the woman's fertility or alter the course of a subsequent pregnancy.

Concern about the effectiveness of the ablative methods has persuaded many gynaecologists to revert to excisional methods. The current preference is to perform a large loop excision of the transformation zone (LLETZ), with ball cautery to the exposed area of the cervix if needed, to achieve haemostasis. The advantage is that the tissue can be examined histologically to exclude invasive cancer, particularly if the suspect areas extend up the cervical canal and their upper limit cannot be identified by colposcopic inspection. The whole transformation zone and some of the cervical canal area is excised. If the procedure is performed by an experienced gynaecologist, there appears to be no adverse effect on the duration of a subsequent pregnancy.

An alternative is for the gynaecologist to use knife conization. Knife conization, usually with suturing to repair the cervix, is associated with a 10% chance of postoperative haemorrhage. If the woman becomes pregnant, there is an increased risk of miscarriage in the second quarter of pregnancy and she may give birth to a preterm baby, as a result

Fig. 38.13 CIN classification		
Grade 1	Mild dysplasia	⎱ Dysplasia of
Grade 2	Moderate dysplasia	⎰ low degree
Grade 3	Severe dysplasia/	⎱ Dysplasia of
	Carcinoma *in situ*	⎰ high degree

of an incompetent cervix. The risk increases with the size of the cone excised. Conversely scarring can cause stenosis of the cervical canal which can prevent the cervix dilating during labour necessitating delivery by caesarean section.

Depending on age, the presence of other gynaecological conditions (for example, myoma or menorrhagia), and personal preferences, some women with CIN 3 may choose hysterectomy.

As mentioned, follow-up is essential. The woman should be reviewed 6 and 12 months after treatment, when a cervical smear is taken and a colposcopic examination is made. If the cytology is negative and the colposcopy normal, annual smears are made from then on. Following hysterectomy for CIN, 6-monthly smears should be made for the first year and, thereafter, every 2 years as abnormal cells may be found in the upper vagina signifying vaginal CIN.

PSYCHOLOGICAL EFFECTS OF CIN ON WOMEN

Many women diagnosed as having CIN become depressed and upset, particularly if a health professional implies that the woman has been sexually promiscuous.

The woman may be concerned that her partner has been or is continuing to be unfaithful. Her attitude to sexual intercourse may change and she may want to avoid sex.

The anxieties and uncertainty should be resolved, as far as possible, by giving the woman a full explanation of CIN and letting her have the opportunity to ask questions. She may also need continued psychological support.

Cervical carcinoma

Carcinoma of the uterine cervix is the second most common gynaecological cancer (after breast cancer). The annual risk for women over the age of 35 years, is 16 per 100,000. The peak incidence is between the ages of 45 and 55 years, with a recent trend towards a younger age. Cervical cancer usually grows outwards becoming a fungating mass; occasionally it grows inwards enlarging the cervix. More than 85% of cervical cancers are squamous cell carcinomas, the remainder being adenocarcinomas which arise from the cells lining the cervical canal or its clefts. With time, the cancer spreads either by direct extension upwards to involve the uterine cavity, downwards to involve the vagina, or via the lymphatic drainage to the external iliac lymph nodes (47% of cases); the obturator lymph node (20%); the hypogastric nodes (7%); or the paracervical nodes (2%). The spread of the cancer detected on clinical examination and CT scan, enables an oncologist to stage the cancer and to recommend treatment on the staging (Fig. 38.15). The higher the stage on the initial examination, the greater is the chance of lymph node involvement and the poorer the prognosis (Fig. 38.16). In early-stage disease (stages Ib and IIa, see later) lymph node metastases are present in 25–30% of cases.

DIAGNOSIS

In its earliest stage, an abnormal smear is the only way to detect cervical cancer as symptoms tend to occur only with

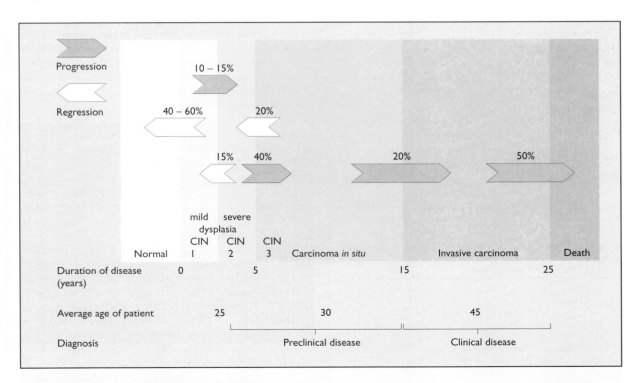

Fig. 38.14 The 'life cycle' of unstable cervical epithelium.

established invasive disease. Irregular bleeding *per vaginam*, particularly after sexual intercourse, or a pink vaginal discharge after urination, demand investigation by a vaginal examination using a speculum and a cervical smear. Diagnosis is confirmed by a cervical wedge biopsy or, if gross evidence of cervical cancer is detected, by biopsy and endocervical curettage.

TREATMENT
The best results of treating of cervical cancer are obtained in oncological units staffed by pelvic surgeons and radiological oncologists. Micro-invasive (stage Ia) cancer is treated by simple total hysterectomy. Stage Ib cancer may be treated either by radical hysterectomy or by radiotherapy. Radical hysterectomy includes removal of the parametrium and pelvic lymphadenectomy, whilst radiotherapy includes a combination of external beam and intra-cavity radiation. Both give similar 5-year survival rates. The choice should be made after a senior doctor has talked with the woman, during which the benefits and drawbacks of each method are discussed. More advanced cervical carcinoma is treated by radiotherapy, although in some centres chemotherapy is being tried.

Fig. 38.15 Staging of carcinoma of the uterine cervix	
Stage 0	Carcinoma *in situ*
Stage I	The carcinoma is confined to the cervix. Ia. Preclinical carcinoma on diagnosis by microscopy. Ib. Invasion >5mm.
Stage II	The carcinoma extends beyond the cervix but has not extended to reach the pelvic wall or the lower vagina. IIa. No obvious parametrial involvement. IIb. The cancer involves the parametrium.
Stage III	The cancer has spread to reach the pelvic wall or the lower third of the vagina.
Stage IV	The cancer has spread beyond the true pelvis or has invaded the bladder.

Fig. 38.16 Squamous carcinoma of the cervix – lymph node involvement and survival rates		
Stage	**Lymph node involvement**	**5-year survival (%)**
0	0	100
Ia	≤1	100
Ib	15	85
IIa	25	75
IIb	35	55
III	55	35
IV	>65	<15

Endometrial carcinoma

Endometrial carcinoma is a disease of women in their middle years, the peak incidence occurring in the 55–65 years of age group. Women whose menopause is delayed beyond the age of 55 years, who are relatively infertile, and overweight or hypertensive are more likely than other women to develop endometrial cancer. This profile suggests that unopposed oestrogen may play a role in the development of the cancer. As discussed on page 224, unopposed oestrogen may lead to endometrial hyperplasia (*Fig. 38.17*). Endometrial hyperplasia has several pathological appearances and, if the pathology shows complex hyperplasia with atypia, 10–25% of women will develop endometrial cancer, unless they are treated.

The tumour may originate in any part of the endometrium, and grows slowly, tending to spread over a part of the endometrium before invading the myometrium. If the growth starts in the lower part of the uterus, the fungating mass may block the cervix and fluid or pus may collect in the uterus (pyometra). Various histological patterns of adenocarcinoma are found on the histological examination of an endometrial biopsy or a curettage. The more undifferentiated the endometrial cells, the worse is the prognosis. The cancer is staged using the International Federation of Obstetrics and Gynaecology (FIGO) classification (*Fig. 38.18*).

CLINICAL FEATURES
The usual symptoms of an endometrial carcinoma are a bloody discharge *per vaginam*, or irregular bleeding, which is slight in amount and recurrent. Some women have a watery vaginal discharge, but this is uncommon. Examination usually shows a normally sized uterus, unless there are associated myomata or a pyometra. Any peri- or postmenopausal woman who has symptoms of irregular bleeding *per vaginam* or a bloody vaginal discharge must

Fig. 38.17 Endometrial hyperplasia.

be examined and endometrial tissue sampled. With the development of the hysteroscope, the uterine cavity can be inspected and a biopsy taken under vision. An alternative is to measure the thickness of the endometrium by transvaginal ultrasonography (*Fig. 38.19*). If the endometrium is less than 5mm thick, endometrial cancer can be excluded. Confirmation is by hysteroscopy and biopsy or by curettage, either using a biopsy curette (this can be done with the woman as an outpatient) or a formal curettage under general anaesthesia. Two biopsy curettes are currently used (Gynnescan and Pipelle). They are introduced through the cervix and rotated in the uterine cavity. The procedures are said to be relatively painless but 60% of women experience discomfort or pain.

SCREENING FOR ENDOMETRIAL CANCER

Some authorities in the USA perform an endometrial biopsy on all postmenopausal women before prescribing hormone replacement treatment. As the prevalence of endometrial cancer in the age group 50–59 years is about 1 in 1000, it is questionable if this invasive procedure is cost-effective.

TREATMENT

Over 75% of cases are diagnosed when the cancer is at an early stage. Total hysterectomy and bilateral oophorectomy is the treatment of choice in these cases. As lymphatic spread is a later development, pelvic lymphadenectomy can be avoided, although the fact that 10% of stage 1 cases have lymph node involvement has led some authorities to advocate pelvic lymphadenectomy for surgical staging and as a

guide to prognosis. The excised uterus is examined histologically and if the myometrium has been invaded to more than half its thickness, either whole pelvis irradiation (50Gy over 5 weeks) or hormone treatment is given. Some gynaecological surgeons arrange for intravaginal irradiation 3–4 weeks after the hysterectomy, giving 40Gy. The objective is to prevent recurrence in the vaginal vault. Problems with this approach are that the vaginal vault may become stenosed, making intercourse uncomfortable, and that bladder or rectal symptoms may occur from radiation damage.

If the patient is unfit for surgery or if the cancer is advanced, hormone treatment may be used as an alternative or an adjuvant. Most medical oncologists give a progestogen, such as medroxyprogesterone acetate 200–400mg orally daily, on a continuous basis. This treatment may cause negative mood change, which is a progestogenic side effect, and may occasionally contribute to thrombophlebitis and thromboembolism.

PROGNOSIS

The prognosis depends on the stage of the disease, the histological grade of the tumour and the age and health of the woman (*Fig. 38.20*).

Women who have received treatment for low-stage endometrial carcinoma and who have severe menopausal symptoms may be prescribed hormone replacement therapy with no increased development of any residual cancer.

Follow-up is recommended at 4 monthly intervals for the first 3 years and annually thereafter. The woman is examined abdominally and vaginally, checked to detect any enlarged lymph nodes and a chest x-ray is taken.

Fig. 38.18 Surgical-pathological staging of endometrial carcinoma (FIGO, 1989)	
Stage	
Ia	Tumour limited to endometrium
Ib	Invasion to <1/2 myometrium
Ic	Invasion to >1/2 myometrium
IIa	Endocervical glandular involvement only
IIb	Cervical stromal invasion
IIIa	Tumour invades serosa and/or adnexae and/or positive peritoneal cytology
IIIb	Vaginal metastases
IIIc	Metastases to pelvic and/or para-aortic lymph nodes
IVa	Tumour invades bladder and/or bowel mucosa
IVb	Distant metastases including intra-abdominal and/or inguinal lymph node

Fig. 38.19 Invasive adenocarcinoma of the uterus after transvaginal ultrasonography.

Stage	Recommended treatment	5-year survival rate (%)
I, GI, 2	Hysterectomy	80
I, G3	Hysterectomy, postoperative radiation	60
II	As for carcinoma of the uterine cervix	50
III	Hormone therapy and megavoltage irradiation of the entire pelvis	30
IV	Hormone therapy	10

Fig. 38.20 The recommended treatment and 5-year survival rate of endometrial cancer related to the stage of the disease

Vulval malignancies

VULVAL INTRA-EPITHELIAL CARCINOMA (VIN)
This condition is being diagnosed increasingly during the colposcopic investigation of women presenting with pruritus vulvae or vulval warts. The best treatment is unknown. The options are watchful expectancy or local excision of the area. Follow-up is important as one-third of patients have recurrent disease.

CARCINOMA OF THE VULVA
Vulval carcinoma accounts for 3% of genital tract cancers and affects elderly women. The growth usually starts as a lump or an ulcer on one labium majus (50% of cases) or on a labium minus (25% of cases). In some cases multiple areas are affected. In recent years, a number of younger women have been presenting with malignant change in a vulval condyloma.

The affected person may have complained of vulval itching for months or years or may have had few symptoms and has only noticed the lump or the ulcer recently.

Clinical
The lesion presents as a hard nodule or an ulcer with a sloughing base and raised edges which may be small or large depending on the duration of the disease (Fig. 38.21). If the cancer is large, lymph node involvement will have occurred in more than 50% of cases.

Treatment is either simple vulvectomy with postoperative irradiation of the inguinal lymph nodes or radical vulvectomy with inguinal, femoral and pelvic lymphadenectomy. Wound necrosis is a troublesome complication after radical vulvectomy and persistent leg oedema occurs in 20% of women.

Fig. 38.21 Vulval carcinoma in the anterior part of the vulva.

Cancer of the ovary

Malignant ovarian tumours are rarely diagnosed early and, in consequence, carry a high mortality. About 6% of ovarian tumours are found to be malignant at surgery, the proportion increasing as a woman grows older.

The tumour may arise in several ways as is shown in *Figure 38.22.*

Primary ovarian carcinoma accounts for about 20% of all gynaecological cancers. In more than 70% of cases the growth has spread beyond the ovaries when first detected. By this time the prospect of 5-year survival of the affected women is less than 25%.

Three per cent of ovarian epithelial cancers appear to have a genetic origin, occurring in several family members. About 40% of current female family members may develop an ovarian cancer. Some authorities suggest a prophylactic bilateral oophorectomy when the woman has completed having children.

CLINICAL

The woman who is usually aged 50 years or more, may notice that her abdomen is becoming larger (from the mass or from ascites), or she may complain of pressure symptoms on her bladder or rectum. Abdominal discomfort and gastrointestinal symptoms may be present. She may have lost weight and have no appetite. In most cases, the symptoms are few and the tumour is detected during a routine examination. Germ cell malignancies can affect women under the age of 30 years. The most common germ cell cancer is dysgerminoma.

MANAGEMENT

Ovarian malignancies should be treated in oncological units, not by a general gynaecologist or a surgeon. The initial management is surgical, as much malignant tissue is removed, including the omentum, as is surgically possible without causing severe damage. The exception to surgery is the dysgerminoma for which radiotherapy appears to be more effective. Following surgery, chemotherapy is initiated including cisplatin (or carboplatin) and paclitaxel (Taxol) taken every 21 days. Some pelvic surgeons make a 'second look' laparotomy after six courses of treatment to assess the response and possibly to 'debulk' persisting or recurrent disease.

Combination chemotherapy is toxic: 60–80% of patients have severe nausea and vomiting during treatment; severe hair loss occurs in 50–60%; peripheral neuropathy in 5–30%; and renal toxicity in 15–60%. Because of the high death rate following a diagnosed ovarian cancer, studies are being made to determine if a cancer can be detected at an early stage in a postmenopausal woman. Currently, transvaginal ultrasound, the measurement of CA 125 antigen and Döppler colour flow mapping (to detect the early angiogenesis which occurs in a malignant tumour) are being investigated. Preliminary results are disappointing.

Telling the patient that she has gynaecological cancer

The fear of cancer is widespread in the population, many people believing that it is a death sentence. If cancer is diagnosed the woman and her family may be devastated. The doctor should understand the patient's fears, and anticipate her possible reaction to the news (anger, distress with crying, silence etc).

Before talking with the woman and, if she wishes, her partner or a near relative, the doctor should have the case records, including test results, available. The discussion should take place in a quiet, private room. The information

Fig. 38.22 A classification of malignant ovarian tumours

Tumour	Type	Proportional incidence of all ovarian tumours (%)
Secondary change in serous cystadenoma, occasionally in a mucinous cystadenoma (includes endometrial carcinoma)	Cystic or semi-solid	5
Rare tumours: Feminizing granulosa-theca cell Virilizing androblastoma Neuter: dysgerminoma Teratoma (embryoma)	Solid	0.5
Secondary carcinoma: Krukenberg, from stomach Adenocarcinoma, from uterus	Solid	0.5

(including providing an honest appraisal of the prognosis) should be given in non-jargon language, and time should be allowed for the information to 'sink in'. The patient's understanding of her condition should be checked in a supportive, empathetic manner, and time given for her to react. If the reaction is anger, the doctor should respond by being sympathetic. If the patient responds by showing shock, or distress or crying, the doctor should let her recover and not try to stop her releasing her emotions. Time should be given for her or her near relative, to ask questions. Most importantly the patient should be offered the opportunity to have a further talk with the doctor as she may be so upset by the news that she is unable to ask questions which concern her.

Psychological implications of gynaecological cancer

During and following treatment for gynaecological cancer many women become depressed, which may adversely affect their relationship with their partner. Surgery of the genital tract, especially if it involves the vagina or vulva threatens the woman's identity. Her vagina may be shortened, her vulva mutilated, she may no longer lubricate when sexually stimulated and she may perceive her sexual activity as inappropriate. Her husband may be concerned that sexual intercourse may damage her or lead to him developing cancer. He may find difficulty in accepting his 'mutilated' wife as a sexual partner. Women who have cervical cancer may be concerned that the disease is a result of past sexual behaviour. These feelings are commonly associated with reduced or absent sexual desire.

Strategies to reduce these psychosexual concerns include preoperative explanations of the effects of surgery or radiotherapy, sexual counselling, and the use of oestrogen vaginal creams, tablets or ovoids when the surgery involves the vagina, or the ovaries are extirpated or irradiated. Sexual explanation and counselling should include information about ways other than sexual intercourse to obtain sexual pleasure, such as cuddling and kissing, oral sex, and sexual organ stimulation by the other partner. The counselling session should include both partners and be conducted in a non-threatening environment with ample time for discussion.

CHAPTER 39

Uterovaginal displacements, damage and prolapse

Uterine displacements

The uterus is an organ which normally pivots about an axis formed by the cardinal ligaments at the level of the internal cervical os. In 90% of women, the uterus is anteflexed and anteverted, lying on the urinary bladder and moving backwards as the bladder fills. In 10% of women, the uterus is retroflexed and may be retroverted (*Fig. 39.1*). This is a developmental occurrence. The uterus is mobile and can be moved by inserting a finger in the posterior vaginal fornix. In spite of anecdotal statements, a mobile retroverted uterus is not a cause of infertility, abortion or backache.

Acquired uterine retroversion may occur, but is less common. It is associated with endometriosis of the uterosacral ligaments or the cul-de-sac; with adhesions resulting from pelvic inflammatory disease; or caused by a tumour in front of the uterus pushing it backwards.

SYMPTOMS

Developmental retroversion is symptomless; only when the retroverted uterus is 'fixed' may symptoms occur. These include the symptoms associated with the underlying cause. In addition, the woman may complain of dyspareunia on deep penetration, pelvic pain and low backache.

A few women who have chronic pelvic pain and are told by their doctor that their uterus is retroverted, will obtain some relief if the uterus is manipulated to become anteverted. They often remain pain-free when the uterus becomes retroverted again, as it usually does.

DIAGNOSIS

A clinical finding that the uterus is retroverted and is accompanied by symptoms, should alert the medical practitioner to determine if the retroversion can be corrected by manipulation (*Fig. 39.2*). If it can, it is not the cause of the symptoms. If it cannot be manipulated it may be the cause of the symptoms.

TREATMENT

In most cases the woman needs reassurance that the retroverted uterus is not the cause of any symptoms she may have and does not require treatment. If the uterus is 'fixed' and the woman has symptoms of deep dyspareunia or chronic pelvic pain, operation may be suggested, but the patient should be told that, although it may correct the position of the uterus, the symptoms may not be relieved permanently. Of the many operations possible the one chosen is to shorten and plicate the round ligaments; at the same time any pelvic pathology is treated.

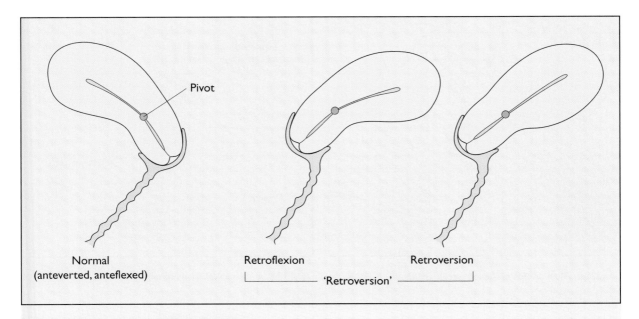

Fig. 39.1 *Retroversion and retroflexion of the uterus.*

Fig. 39.2 Manipulation of the retroverted uterus.

Uterovaginal damage and injuries

Injury to the vulvovaginal area may occur, for example if a girl or woman falls astride some object or is kicked. The vagina may be damaged or a haematoma may form in the vulva (*Fig. 39.3*). Injury may also occur if a young girl or a postmenopausal woman is sexually assaulted.

During the first sexual intercourse, the hymen is stretched and torn and a small amount of bleeding results; very occasionally more severe bleeding occurs if a large blood vessel is damaged.

Injury resulting from childbirth is discussed on pages 69 and 84. Occasionally a vaginal tear is not sutured immediately, and the woman attends a medical practitioner some time later. On inspection the vaginal entrance is seen to gape and the perineal muscles are separated (*Fig. 39.4*). The woman may complain that water enters her vagina when she bathes, or that vaginal flatus occurs.

Vaginal burns may occur following a very hot vaginal douche, or the deliberate insertion of a caustic agent, such as rock salt, to procure an abortion or, in a few cultures, following tightening of the vagina after childbirth to make sexual intercourse more satisfying to the man.

Cervical damage may occur during rough cervical dilatation. The laceration is usually small but may extend from one or other lateral angle of the external cervical os. This may cause marked bleeding. Cervical damage may also occur during childbirth and is discussed on pages 86–87.

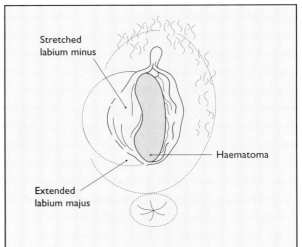

Stretched labium minus

Extended labium majus

Haematoma

Fig. 39.3 A large vulval haematoma.

Genital tract fistulae

Genital tract fistulae occasionally follow childbirth but, in developed countries, they usually result from a complication of surgery or following radiotherapy. Fistulae are very uncommon in the developed countries. They may develop between the vagina and uterus and any adjacent organ. The most frequently encountered fistulae lie between the vagina and the bladder (vesicovaginal fistula) or between the vagina and rectum (rectovaginal fistula).

Obstetrical and surgical fistulae occur immediately after the procedure or 5–14 days after the operation, when the traumatized ischaemic tissue sloughs. The woman complains of continuous leakage of urine in cases of a vesicovaginal fistula, or faeces in the case of a rectovaginal fistula. If the fistula is large it can be seen on vaginal inspection with a Sims speculum, the woman lying in the left lateral position. Small fistulae may require tests to pinpoint the damaged area. One such test is shown in *Figure 39.5*. Closure of small vesicovaginal fistulae may occur if the bladder is drained continuously for 14 days, but rectovaginal fistulae and larger fistulae require surgery.

Uterovaginal prolapse

Uterovaginal prolapse is defined as a descent of the uterus or vagina. A vaginal prolapse may occur independently of any uterine descent, but a prolapsed uterus always carries some part of the upper vagina with it.

To understand how uterovaginal prolapse occurs requires some knowledge about the supports of the uterus. The uterus is supported in the midpelvis by three structures. These are:

* The vagina, the walls of which lie in apposition and are muscular.
* The transcervical (cardinal) ligaments, which stretch from each pelvic wall and attach to the uterus at the level of the supravaginal cervix. They are not ligaments in the true sense as they are composed of a felted mass of collagenous connective tissue through which blood vessels pass to supply the uterus and bladder (*Fig. 39.6*). The

Fig. 39.4 Marked perineal deficiency.

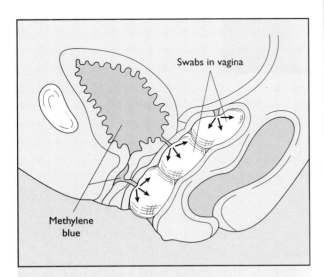

Fig. 39.5 Detecting a vesicovaginal fistula.

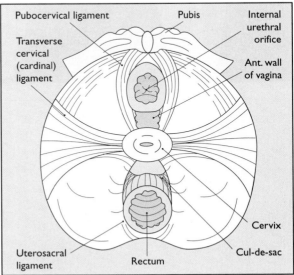

Fig. 39.6 The transverse cervical ligament.

cardinal ligaments act as the middle support of the uterus and their function can be explained in terms of chicken wire. If the strain is not too great the ligaments have considerable tensile strength, but if the strain is increased or the ligaments are damaged, they stretch (*Fig. 39.7*). Posteriorly, on each side, condensations of the tissue form the uterosacral ligament.

- The upper supports of the uterus, i.e. the relatively weak, round ligaments, which operate mostly by maintaining the uterus in an anteverted position so that the increase in intra-abdominal pressure on straining forces the uterus onto the bladder rather than directly down towards the vulva.

Acting in conjunction, these supports prevent uterine prolapse (*Fig. 39.8*). However, this state of affairs may be altered if the supports are stretched during childbirth. This may occur if the woman tries to expel the fetus before the cervix is fully dilated, strains for a long time in the second stage of labour, or if undue force is used to expel the placenta. In these circumstances the cardinal ligament may be stretched, making a uterine prolapse more likely. In consequence prolapse is more common in women who have had several children and are obese.

The prolapse may only become apparent after the menopause when, deprived of oestrogen, the collagen tissue of the ligaments diminishes and the vaginal muscle becomes weaker, permitting the prolapse to occur.

A further way in which prolapse occurs in a very few nulliparous women, is through the supporting tissues failing to develop properly.

DEGREES OF UTERINE PROLAPSE

For descriptive purposes uterovaginal prolapse is divided into three degrees of increasing severity (*Fig. 39.9*). In each of the three degrees the cervix elongates and may become congested or oedematous. When the cervix protrudes from the vagina as in the 3rd degree of prolapse, the cervical epithelium becomes dry and its superficial layers are keratinized.

Uterovaginal prolapse is more common in the later reproductive years and after the menopause. In most cases it is due to damage to the supporting tissues and pudendal nerve damage occurring during childbirth, but not

Fig. 39.7 The 'chicken wire' analogy. In (a) the areolar tissue is not stretched; in (b), because of the uterine descent, condensation of the tissue occurs, with the appearance of a ligament.

Fig. 39.8 Mechanism of prolapse – if the 'holding apparatus', or the 'supporting apparatus' is stretched, some descent of the uterus, or of the vagina, will occur, particularly if the intra-abdominal pressure is increased.

apparent until the tissues atrophy in middle age. An additional cause may be chronic constipation leading to straining to evacuate stools.

With better obstetric care the frequency of uterovaginal prolapse is diminishing and severe cases are not so often seen.

PROLAPSE OF THE ANTERIOR VAGINAL WALL (CYSTOCELE)

This occurs during childbirth when the fibres of the levator ani muscle, which supports the vagina, are stretched.

The weakened anterior vaginal wall bulges into the vagina, bringing the adjacent bladder with it (*Fig. 39.10*).

PROLAPSE OF THE POSTERIOR VAGINAL WALL (RECTOCELE)

In this situation the supporting tissues of the distal posterior wall, including the perineal muscles, are stretched or damaged during the delivery of the baby. With diminished support, the posterior vaginal wall, together with the anterior rectal wall, bulges into the vagina (*Fig. 39.11*).

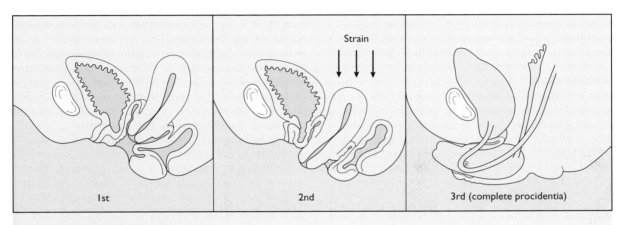

Ist   Strain   2nd   3rd (complete procidentia)

Fig. 39.9 Degrees of uterovaginal prolapse.

Fig. 39.10 Cystocele.

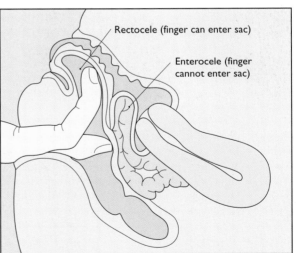

Rectocele (finger can enter sac)

Enterocele (finger cannot enter sac)

Fig. 39.11 Enterocele and rectocele.

If the supports of the proximal vaginal wall are weakened (for example after hysterectomy) it may bulge into the vagina, often containing bowel. This is termed an enterocele.

SYMPTOMS AND DIAGNOSIS

Many women have no symptoms but are concerned that 'something is bulging in my vagina'. Some women feel dragging pains in the lower pelvis, and have difficulty or discomfort when they try to micturate or defaecate. Other women are mildly incontinent.

The type and degree of uterovaginal prolapse can be diagnosed by looking at the woman's vulvovaginal area when she coughs or strains. A vaginal examination using a Sims speculum will confirm the prolapse. A rectal examination may be needed to differentiate a rectocele from an enterocele.

TREATMENT

Treatment depends on the age of the woman, her desire to have further children and the degree of the prolapse. Younger women with mild degrees of symptomless prolapse can delay treatment until the prolapse worsens or the menopause is reached. She should be taught pelvic floor exercises (see page 307) which alone may control her symptoms. It is preferable not to treat a prolapse surgically if the woman wishes to have a further child, as the delivery must then be by caesarean section to avoid damage to the repair. If the woman has a cystocele, a midstream urine sample should be taken to exclude bacteriuria. If the urine is sterile, surgery is not required unless the woman desires it. She should be checked periodically.

If the prolapse is marked and is causing symptoms, surgery can be recommended. There are two choices, which should be discussed with the woman. The first is vaginal hysterectomy and vaginal repair. The second is the Manchester operation, which involves shortening the cervix and the cardinal ligaments and plicating them in front of the shortened cervix (to keep the uterus anteverted) and then performing a vaginal repair. If urinary incontinence is present it should be treated.

Elderly women should be given oestrogen for 4–6 weeks before the operation to improve the quality of the vaginal tissues. Old frail women, or women who refuse an operation, may choose to have a polythene ring pessary introduced into the vagina. The size chosen should prevent descent of the vaginal walls or the uterus and be comfortable. The woman should have the ring pessary removed at intervals for cleaning and then replaced.

The treatment of a cystocele or a rectocele consists of repairing the vagina by excising a triangular piece of the anterior or posterior vaginal wall, depending on whether a cystocele or a rectocele is present, pushing the bladder or rectum proximally, and suturing the supporting muscles beneath it and then rejoining the cut edges of the vagina.

CHAPTER 40

The urinary tract and its relationship to gynaecology

The close connection of the bladder to the vagina and the short urethra give rise to more problems in a woman's urinary tract than in a man's. The anatomy of the urinary tract is described on page 337. The function of the urinary tract is to permit waste products of metabolism to be removed from the body in the urinary flow. For this reason the mechanics of micturition will be discussed first.

Mechanics of voluntary micturition

The bladder fills as urine trickles down the ureters. To accommodate the urine, the bladder distends, and it can accommodate 300–400ml of urine without any increase in the resting intravesical pressure, which remains below $10cmH_2O$. In the resting state the urethro-vesical junction is flat and there is an angle of about 90° between the bladder and the urethra (the urethro-vesical angle) (Fig. 40.1a).

Continence is maintained because of the inherent tone of the urethra and by the muscles which envelop the urethro-vesical junction and the proximal urethra, which keep the intraurethral pressure $7–10cmH_2O$ higher than the pressure within the bladder.

When more than 350ml of urine distends the bladder, cholinergic muscarinic stretch receptors in the bladder wall are stimulated. This causes the detrusor muscle to contract and the intravesical pressure rises. Paradoxically, the extension of the detrusor muscle which surrounds the proximal urethra in a spiral fashion relaxes, with the result that the intraurethral pressure falls below the intravesical pressure. By the age of 5 years, most children have learned to inhibit the detrusor contractions and to keep the urethra closed, so that micturition can be delayed until an appropriate time. In some women, this higher centre control cannot be maintained and micturition occurs inappropriately. A second line of defence against involuntary micturition is provided by the muscles forming the external urethral sphincter and the fibres of the pubococcygeal muscle which surround and support the distal urethra.

When the person is ready to pass urine, the detrusor muscle is permitted to contract strongly, which raises the intravesical pressure above the intraurethral pressure. The detrusor contractions also cause funnelling of the bladder base and obliterate the urethrovesical angle (see Fig. 40.1b).

At the same time, the person contracts the abdominal muscles which raise the intravesical pressure further. These changes and the relaxation of the proximal urethral muscle permit urine to pass into the urethra. The person now relaxes the muscles surrounding the distal urethra, and urine is voided until the bladder is empty. When this occurs the detrusor ceases to be stimulated and relaxes, and the urethro-vesical angle is restored. The proximal urethra contracts from its distal end to the urethro-vesical junction, 'milking' back a few drops of urine into the bladder. Finally, the external sphincter closes.

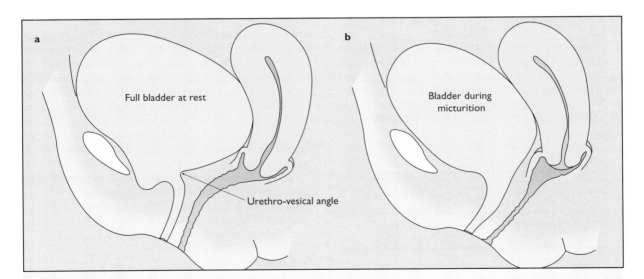

Fig. 40.1 Tracing from radiographs of the bladder and urethra. (a) At rest; (b) during micturition.

Urinary incontinence (involuntary micturition)

As women grow older the incidence of urinary incontinence increases, often causing social isolation or psychological problems. In the age group 35–50 years, 5% of women are incontinent at least once each week. By the age of 60 years, 15–20% of women complain of urinary incontinence, and by the age of 80 years 1 woman in 4 is incontinent.

In women two main and two subsidiary forms of urinary incontinence occur. The two main forms are:

- *Urge incontinence.*
- *Urethral sphincter incontinence* (genuine stress incontinence).

The two subsidiary forms are:

- *Reflex incontinence.*
- *Overflow incontinence.*

Of the subsidiary forms, *reflex incontinence* is an involuntary loss of urine due to abnormal reflex activity in the spinal cord in the absence of a desire to pass urine. *Overflow incontinence* (urinary retention with overflow) occurs in:

- Motor neurone disease.
- Urethral obstruction, which is rare in women.
- Cases of chronic bladder distension.

The proportion of women complaining of the two main forms of incontinence is not known. The best estimates are shown in *Figure 40.2*.

URGE INCONTINENCE (THE UNSTABLE BLADDER)

In this disorder the detrusor muscle contracts involuntarily. There are two categories of urge incontinence. In the first, *sensory incontinence*, the woman passes urine, not because of involuntary detrusor activity but because it hurts if she does not empty her bladder. The woman has to micturate frequently, often several times at night as well as during the day, and may have dysuria. In some cases there is obvious urinary tract infection. In others no evidence of this is found.

In the second category, *motor urgency (detrusor instability)*, the urge to micturate before the bladder is full occurs at variable intervals and variable amounts of urine are voided. This may be accompanied by urinary frequency and incontinence if the woman is unable to reach a toilet. At night she may wet the bed. Pain on micturition is not a feature.

Urge incontinence is a psychosomatic, not a psychological problem, as women with the condition are no more likely to demonstrate psychiatric morbidity than are other incontinent women.

URETHRAL SPHINCTER INCONTINENCE

In urethral sphincter incontinence, involuntary loss of urine occurs when the intravesical pressure exceeds the intra-urethral pressure in the absence of detrusor activity. Two defects are thought to be present. The first is that the proximal urethra has been displaced downwards through the urogenital diaphragm. When the abdominal pressure rises, as occurs when a woman sneezes, coughs or is jolted, the pressure is not transmitted to the urethra, with the result that the intravesicular pressure rises while the intraurethral pressure does not. The second mechanism is that, either because of defective development of the urethral supporting muscles or damage to the bladder neck supports during childbirth, when the bladder is at rest, its base is funnelled, not flat. This impairs the normal closure mechanism at the urethro-vesical junction.

The combined effect of these mechanisms is to increase the intravesical pressure above the intraurethral pressure in the absence of a voluntary pressure increase. This results in a leak of urine into the urethra when only a small increase in intra-abdominal pressure occurs.

Clinical findings

The mechanisms explain the clinical findings, which are that the woman complains that a small amount of urine leaks if she laughs, coughs or jumps. The leak can be confirmed if her doctor asks her to cough when she has a full bladder.

DIAGNOSTIC MEASURES TO DETERMINE THE CAUSE OF THE INCONTINENCE

A woman presenting with a complaint of urinary incontinence requires careful examination. The social inconvenience caused by the incontinence should be evaluated. The woman should be asked if she is taking any medications, as some drugs (for example, tricyclics, prazosin and lithium) may cause symptoms of urinary incontinence. General medical conditions, such as Parkinsonism, multiple sclerosis and diabetic neuropathy must be looked for and excluded, as should local bladder causes, such as bladder stone or pressure on the bladder from a myoma. The physical examination should include assessment of the perineal reflexes of segments S1–S4, and the anal sphincter tone should be tested. A specimen of midstream urine should be obtained and sent to a laboratory to exclude the possibility of bladder infections.

To try to identify the main (or the only cause) of the incontinence, tests should be arranged.

Pad test

The woman is asked to place a weighed pad (with a waterproof backing) over her vulva. Then she drinks 500ml of

---

Type of incontinence	Age (years)	
	<70	**>70**
Urethral sphincter	50	26
Urge incontinence	20	33
Mixed	30	41

Fig. 40.2 Percentage prevalence of the types of urinary incontinence

sodium-free liquid over a 15-minute period. For the next 30 minutes, she performs a range of activities such as climbing a flight of stairs, walking, standing up from sitting and washing her hands under running water. The pad is then removed and weighed again, any weight difference being urinary loss. A more sophisticated pad test, which demands considerable patient compliance, is to test for 48 hours, the woman keeping the pads and bringing them to the doctor for weighing.

Urinary diary

If urge incontinence is suspected, the woman is asked to record her daily fluid intake and output each time she drinks or passes urine.

Urodynamic studies

Because the history gives a poor discrimation between the two main types of incontinence, urodynamic studies are used to provide a definitive diagnosis. This is especially important if a woman has had previous surgery for urinary incontinence. Urge incontinence and urethral sphincter incontinence can co-exist and urodynamic studies allow an assessment of which is dominant and hence whether treatment should be primarily medical or surgical. Inappropriate surgery which obstructs urinary outflow will cause even greater detrusor instability and hence the importance of reaching the right diagnosis before embarking on any form of surgery.

Urodynamic studies measure the change in intravesical and intraurethral pressure as fluid is instilled into the bladder. In urge incontinence the intravesical pressure rises early and the capacity of the bladder is diminished, in urethral sphincter incontinence, the bladder capacity is usually normal and the pressure does not rise until just before capacity is reached.

TREATMENT
Urge incontinence

Several strategies are recommended but the success rate is variable. A bladder drill may help. The woman tries to increase the time between episodes of micturition, no matter how difficult she finds it. The objective is to retrain her bladder to contain more urine before detrusor activity is stimulated. Bladder drill takes time and application. Considerable support and help, preferably from a trained person, is needed.

Drugs may also be helpful. As detrusor activity is under cholinergic control, anticholinergic drugs are chosen. The currently preferred drug is oxybutynin (2.5–5.0mg three times a day). A number of women cannot take oxybutynin because of the anticholinergic effects of dry mouth, dry skin, blurred vision or constipation. These women may find relief if they take dicyclomine 30mg four times a day. Bladder retraining programmes for urge incontinence have a success rate of 80–90%.

Urethral sphincter incontinence

Unless the incontinence is severe, the choice of medical or surgical treatment should be offered to the patient. Obese women should try to reduce their weight as this has been found to relieve incontinence in some women. A chronic cough should also be treated. Postmenopausal women need additional treatment, especially if they have recurrent urinary tract symptoms. These symptoms occur because of atrophy of the urethral mucosa. The women should be treated for 2–3 months with an oestrogen vaginal pessary, ovoid or cream, as well as antibiotics if indicated. Pelvic floor exercises should be initiated (Fig. 40.3). The exercises must be continued for several months. An alternative, which many women may find more convenient, is the use of vaginal cones. Weighted vaginal cones (in sets of 5 weighing 20–90g) are purchased. The woman inserts the lightest cone into her vagina. It is kept in by contraction of the levator ani muscle. She progresses from the lightest cone to the heaviest.

These measures effectively relieve urinary sphincter incontinence in up to 60% of affected women. If they fail or the woman chooses surgery, several surgical approaches are possible. Most gynaecologists prefer an operation which elevates the bladder neck so that it lies within the abdominal pressure zone (Fig. 40.4) and provides support under the urethrovesical junction. One example is shown in Figure 40.5.

Fig. 40.3 Pelvic floor exercises

These exercises help a woman strengthen the muscles which act as a sling to keep the bladder, the genital organs and the rectum in their correct position.

She should try to do the exercises at least once an hour when awake, for the rest of her life.

At first the exercises may be a little tiring but with perseverence she will find them easy to do. The pelvic floor exercises only take about two minutes of each hour and relieve urinary problems.

The exercises are easy to learn. No one can detect that a woman is doing them so they may be done in company, when watching TV, washing the dishes, cleaning the house, at work, etc.

The exercises have three components:

1. When she is sitting down the woman should contract the pelvic floor muscles, as if trying to lift the genital organs from the seat. The contraction should be held for a slowly counted 5 seconds. After each contraction relax. Repeat the exercise 10 times.

2. The woman should stand up and contract the pelvic floor muscles as if she were trying to stop the flow of urine midstream, or if she were tightening her vagina. Hold the contraction for 5 seconds, then relax. Repeat the exercise 10 times.

3. Finally do a fast version of the exercise, contracting and relaxing every second, 10 times.

Women can check their progress if they wish and can make sure that they are contracting the right muscles by inserting a finger into the vagina and feeling the strength of the contraction.

If the exercises are followed as described, after a week or two she will be pleased with the improvement of the grip.

The operations have similar success rates of over 90% in the immediate postoperative years, but long-term studies show that 6 years after the operation only 75% of women are continent and 15–20% have detrusor instability. Uterovaginal

prolapse is increased among some treated women. Whether this is due to the operation or to a general weakness of the uterovaginal supports, which also caused the incontinence, is not known.

If surgery fails to elevate the bladder neck, glutaraldehyde crosslinked bovine collagen (GAX-collagen), may be injected into the tissues on each side of the bladder neck.

Women who are frail or who do not want surgery may be helped by using a bladder-neck support prothesis. The device has two prongs which elevate the urethrovaginal junction to its normal anatomic position (*Fig 40.6*), without compressing the urethra. The device is removed at intervals for cleaning or if the woman has sexual intercourse. The appropriately sized prothesis must be fitted by a doctor. A success rate of more than 80% is claimed.

Urinary tract infection

The short urethra and its intimate relationship with the vagina increases the chance that a woman will develop urinary tract infection. When the woman becomes sexually active, penile thrusting may move bacteria which have colonized the lower urethra upwards to infect the bladder. This may lead to symptomatic infection or to symptomless bacteriuria (more than 100,000 organisms per ml of urine), which affects 3–8% of sexually active women. Provided that the woman empties her bladder regularly, the condition is without consequence, but should urinary stasis occur, as in pregnancy, the bacteria may grow in the urine causing clinical acute infection. Initially, the infection is confined to the bladder causing *cystitis*, but the infection may spread, either along the ureter or via the lymphatics to infect the kidney, causing *pyelonephritis*.

Fig. 40.4 *The effect of the position of the bladder neck on stress incontinence. In (a) the urethrovesical junction occupies a normal position. An increase in abdominal pressure acts equally on the detrusor pressure and on the bladder neck pressure, with the result that the pressure gradient is maintained and a positive 'closure' pressure is present. In (b) the urethrovesical junction lies outwith the effects of abdominal pressure as the junction is below the pelvic floor. An increase in abdominal pressure is transmitted only to the detrusor pressure, which exceeds momentarily the intraurethral pressure. The positive closure pressure is lost and the patient passes a small amount of urine.*

Fig. 40.5 *Modified colposuspension (retropubic approach). Sutures are placed between the paravaginal fascia and the ileopectineal ligaments. These sutures elevate the bladder neck. The sutures on the right have been tied; those on the left are ready to be tied. During exertion the intra-abdominal pressure rises and presses the urethra against the symphysis pubis, thus controlling the incontinence.*

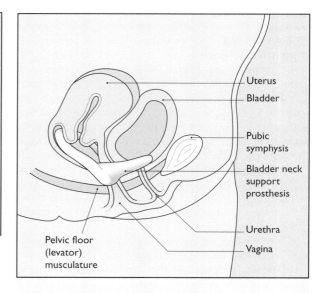

Fig. 40.6 *A bladder neck support prosthesis.*

CLINICAL ASPECTS

The symptoms of lower urinary tract infection (UTI) are frequency of micturition and dysuria; whilst if the kidneys are involved, the woman will be febrile and may have rigors and loin pain.

INVESTIGATIONS

The woman should be asked if she has had previous attacks of UTI and whether she has an irritating vaginal discharge which, if present, should be investigated. Her recent sexual activity should be explored and a urethral discharge looked for. A midstream specimen of urine should be obtained and sent for examination and culture.

TREATMENT

Antibiotics are prescribed. The antibiotic chosen depends on local conditions. Norfloxacin 800mg in a single dose, or Augmentin are currently recommended. If the patient has pyelonephritis aggressive treatment is needed. Parenteral cephalexin 1g, followed by 500mg 6-hourly, is appropriate therapy.

The urethral syndrome

In this syndrome, the woman complains of dysuria, frequency and pain, which usually start 12–36 hours after sexual intercourse. The symptoms last for 1–4 days and recur when sexual intercourse is resumed, although not every time. If the symptoms are severe and recur frequently they can cause a considerable disruption to the relationship and often sexual frustration.

Investigation includes taking a careful history. Vaginal swabs should be taken as some women with the syndrome are found to have vaginitis. A midstream specimen of urine is also taken. This either fails to show any bacterial growth, or a concentration of bacteria of less than 100 organisms per ml.

TREATMENT

Many women are cured if they drink 500ml of water before intercourse, and empty the bladder completely 20–30 minutes after having sex. If this simple measure fails to cure the condition, amoxycillin 250mg taken after each act of sexual intercourse may be tried or the woman may be prescribed trimethoprim 100mg or nitrofurantin 50mg, each taken daily. (Nitrofurantin should not be taken for more than 6 months because of the possible development of fibrotic alveolitis.) In the past, the condition was believed to be caused by trigonitis, which was treated by cauterizing the trigone. However, this treatment has been outmoded.

Urethral problems

URETHRAL PROLAPSE

In the *acute form*, the entire circumference of the urethra suddenly everts and becomes engorged, as the venous return is impeded (Fig. 40.7a). The woman, who is usually elderly, complains of pain, dysuria and frequency. The immediate treatment is to reduce the prolapse and insert a catheter. Surgery may be offered later.

In the *chronic form*, atrophy of the urethral tissues may permit the external urinary meatus to gape, and allow the posterior urethral wall to prolapse (see Fig. 40.7b). The prolapse appears as a small red swelling and is painless. If it becomes infected, it becomes larger and painful. Treatment consists of applying an antiseptic ointment and an oestrogen cream. If the symptoms persist, surgery should be suggested.

URETHRAL CARUNCLE

This is a pedunculated polyp, arising from the posterior margin of the urinary meatus (see Fig. 40.7c). It is vascular, dull red in colour and tender. The patient complains of pain, frequency and dysuria. Treatment consists of excising the caruncle and cauterizing its bed.

| a | b | | c |
| Acute | | Chronic | Caruncle |

Fig. 40.7 Urethral prolapse and urethral caruncle.

CHAPTER 41

The breast

The adult breast is of various sizes and is divided into 15–25 lobes separated from each other by fibrous septa which radiate from the nipple. Each lobe has its own duct system which terminates in a dilated area beneath the nipple and then opens on to the surface of the nipple as a punctate orifice. Each lobe is divided into lobules, each of which contains 10–100 acini surrounded by fatty tissue, lymphatics and blood vessels.

During the menstrual cycle, the female breast undergoes cyclical changes induced by oestradiol and progesterone. Oestradiol induces growth of the acini and, combined with progesterone in the luteal phase of the menstrual cycle, causes duct development, increased vascular congestion, and fluid transudation into the breast tissues. The result is that in the late luteal phase the breasts are fuller, heavier and may be painful.

Disorders of size and shape

Current fashion decrees that to be beautiful a woman's breasts should be large (but not too large), full and well supported. Many women have small breasts and some have breasts which are large and pendulous. A woman who has breasts which she perceives as too small or too large may seek medical aid. In most cases, the woman is secreting normal quantities of oestrogen, so oestrogen ointments or creams will not increase breast size nor will any hormone decrease breast size.

SMALL BREASTS

The size of the breasts may appear larger if the woman has a good posture and contracts her pectoral muscles. Increase in breast size may be obtained by inserting a shaped 'form' behind the breast tissue and in front of the pectoral muscle, via an incision at the lower margin of the breast. Until 1992, the form was filled with silicone but, with recent concern that silicone may leak and cause damage, this has now been prohibited. A saline-filled implant may be chosen, but this too may cause problems. Augmentation mammaplasty should only be undertaken by an experienced cosmetic surgeon.

LARGE BREASTS

Large, pendulous breasts not only appear unattractive (or so some women believe) but may cause shoulder pain. Treatment consists of wearing a supporting bra or undergoing a reduction mammaplasty.

Breast diseases

In some women, the normal cyclical enlargement of the breasts is exaggerated, with the result that the duct systems increase in size and the breasts become tender and nodular. The change may affect one segment of each breast, usually the upper, outer segment, but may involve all segments.

The condition is termed benign breast disease, which has replaced the previous diagnostic terms of mazoplasia, fibroadenosis and chronic mastitis. Benign breast disease may be localized or diffuse. Its aetiology is not known.

LOCALIZED BREAST DISEASE

This type of breast disease is usually found among women aged 25–45 years and in premenopausal women when single large cysts are found. The woman has few if any symptoms, but the discovery of the breast lump causes fear of cancer. The breast should be examined carefully, an ultrasound image made and a mammogram arranged. Once cancer has been excluded, treatment is reassurance.

DIFFUSE BREAST DISEASE

This form is found most often in women aged 30–50 years. The symptoms vary from mild discomfort to severe tenderness and pain. They are worse in the luteal phase of the menstrual cycle, but may persist throughout. Palpation of the breasts reveals coarse nodular areas as if bundles of string were in the breast.

There appears to be a considerable psychological element in the cause of breast tenderness and pain. Many of the women have or have had chronic pelvic pain and premenstrual syndrome (PMS). For this reason, it is often helpful to explore the woman's lifestyle and to talk about relationship problems. As in the management of PMS, it often helps if the woman keeps a daily diary of her symptoms, in terms of type, severity and duration, before any treatment is offered. This is because treatment is not very effective, although some women find relief by wearing a well-fitting bra day and night. Some authorities claim that a low-fat diet reduces the problem, but there is no clear evidence that this is true.

By the time that the woman seeks medical help, she will probably have tried reducing her caffeine intake and dieting and have purchased over-the-counter medications, such as vitamin B_1 and evening primrose oil, or have been prescribed diuretics. Double-blind studies using these medications have shown them to have no benefit over placebo, which emphasizes the psychosomatic nature of the complaint.

If the breast tenderness and pain is severe and the above treatments have been used, the woman may choose to try a hormonal approach.

One such approach consists of prescribing one of two anti-oestrogenic, antiprogestogenic, androgenic drugs, danazol or gestrinone, both of which reduce follicle-stimulating hormone secretion with consequent falls in oestrogen and progesterone levels. The drugs relieve the pain either completely or partially in 40–50% of users. Danazol is given in a dose of 200mg twice daily from day 12 to day 26 of the menstrual cycle, or continually for 6 months in a dose of 200mg daily. Gestrinone is given in a dose of 2.5mg twice weekly for 3 months or longer. Unfortunately both drugs have androgenic side effects, as discussed on pages 273–274.

A second hormonal treatment entails prescribing dydrogesterone 10mg daily from day 12 to day 26 of the menstrual cycle on the presumption that the cause of the disease is progesterone deficiency. A third consists of prescribing the prolactin antagonist, bromocriptine 2.5–5.0mg daily throughout the menstrual cycle. About 8% of women treated stop using bromocriptine because of side effects, usually nausea.

No method of treatment seems superior to any other, and if one fails to relieve the symptoms another may be suggested. Studies have shown that neither breast pain nor discomfort is relieved by any of the available treatments in one-third of patients.

Patients should be given a full, clear explanation of the possibility that treatment will not be successful and the opportunity to talk with their doctor.

A recent study has found that a woman who has benign breast disease has a slightly increased risk of developing breast cancer in the premenopause. It would be wise to encourage such women to have mammograms regularly from the age of 40 years.

Duct ecstasia

The pain is localized to an area below the areola or an inner quadrant of the breast, may occur at any time during the menstrual cycle and is increased in cold weather. Flame-shaped shadows may show on mammography. Treatment entails exercising the affected wedge-shaped area.

Fibroadenoma of the breast

Benign encapsulated tumours may arise in the breasts of women aged less than 30 years. Fibroadenomas are symptomless and are detected by accident or by breast self-examination. The lump is smooth and very mobile; it has been called a 'breast mouse'. Treatment consists of excising the fibroadenoma.

The Tietze syndrome

Some women complain of breast pain which is, in reality, due to an enlarged costochondral junction of one of the ribs,

usually the second rib. The pain is localized, chronic and not related to the premenstruum. There is no effective treatment.

Breast cancer

Breast cancer is the second most common cancer in women, and affects one woman in 14, usually after the age of 50 years. Early detection is the only way to control the disease as, by the time the cancer can be palpated easily, spread is likely to have occurred.

For this reason, programmes to persuade women to learn and practise breast self-examination have been developed in many countries (see pages 1–2). In addition, health authorities recommend that women over the age of 35 years have an annual breast examination by a doctor. This should be supplemented by mammography between the ages of 40 and 45 years, then annually from the age of 50 years (*Figs. 41.1a* and *b*). Two views should be taken as they increase the detection of breast cancer and reduce recall rates. About 95% of women who have mammographic and clinical screening will have no evidence of breast cancer, 5% will require further investigation, and 1% will need a breast biopsy to establish or exclude breast cancer.

The aetiology of breast cancer has not been elucidated. A genetic factor exists as breast cancer tends to be found in families. Childbearing before the age of 30 years seems to be protective.

TREATMENT

Early breast cancer is best treated by breast-conserving surgery and radiation therapy to the axilla. The effectiveness of adjuvant treatment using chemotherapy or tamoxifen is being studied. A recent meta-analysis of over 75,000 women with early breast cancer has shown that women who received additional treatment following surgery had a higher 5- and 10-year survival rate. For women under the age of 50 years, adjuvant chemotherapy for 6 months, tamoxifen for 2 years or ovarian ablation had approximately equal efficacy in prolonging survival. The treatments increased the 10-year survival rate by 10%. For women over 50 years old, tamoxifen or chemotherapy increased the survival at 10 years by 12%. Tamoxifen had fewer adverse effects.

More advanced breast carcinoma is treated by modified radical mastectomy or radiotherapy. Survival is increased in postmenopausal women younger than 65 years, who have positive lymph nodes and are oestrogen receptor positive, if they are given chemotherapy initially, followed by tamoxifen for 2–5 years. If the woman is older than 65 years, chemotherapy may be omitted. Women who have positive nodes but are receptor negative should be prescribed chemotherapy, whilst women who have negative nodes but are receptor positive should take tamoxifen for 2–5 years.

These treatments eliminate oestrogen secretion with the result that the patient is likely to suffer severe menopausal symptoms (hot flushes, dry vagina, bone

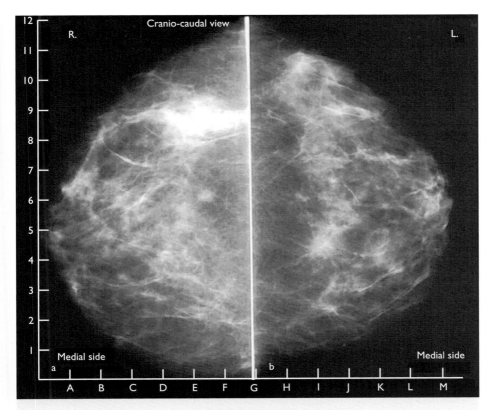

Fig. 41.1 *(a) A mammogram of a breast containing a small carcinoma at co-ordinates E6. (b) A mammogram of a normal breast.*

loss), which may interfere with her social and sexual life. For this reason, each patient should be given sufficient information to enable her to make an informed choice. The current view is that hormone replacement therapy can be given safely and does not increase the risk of recurrence.

PSYCHOSOCIAL AND PHYSICAL ASPECTS OF BREAST CANCER

Following breast-conserving surgery or a modified radical mastectomy, the majority of women have no psychiatric or sexual problems, provided a full explanation of the extent of and problems associated with surgery has been given by the surgeon. Breast conservation is marginally better in preserving body image and, perhaps, sexual enjoyment. About 25% of women have significant depression or anxiety.

An increasing number of women of premenopausal age are receiving chemotherapy or anti-oestrogen treatment after surgery, so menopausal symptoms are causing more problems because of hot flushes and failure of vaginal lubrication. In addition, some women find difficulty in accepting the alopecia, weight changes and pallor following chemotherapy. The anti-oestrogen, tamoxifen, appears to cause fewer menopausal symptoms, possibly because it has mild oestrogenic effects on the vagina.

Most women, following treatment for breast cancer, are helped if they (and their partners) can talk with an experienced clinician about the problems they may develop. Questions will relate to how each partner sees the woman's body (how to find comfortable ways to have sex and to use a water-based lubricant to avoid vaginal dryness) and what sexual enjoyment other than sexual intercourse can be experienced by the couple.

CHAPTER 42

Gynaecological problems in childhood and adolescence

Intersex

The first question a mother asks after her baby has been born is 'Is it a boy or a girl?' The answer is given after looking at the infant's genitals, but in 2 in 10,000 neonates the genital sex is ambiguous and the child is judged as being intersex.

Most neonates with ambiguous genitals are genetically female and have congenital adrenal hyperplasia. A few have an adrenal tumour or drug-induced virilism. In rare cases, the neonate is a hermaphrodite, having a testis, an ovary and ambiguous external genitals.

CONGENITAL ADRENAL HYPERPLASIA (CAH)

This condition affects 1 in 10,000 neonates and is due to a group of enzyme defects which prevent the synthesis of cortisone from progesterone. The lack of circulating cortisone permits the hypothalamus–pituitary to release quantities of corticotrophins which stimulate the adrenal gland to secrete androgens, with resulting virilization of the external genitals (Fig. 42.1).

The most common enzyme defect is C-21-hydroxylase deficiency (found in more than 90% of cases). In three-quarters of cases, ambiguous external genitals are the only sign of the condition, but in a quarter of cases aldosterone production is lost and the patient has a salt-losing syndrome.

Any child with ambiguous genitals should be investigated for CAH, by determining the chromosomal sex and by measuring the 17-hydroxyprogesterone level, a level of more than 7mmol/L confirming the diagnosis and checking the serum electrolytes. Treatment should be effected urgently or death may supervene from salt loss. The infant is treated with cortisone or one of its derivatives and careful follow-up is essential, but surgical correction of the external genitals should be delayed for 3–4 years.

OTHER CAUSES OF INTERSEX

Other varieties of intersexuality are not diagnosed until after puberty, when menstruation fails to start. They include *gonadal dysgenesis* (Turner's syndrome); *testicular feminization* (androgen insensitivity syndrome) and *Klinefelter's syndrome* (seminiferous tubular dysgenesis).

GONADAL DYSGENESIS

Two varieties of this condition exist. They are pure gonadal dysgenesis and Turner's syndrome.

Pure gonadal dysgenesis

In this disorder, genital hypoplasia is detected in a girl who has normal breast development. A chromosomal analysis shows a mosaic 46, XO/XX.

Turner's syndrome

The adolescent girl is short in stature having failed to experience a marked prepubertal growth spurt. She may have a webbed neck or other deformities (Fig. 42.2). She seeks medical help when she fails to menstruate and investigations show that she has raised follicle-stimulating hormone (FSH) and luteinizing hormone (LH) levels and a chromosome analysis reveals a karyotype of 46, XO. Treatment is undertaken by a paediatrician who will prescribe hormone replacement treatment (see page 321) to help the development of her breasts and genital tract and to prevent osteoporosis in later life. As the ovaries contain no follicles,

Fig. 42.1 Ambiguous external genitalia due to the adrenogenital syndrome.

the girl is sterile. She is helped by counselling. She needs to be reassured of the benefits of hormone replacement, and helped to accept her short stature and sterility. The counsellor should stress that neither of these should reduce her sexuality and sexual enjoyment.

TESTICULAR FEMINIZATION

Physically, the person is female with female external characteristics, including good breast development (Fig. 42.3) and has been reared as a girl. She and her parents are concerned when she fails to menstruate. Examination shows that she has a short vagina which ends blindly. Her karyotype is 46, XY, as she is genetically male. The gonads are in the abdominal cavity or in a hernial sac. They synthesize testosterone but the body tissues lack alpha reductase enzyme to convert it to dihydroxytestosterone and receptor cells in genital tract tissues and skin may be missing. As the testes may become malignant they should be removed and hormonal replacement treatment given.

KLINEFELTER'S SYNDROME

The person is a tall, phenotypical male whose puberty is delayed and who has a small penis and testes. The chromosome count is 47, XXY or 46, XY/XXY. The person may have a low libido. The young man needs sympathetic support, counselling and encouragement to become more assertive. Testosterone implants may improve his libido, but his small penis may prevent him from forming a full sexual relationship.

The 'genital crisis'

In a few female infants, because of tissue sensitivity, maternal oestrogen thickens the vaginal and uterine epithelium. After birth, the oestrogen is withdrawn and the child has a small withdrawal bleed *per vaginam*, the so-called 'genital crisis'. Similarly, a few female infants may secrete a small amount of watery milk. The parents require assurance.

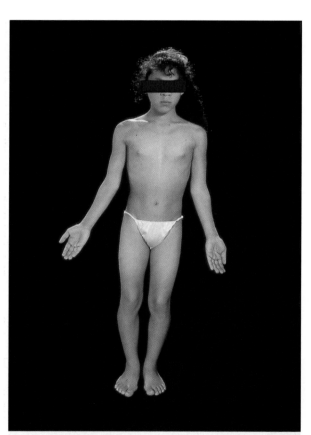

Fig. 42.2 *Gonadal dysgenesis (Turner's syndrome). The patient is of short stature and has a 'webbed' neck. Pelvic examination showed a vagina and a rudimentary uterus, but palpable gonads.*

Fig. 42.3 *Incomplete testicular feminization.*

Fusion of the labia minora

The labia may be seen to be adherent at the neonatal examination or this may occur when the girl is a toddler. The treatment is to separate the labia with the fingers and for the mother to apply an oestrogen cream to the separated labia for 2–3 weeks to encourage epithelialization.

Vulvovaginitis in prepubertal children

Vulvovaginitis may occur at any age. The child is brought by the mother complaining of an inflamed, tender vulva and, perhaps, a vaginal discharge. The causes are listed in *Figure 42.4*. The vulval area should be inspected and an anal swab taken for pin and thread worms. A swab should be taken from the vagina. If an intravaginal foreign body is suspected and cannot easily be detected the child should be referred to a gynaecologist who deals with children, for examination with a vaginoscope.

Treatment consists of:
* Treating an identified specific cause appropriately.
* Encouraging vulval general cleanliness (and the avoidance of soap), followed by careful vulval drying and the wearing of cotton panties day and night.

If the condition persists for more than 2 weeks, in spite of these treatments, oestrogen cream may be applied to the vulva and vaginal introitus twice daily for 5 days.

Precocious puberty

Precocious puberty indicates that sexual maturation has occurred before the age of 9 years. Most cases are constitutional in origin but ovarian or adrenal hormone-secreting tumours must be excluded. The investigations include:
* Full history and physical examination.
* Bone age studies.
* Ultrasound, CT scan or MRI to exclude an ovarian or an adrenal tumour, and a brain scan.

Management is psychological and endocrinological. The girl (and her parents) need considerable psychological support as the girl perceives herself as different from her peers and may be teased. If the girl's bone age is advanced, she will be taller initially but, as the epiphyses fuse earlier, she will ultimately be shorter than her peers. Several hormone treatments are being tested to treat precocious puberty. The most promising is a gonadotrophin-releasing hormone (GnRH) analogue given daily by nasal sniffs or as a depot preparation each month, to reverse the physical changes.

Physical changes of puberty and early adolescence

The endocrinological changes which occur before and after puberty were detailed in Chapter 2, Ovulation and the menstrual cycle. These changes manifest in physical changes (*Fig. 42.5*). If they do not parallel, fairly closely, the changes in their peers, some girls become anxious and seek reassurance. Other girls develop an eating disorder.

Fig. 42.5 Time of appearance of sexual characteristics in Australian girls

Age	Characteristics
9–10	Growth of bony pelvis begins Fat deposition initiates beginnings of female contour Budding of the nipples
10–11	Budding of the breasts Appearance of pubic hair (androgens are responsible for pubic and axillary hair)
11–13	Growth of internal and external genitalia Glycogen content of the vagina increases; the height of the epithelium increases with change in cell type, and the pH is lowered. Occasionally a vaginal discharge is noted
12–14	Pigmentation of the nipples Growth and rounding of the breasts
13–15	Axillary hair appears Menarche occurs (mean 13 years, range 9–16) Pubic hair increases in amount Acne present in 60% of adolescents
16–18	Cessation of skeletal growth

Fig. 42.4 Vulvovaginitis: causes

	Percentage
1. Non-specific	60
2. Specific	
a) Bacterial E. coli 12, N. gonorrhoeae 2, Other 6	20
b) Fungal (Candida)	10
c) Protozoal (trichomonad)	5
d) Foreign body	5
e) Helminthic/viral	1

Fig. 42.6 Primary amenorrhoea	
	Percentage of cases
Gonadal dysgenesis (inc. Turner's syndrome)	45
Congenital absence of uterus or vagina	15
Low body weight (inc. anorexia nervosa and severe malnutrition)	10
Congenital adrenal virilism	5
Testicular feminization	5
Other (inc. hypothyroidism in 4%; systemic disease 4%)	15
Hypogonadotrophic hypogonadism, (usually constitutional delayed menarche)	5

By the age of 17 years over 99% of adolescents will have reached menarche. Delay after this age may be constitutional or have a recent cause (Fig. 42.6). Investigations include:

- A full careful history.
- A full physical examination including a pelvic examination.

The history and examination may indicate special examinations, for example: measurement of FSH; imaging of the skull or the pelvic organs; nuclear sex chromatin; laparoscopy. Treatment is discussed in Chapter 29, Disorders of menstruation.

Menstrual disturbances in adolescence

Menstrual disturbances have been discussed in Chapter 29, Disorders of menstruation. As mentioned, in the first 2 years after the menarche, some young women experience oligomenorrhoea, whilst in others menstruation occurs at longer or shorter intervals. Unless the disorder persists, treatment consists of reassuring the young women that it will settle.

Later in the teenaged years, dysfunctional uterine bleeding affects a small number of young women. Many of the invasive investigations listed for older women are inappropriate for teenagers. For example, diagnostic curettage is invasive and usually not necessary. Treatment using hormones is the main modality, as endometrial ablation and hysterectomy are inappropriate. Hormonal treatment or treatment with NSAIDs, e.g. mefanamic acid, for 3–6 months usually controls the menstrual disturbance, after which reciprocity of the hypothalamic–pituitary–ovarian axis re-establishes itself, but in 5% of affected adolescents, the dysfunctional uterine bleedings recur. If the menstrual disturbance does not resolve quickly with the suggested treatment, a screen for coagulation abnormalities is indicated.

Dysmenorrhoea affects many adolescent women and is considered on page 232.

CHAPTER 43

A woman's middle years: menopause

A woman's middle years extend from the age of 40 to 65 years. The most important landmark during this time is the menopause. Menopause means the cessation of menstruation, but the term is commonly used to include the perimenopausal years and the 10 or more years following the cessation of menstruation. The period is more correctly called the climacteric.

From the mean age of 40 (±5) years a woman's ovaries become less receptive to the effects of follicle-stimulating hormone (FSH) and luteinizing hormone (LH), either because the number of receptor binding sites on each follicle are decreasing or because increasing numbers of follicles are disappearing, or because of both. The effect is that oestrogen secretion declines and fluctuates and anovulation becomes more frequent. The fluctuations are a major factor in causing the menstrual disturbances which occur in some women in the years preceding the menopause (see Chapter 29, Disorders of menstruation). The negative feedback to the hypothalamus and pituitary gland is less effective with the result that FSH levels begin to rise. The release of FSH is also increased by the falling levels of inhibin secreted by the ovarian follicles.

As the years pass, fewer follicles are left in the ovaries and the level of oestrogen begins to fall more rapidly. When this occurs, FSH levels continue to rise as do LH levels, reaching a peak in the immediate postmenopause. The high circulating levels of gonadotrophins persist from this time on.

The remaining ovarian follicles become increasingly resistant to the higher FSH levels and oestrogen secretion is reduced still further until oligomenorrhoea, and later, amenorrhoea result. If the amenorrhoea persists for 6 months, with or without menopausal symptoms, the menopause has been reached. If the clinician is doubtful if the menopause has occurred, it can be confirmed by measuring serum FSH on several occasions. A level of more than 40IU/L indicates menopause (Fig. 43.1). The measurement of oestrogen levels is not helpful, as the levels of oestrone, oestradiol and oestriol fluctuate even after the menopause, particularly in the first 12 months. A change in the ratio of oestradiol:oestrone occurs, oestrone becoming the dominant circulating

oestrogen. After the menopause, any circulating oestrogen detected is synthesized in the peripheral fat by aromatization of androstenedione, derived mainly from the adrenal cortex, with some from the ovarian stroma.

Changes in the genital tract after the menopause

The decline in circulating oestrogen to low levels after the menopause leads to atrophy of the organs of the genital tract and the breasts (Fig. 43.2). The *ovaries*, the *Fallopian tubes* and the *uterus* become progressively atrophic. In the uterus, the muscle fibres are converted into fibrous tissue and any myomata present atrophy. The *vaginal epithelium* becomes thinner and less rugose and intermediate cells replace superficial cells. The vaginal secretions diminish as does the vaginal acidity, and pathogenic organisms grow more easily. The *urethral mucosa* may become atrophic. In some women, urinary symptoms of frequency, dysuria and incontinence result (see Chapter 40, The urinary tract and its relation to gynaecology). The *pelvic floor muscles* lose their tone as their blood supply is reduced; relaxation of the muscles increases and uterovaginal prolapse may become evident (Chapter 39, Uterovaginal displacements, damage and prolapse). The external genitals slowly become atrophic and, in old age, the labia majora may lose their fat, revealing the labia minora.

Symptoms of the climacteric

The symptoms experienced by menopausal women result from the low levels of oestrogen. The two true menopausal symptoms are hot flushes and the vaginal symptoms of 'burning', dryness and dyspareunia. Not all women experience these symptoms. Studies show that about 25% of women have no symptoms and do not find the menopause disturbing in any way. Thirty-five per cent of women have mild or moderate symptoms and usually do not visit a doctor. The remaining 40% of women have severe menopausal symptoms. The severity of the symptoms is related (loosely) to the circulating level of oestradiol, and usually they occur if the level is less than 60pmol/L.

The hot flushes occurring at night lead to sweating and insomnia, with fatigue the next day. Many other physical and psychological symptoms (such as aching painful joints, headaches, palpitations, dizziness, irritability, lack of concentration, anxiety and depression) are experienced but most do not depend exclusively, or at all, on oestrogen deprivation.

Psychosocial factors are also involved. A woman who complains of severe premenstrual syndrome is more likely

Fig. 43.1 Postmenopausal plasma hormone levels measured one year after the menopause	
FSH (IU/L)	90–110
LH (IU/L)	60–70
Oestradiol (pmol/L)	30–100
Oestrone (pmol/L)	100–150
Total testosterone (nmol/L)	1–3
Free testosterone (pmol/L)	3–9
Dihydrotestosterone (pmol/L)	100–300

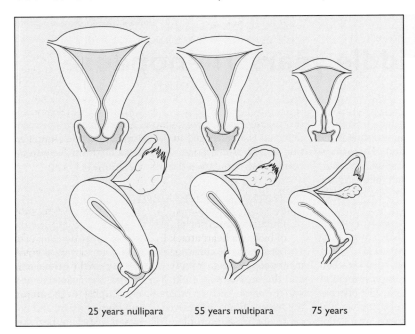

Fig. 43.2 The reduction in the size of the uterus in old age.

25 years nullipara   55 years multipara   75 years

to complain of menopausal symptoms than are women who are depressed or have family conflicts.

HOT FLUSHES

During a hot flush (hot flash in the USA), the woman experiences a feeling of heat centred on her face, which spreads to her neck and chest and may become generalized. This flushing is associated with peripheral vasodilatation and a temporary rise in body temperature of 3°C. The cause of the hot flush is unknown.

Each hot flush lasts for 1–3 minutes and is often accompanied by sweating. Hot flushes may occur many times during the day and night. If they occur at night when the woman is in bed, sweating tends to be profuse and sleep is disturbed; the next day she may feel fatigued.

Hot flushes may begin in the months before the menopause, but are worse after it, reaching a peak incidence 1–2 years after the menopause. Approximately one-third of climacteric women experience no or mild symptoms, one-third have moderate symptoms but usually do not seek medical advice and one-third have severe disabling symptoms. The hot flushes may persist for a number of years after the menopause.

VAGINAL DRYNESS

The vaginal symptoms owing to oestrogen deprivation tend to occur later in the climacteric, if they occur at all. Vaginal dryness and 'burning' are usually reported, but some women experience marked dyspareunia, which may affect their relationship with their partner considerably. Women who have regular sexual intercourse are less likely to develop dyspareunia.

OTHER SYMPTOMS

Urogenital atrophy leads to urinary incontinence and recurrent urinary tract infections (see page 307). For these conditions vaginal oestrogen therapy is recommended

Of many other symptoms listed as 'due' to the menopause, few are. Some menopausal women lose interest in sex, but this may be as much a function of their poor relationship as due to a hormonal deficiency. Contrary to popular belief, depression is no more common in the menopausal years than at other times. As a woman grows older her skin becomes less elastic, particularly if it is photodamaged. Lack of oestrogen in the postmenopausal years makes the wrinkling and dryness more apparent; however, this may respond, to some degree, to hormonal treatment.

Long-term effects of oestrogen deficiency

As well as symptoms occurring at or soon after the menopause, the long-term effects of oestrogen deficiency occur which reduce life expectancy and the quality of life. These are an increased risk of ischaemic heart disease and osteoporosis.

ISCHAEMIC HEART DISEASE

At all ages of life, women have a lower mortality from cardiovascular disease than men, but in the postmenopausal years the gap closes. These observations suggest that oestrogen offers a woman some degree of protection against developing heart disease.

OSTEOPOROSIS

As women and men grow older, there is an increased tendency for their bones to become osteopenic and spinal fractures occur, leading to some symptoms of backache and a reduction in height. Other women sustain fractures of the wrist or hip from falls that would previously have been trivial. These women are likely to have osteoporosis. Postmenopausal women, deprived of oestrogen, develop osteoporosis earlier in life than men, who are protected at least until the age of 75 years by circulating testosterone.

Psychological symptoms of the climacteric

The perception of the menopause as threatening is culture-based. In some societies, women welcome the menopause as they are no longer able to bear children, and have greater freedom. In many Western cultures, where the stress is on youth, the menopause is often perceived negatively. Relationships with a partner and children may have deteriorated, the woman may be anxious about the future, or she may feel that she is becoming less attractive.

Sexuality after the menopause

Sexual desire and drive are unchanged in 60% of post-menopausal women, at least up to the age of 65–70 years. Sexual desire and drive are increased in 20% and reduced in 20% of postmenopausal women. The most important influence on a postmenopausal woman's sexuality is the pattern established in the reproductive years: if it was good then it will continue to be good! As men grow older, however, their sexual desire and response changes. The man may desire sex less often, it takes longer to stimulate him and his erection is less firm and prolonged. Doctors who are consulted about a sexual problem by a postmenopausal woman may have to explain the changes. As women live longer than men, more elderly women have no partner and may seek 'permission' from a doctor if they use self-stimulatory methods to obtain sexual pleasure.

Management of the climacteric

The management of menopausal women includes:
- Providing an explanation of the changes which are occurring.
- Giving advice about nutrition and diet and answering concerns about weight.
- Recommending that the woman exercises for 30 minutes three times a week. Most experts suggest brisk walking, but she should choose an exercise she enjoys.
- Discussing the benefits of hormone (oestrogen) replacement treatment.

HORMONE REPLACEMENT TREATMENT/THERAPY (HRT)

Before prescribing HRT, the doctor should make a general medical check, if this has not been made in the previous year. The physical examination should include: an estimation of the body mass index; a breast examination, including a mammogram; a measurement of the blood pressure; and a vaginal examination, including a Pap smear.

There are compelling data which show for a menopausal woman, small daily doses of an oestrogen, with progestogen added if she has not had a hysterectomy, will:
- Relieve the flushes and vaginal symptoms.
- Induce a feeling of well-being.
- Providing she is prepared to take HRT for a long time, preferably until she is 70 years or older, reduce the risk of having a heart attack by 30–50%, provided she takes the other measures recommended i.e. stopping smoking; eating a prudent diet; and taking regular enjoyable exercise, such as walking.
- Prevent bone loss and consequently delay the onset of osteoporosis.
- Probably improve the thickness of the skin, reduce wrinkles and make the skin less dry.
- Probably reduce or delay her chance of developing Alzheimer's disease.

Contra-indications to the use of HRT

A few women should not use HRT. These include women who have a history of a recent thromboembolism, women with acute or chronic liver disease, women who have undiagnosed uterine bleeding and some women who are diabetic, unless they are monitored carefully. A recent scare linking HRT with an increased risk of breast cancer has added to women's concern. The report suggested that if HRT is taken for more than 5 years the risk of developing breast cancer increases from 1.6 to 3% over 5 years. Subsequent studies cast doubt about these findings, suggesting that the increase is only found if the woman's mother or sister had breast cancer before the age of 45 years.

Studies in several countries show that fewer than 20% of women are prepared at this time to take HRT for longer than 3–5 years. There are several reasons: 'Hormone treatment is unnatural and you only need HRT if you have severe symptoms; it makes the menstrual periods return or may cause irregular uterine bleeding; it causes high blood pressure and weight gain'. Talking with the patient may resolve these concerns.

The current evidence is that the benefits of HRT, even in asymptomatic women, are greater than its disadvantages, and a campaign to persuade women to take HRT would improve women's health, but must be handled carefully.

Treatment choices

There are several choices of oestrogen replacement treatment. The woman may choose, for example, to take a daily oestrogen tablet, apply an oestrogen transdermal patch every third day, or to use an oestrogenic vaginal ring which releases very small amounts of oestrogen to control vaginal symptoms or larger amounts to control menopausal symptoms. The advantage of this method is that the control is in the woman's hands. The dose of oestrogen is adjusted so that the symptoms are relieved. A few women, particularly those who have had a hysterectomy, choose to have an oestradiol implant every 6 months.

If the woman has not had a hysterectomy, unopposed oestrogen treatment increases the risk that she will develop an endometrial carcinoma (from 1 per 1000 women per year to 3–4 per 1000 per year). Women who have retained their uterus should be prescribed a progestogen for the first 12 days of each month or every third month. During the time the woman takes the progestogen she may experience symptoms similar to those of the premenstrual syndrome, and at the end of the course usually she will have a withdrawal bleed, which lasts 3-4 days. The effects of progestogen and the withdrawal bleeds deter many women from taking HRT, in spite of the clear benefits of the treatment. Two strategies are available to overcome the problem. The first is for the woman to be prescribed a combination of oestrogen and progestogen to be taken each day; the second is for the woman to take tibolone (Livial) daily. In each case irregular bleeding may be expected for the first 4-6 months of treatment but after that amenorrhoea is a usual finding.

If the woman's main problem is atrophic vaginitis, oestrogen pessaries or cream may be preferred, at least until the symptoms are relieved.

Should irregular bleeding occur during HRT, the woman should have an endometrial biopsy or curettage performed or a transvaginal ultrasound image of the endometrium, even if the clinical diagnosis indicates that the woman has atrophic vaginitis or a cervical polyp. If the ultrasound image detects that the endometrial thickness is less than 5mm, endometrial adenocarcinoma is unlikely to be present. If the endometrium is 5mm or more thick, a hysteroscopic examination of the uterine cavity and an endometrial biopsy (or a curettage) should be made.

Postmenopausal bleeding

Irregular bleeding *per vaginam* may also occur in women not taking HRT. The causes are listed in *Fig. 43.3*. As 15% of women who have postmenopausal bleeding will be found to have a malignancy, investigations include inspection of the vagina, a Pap smear and an endometrial curettage or biopsy, even if the clinical diagnosis appears to be atrophic vaginitis or a cervical polyp. Treatment depends on the cause.

Osteoporosis

Osteoporosis is defined as a reduced bone mass per unit volume and, in clinical practice, as the relation to the degree to which bone mineral density is reduced. There are several types of osteoporosis (*Fig. 43.4*) but that which concerns women most is postmenopausal osteoporosis. The WHO has provided diagnostic criteria for the categories of osteoporosis (*Fig. 43.5*).

Osteoporosis is becoming a major health problem for women as they are living longer. Data from several countries show that between 30 and 50% of women will have an osteoporotic fracture if they live into their 70s. Up to the age of 70 years, vertebral fractures leading to collapse of some vertebrae and Colles' fracture of the wrist are the most common fractures. After the age of 70 years, hip fractures increase in frequency because older women have a greater chance of falling. In Australia, for example, over 10,000 hip fractures in a population of 16 million were reported in 1986, and the number is increasing.

The chance that a woman will develop osteoporosis depends on genetic inheritance, her peak bone mineral density (which is reached between the age of 15 and 25 years), and the rate at which she loses bone. Until the age of 40 years, bone loss is balanced by bone formation; after the age of 40 years, about 0.5% of the bone mass is lost annually (*Fig. 43.6*). Following the menopause, bone loss varies from 1 to 7% a year depending on the individual, averaging 3% a year. This amount of bone loss continues for 10 years and then reduces to between 0.5 and 1.0% per year.

Fig. 43.3 Causes of postmenopausal bleeding (800 reported cases)

	Percentage
No demonstrable lesion	25
Oestrogen therapy	20
Atrophic vaginitis	15
Endometrial adenocarcinoma	15
Endometrial polyp or hyperplasia	15
Cervical carcinoma	4
Benign cervical lesions (polyps)	4
Ovarian tumour (mostly malignant)	1
Bleeding from urinary tract	1

Fig. 43.4 Classification of osteoporosis

Primary osteoporosis

Postmenopausal
Senile

Secondary osteoporosis

Endocrine: Cushing's syndrome, thyrotoxicosis, hypogonadism, hyperparathyroidism, anorexia nervosa, exercise-induced amenorrhoea
Drugs: Corticosteroids, heparin, anticonvulsants

CLINICAL FEATURES OF OSTEOPOROSIS

The clinical features of vertebral body fractures, producing wedge-shaped vertebrae, are height loss, 'Dowagers Hump' and backache, which may be severe, and may occur suddenly after bending. However, most vertebral fractures are asymptomatic. In many cases, the diagnosis of osteoporosis can be made clinically but greater accuracy in determining the severity of the disease is obtained if a bone mineral scan is made, preferably using a dual energy X-ray absorbiometry machine (DEXA).

Once osteoporosis has been established, treatment is not particularly effective. The strategy must be to prevent or delay its onset.

PREVENTION OF OSTEOPOROSIS

Adolescent and young adult women should be persuaded to take at least 800mg of calcium a day preferably in food. Two or three servings of milk, cheese or yoghurt will provide this amount, and the teenaged woman may thus achieve her peak bone mass. Her doctor should explain that if she chooses low-fat dairy products she will not become fat, a matter of considerable concern to teenagers. Adolescent women should also take regular moderate exercise, and avoid smoking.

Young women who are amenorrhoeic for more than 6 months (for example women who have anorexia nervosa or who are compulsive exercisers) should be prescribed an oestrogen, the contraceptive pill being a good choice.

A *mature woman* should take the following measures to try to prevent osteoporosis:
* Take calcium 1–1.5 g a day in food or as a supplement.
* Take regular exercise, such as walking for 30 minutes three times a week.
* Avoid smoking.
* Reduce salt intake. No salt to be sprinkled over food.

A *postmenopausal woman* should also consider starting to take HRT, as oestrogen effectively prevents bone loss. If HRT is contra-indicated, or she chooses not to take the hormones, an alternative is to take one of the bisphosphonates. Before starting this treatment a more accurate prognosis can be obtained if her bone mineral density is measured using the DEXA machine. Depending on the result of DEXA, she should be advised whether she needs treatment or to wait and repeat the DEXA 2 years later (see *Fig. 43.4*). It is unclear if exercise helps to decrease the rate of bone loss, but it may increase bone strength and reduce the chance of falls. An approach to the management of established osteoporosis is given in *Figure 43.7*.

ESTABLISHED OSTEOPOROSIS

Once clinical osteoporosis has been diagnosed, either by bone densitometry or following a fracture, treatment is more

Fig. 43.5 Bone mineral density and osteoporosis.

Fig. 43.6 Osteoporosis: bone from the iliac crest of a 20-year-old woman (a) compared with that of a 60-year-old woman (b).

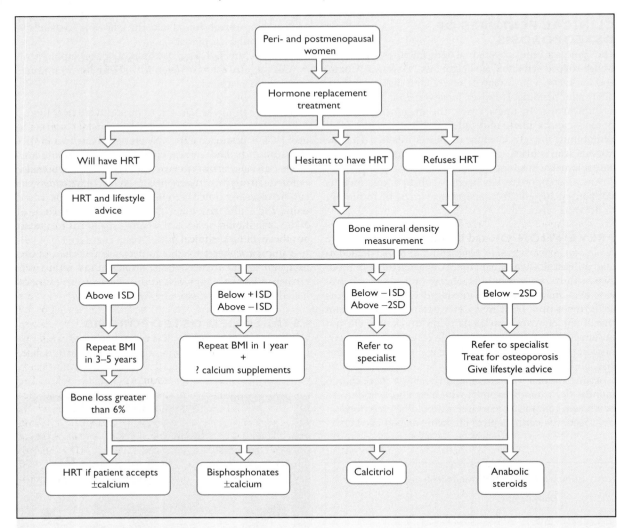

Fig. 43.7 Osteoporosis: management.

difficult. Drugs used to treat established osteoporosis act either by preventing bone resorption or by stimulating bone formation. Drugs preventing bone resorption such as those used in HRT (which also increases bone formation), bisphosphonates (pamidronate, alendronate or etidronate with intermittent calcium), calcitonin or calcitriol are being investigated. The anabolic steroid nandrolone decanoate, (Deca-Durabolin), which stimulates bone formation and prevents resorption to some extent, is also under study. Until the benefits and adverse effects of these drugs have been evaluated, prevention holds the most promise for reducing the adverse health effects of osteoporosis.

CHAPTER 44

Anatomy of the female genital tract

By the time students study gynaecology, they have been well grounded in the disciplines of anatomy and physiology, and only a brief review of the anatomy of the female genital tract will be made here.

The vulva

The *labia majora* are two large folds containing sebaceous and sweat glands embedded in adipose and connective tissue and covered by skin (*Fig. 44.1*). They form the lateral boundaries of the vulval cleft, and are the homologues of the scrotum. Anteriorly, they unite in an adipose pad over the symphysis pubis, to form the mons veneris. In the adult, the mons is covered with hair, which terminates cephalically in a horizontal upper border. Hair also grows on the outer, but not the inner, surface of the labia majora. Posteriorly, the labia majora unite to form the posterior commissure. In childhood, the labia majora contain little adipose tissue, and, in older age, the adipose tissue disappears. At the extremes of life, therefore, the labia majora are relatively small.

The *labia minora* are flat, delicate folds of skin containing connective tissue and some sebaceous glands, but no adipose tissue. On their medial aspect the keratinized epithelium of the skin changes into poorly keratinized squamous epithelium, containing many sebaceous glands. Anteriorly, the labia minora split into two parts, one passing over the clitoris to form the prepuce of the organ, the other passing beneath to form the homologue of the frenulum of the male. Posteriorly, they fuse to form the fourchette, which is always torn during parturition. In the reproductive years, the labia minora are hidden by the labia majora, but in childhood and old age they appear to be more prominent as the labia majora are relatively small. The size of the labia minora varies considerably in different women, but this is of little clinical importance.

The proximal two-thirds of the internal surface of the labia minora and all the tissues internal to them are derived from the endoderm. The distal third of the internal surface of the labia minora and all of the vulva external to this are derived from the ectoderm and the histology is that of the skin. The junction between the endodermal-derived tissues and the ectodermal-derived tissues is termed Hart's line.

The cleft between the labia minora is called the *vestibule*, and contains the *external urethral meatus* and the *hymen*, which lies just inside and surrounds the vaginal orifice. The vestibule is surmounted by the *clitoris*, which is the homologue of the penis, and is composed of erectile tissue. As with the penis, it becomes enlarged and stiffens during sexual excitement. The clitoris is one of the major erotic zones of the woman. Only the glans and prepuce of the clitoris are normally visible, but the corpus can be palpated along the lower surface of the symphysis pubis as a cord-like structure.

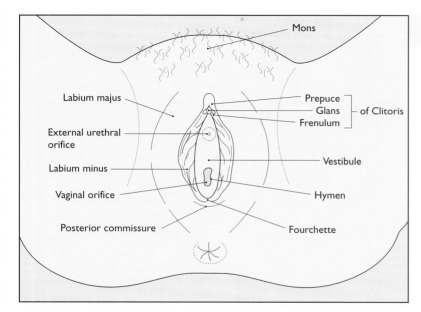

Labium majus

External urethral orifice

Labium minus

Vaginal orifice

Posterior commissure

Mons

Prepuce
Glans } of Clitoris
Frenulum

Vestibule

Hymen

Fourchette

Fig. 44.1 The vulva of a virgin.

The *hymen* is a thin, incomplete membrane surrounding the vaginal orifice, and has one or more apertures in it, which allow menstrual blood to escape. The apertures are of various shapes and sizes and the hymen varies considerably in elasticity, but is generally torn during a first coitus. An 'intact' hymen is considered a sign of virginity, but this is not reliable as in some cases coitus fails to cause a tear, and in others the hymen may be torn by digital interference. In attempting to make a decision regarding virginity, palpation to feel a circular ridge of hymenal tissue is more accurate than inspection. Although the hymen is relatively avascular, tearing at first coitus may be accompanied by a small amount of bleeding, which ceases rapidly. Childbirth causes a much greater tearing of the hymen, and after parturition only a few tags remain. These are carunculae myrtiformes (*Fig. 44.2*). Just lateral to the hymen, surrounding the vaginal orifice on each side, and deep to the bulbocavernosus muscle (the sphincter vaginae), are two collections of erectile tissue – the *vestibular bulbs*. Embedded in the posterolateral parts of the bulbs, on each side is Bartholin's gland (*Fig. 44.3*), which is the homologue of Cowper's gland in the male. The gland is pea-sized and not palpable unless infected. It is connected to the posterior part of the vestibule, between the hymen and the fourchette, by a duct some 2cm in length. It is lined by columnar cells, which secrete a mucoid substance during sexual excitement.

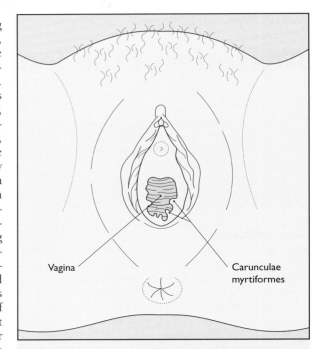

Vagina

Carunculae myrtiformes

Fig. 44.2 The vulva of a parous woman.

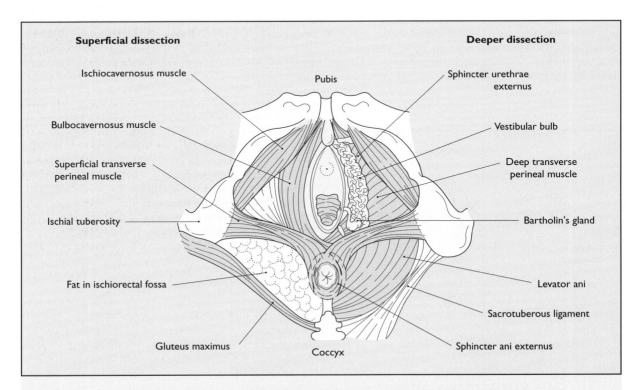

Superficial dissection

Deeper dissection

Ischiocavernosus muscle

Pubis

Sphincter urethrae externus

Bulbocavernosus muscle

Vestibular bulb

Superficial transverse perineal muscle

Deep transverse perineal muscle

Ischial tuberosity

Bartholin's gland

Fat in ischiorectal fossa

Levator ani

Sacrotuberous ligament

Gluteus maximus

Coccyx

Sphincter ani externus

Fig. 44.3 Dissection of the perineum to show the superficial muscles, the position of Bartholin's gland and the vestibular bulb.

VASCULAR AND NERVE SUPPLY
Arteries
The external genitalia are very vascular, and are supplied by branches of the internal pudendal arteries, which originate from the internal iliac arteries, and by the external pudendal arteries, deriving from the femoral arteries.

Veins
The veins of the vulva form large venous plexuses, which become dilated during sexual excitement, and to an even greater degree during pregnancy, when varicosities are not uncommon. Most of the veins accompany the corresponding arteries, but those draining the clitoris join the vaginal and vesical venous plexuses.

Lymphatics
Lymphatic vessels form an interconnecting meshwork which extends through the labia minora, the prepuce, the fourchette and the vaginal introitus. These vessels join to form 'trunks'. The anterior trunks join with a lymphatic meshwork over the mons (which also drains the glans of the clitoris). The anterior collecting trunks pass to reach the ipsilateral and contralateral superficial femoral nodes. The lymphatics from the labia majora also form trunks and pass to the superficial femoral nodes. There are

connections between the superficial and the deep femoral nodes, which then connect with the nodes along the external iliac vessels.

The lymphatics from the clitoral shaft (which interconnect with those of the glans) pass directly to internal iliac nodes in the pelvis (*Fig. 44.4*). The lymphatics anastomose with those of the opposite side, and consequently bilateral or contralateral involvement is not uncommon in malignant tumours of the vulva. The vulval lymphatics also anastomose with the lymphatics of the lower third of the vagina, which drain into the external iliac nodes.

Nerve supply
The nerve supply of the vulva is described on page 88.

The vagina

The vagina is a fibromuscular sheath, extending upwards and backwards from the vestibule, at an angle of about 85° to the horizontal, and parallel with the plane of pelvic brim when the woman is standing erect (*Fig. 44.5*). The walls of the vagina, as well as being muscular, contain a well-developed venous plexus. Normally the walls are in apposition, the vagina being a potential cavity, and having an H-shape in cross-section in the middle third (*Fig. 44.6*). In the lower third, the widest diameter of the vagina is the anteroposterior diameter, but above this the widest diameter is the transverse diameter. Knowledge of this is of importance when introducing a vaginal bivalve speculum. Because of the well-developed walls, the lining epithelium tends to be lifted into ridges, or rugae, which run in a circumferential manner from two longitudinal columns running sagittally the length of the anterior and posterior vaginal walls. The formation of rugae in this manner, permits the great distension without damage of which the vagina is capable. The length of the anterior vaginal wall is about 7cm, and its upper end is invaginated by the cervix. Because of this, the posterior vaginal wall, which ends blindly, is about 2cm longer. The vaginal vault is divided into four areas, which are related to the projecting cervix. These are the shallow *anterior fornix*, the capacious *posterior fornix* and the shallow *lateral fornices*. Although the vagina varies considerably in length and width, its functional size is largely determined by the tone in its muscular wall and the contractions of the surrounding muscles. These are under voluntary control. Unless the vagina has been injured or shortened at operation, anatomical variations in size do not cause difficulty or pain (dyspareunia) during coitus; most cases of dyspareunia are psychosomatic in origin.

The vagina is surrounded by several important structures. The anterior wall is in contact with the urethra, to which it is closely bound, and above this with the base of the bladder. Posteriorly, the lower one-third is separated from the rectum by the complex of muscles and fascia which constitutes the perineal body but, above, is in direct contact with the rectum. The upper one-quarter, including the posterior fornix, is covered by the peritoneum of the

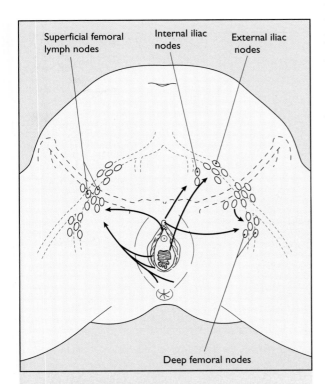

Fig. 44.4 *The distribution of the lymphatics of the vulva. Extensive intercommunications exists between the lymphatics of each side.*

Superficial femoral lymph nodes

Internal iliac nodes

External iliac nodes

Deep femoral nodes

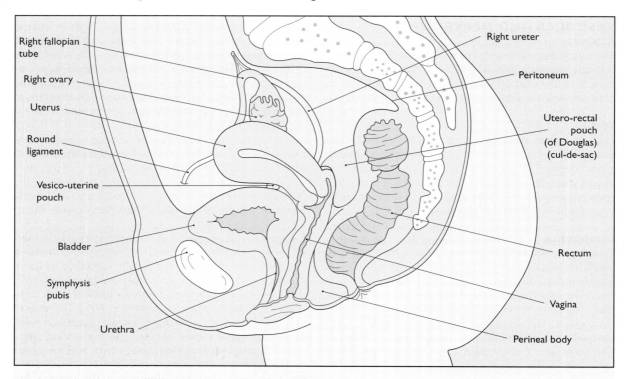

Fig. 44.5 *Sagittal section of the pelvis, with the woman in the erect position.*

Fig. 44.6 *The vagina in cross-section. Note the greater length of the posterior wall and the H-shape on a cross-section. It can be seen that the vaginal walls are normally in apposition.*

utero-rectal pouch (pouch of Douglas or cul-de-sac). The upper third of the lateral walls are in intimate contact with the pelvic connective tissue, and the fornices abut the parametrium, which contains a rich venous plexus. Lying about 1cm above each lateral fornix are the uterine artery and the ureter (*Fig. 44.7*). In the middle third, the lateral wall blends with the levator ani muscles, which together with the muscular vagina form one of the supports of the uterus. In the lower third, the walls are related to the bulbocavernosus muscle, the bulb of the vestibule and Bartholin's glands.

HISTOLOGY

The vagina is lined with stratified, squamous, non-keratinized epithelium, some 10–30 cells deep, which rests upon a basement membrane and is continuous at the upper end with an identical epithelium covering the vaginal portion of the cervix. Should the epithelium be exposed to the dry external atmosphere, keratinization occurs. The cells are all derived by differentiation from the basal cells which lie upon the basement membrane. Three main cell types are described; parabasal cells, intermediate cells and superficial cells. The superficial cells, and some intermediate cells, contain glycogen. The entire epithelium shows cyclic changes during the menstrual cycle, and in pregnancy, and cellular development and differentiation is controlled by the ratio of circulating oestrogens, progesterone and androgens (*Fig. 44.8*). The cells do not secrete mucus, but secretions seep between the cells to moisten the vagina, and the superficial cells are constantly exfoliated. The exfoliated cells release the contained glycogen, which is acted upon by Döderlein's bacilli, a normal inhabitant of the vagina, to produce lactic acid. This causes the normal acidity of the vagina, and explains the relative resistance of the vagina to infection. The vaginal epithelial cells can also absorb drugs, particularly oestrogens.

The epithelium rests upon a connective tissue layer containing elastic tissue, nerves, lymphatics and blood vessels, and external to this are the thick layers of interdigitating muscle fibres, which cross in a spiral manner, the main direction being oblique rather than circular. Outside the muscle is a well-developed sheath of connective tissue, which is condensed, anteriorly, to form the so-called pubocervical (or vesicovaginal) fascia, and, posteriorly, to form the rectovaginal fascia. The condensed connective tissue fuses with, and is part of, the visceral layer of the pelvic fascia.

VASCULAR CONNECTIONS

The arterial blood supply is from the vaginal and uterine arteries, which are branches of the internal iliac artery, and which form a plexus around the vagina. A median artery arises from this plexus on the anterior and on the posterior walls. The arteries are called azygous vaginal arteries (*Fig. 44.9*). The venous drainage, which goes to the internal iliac veins, is from a rich venous plexus situated on the muscular

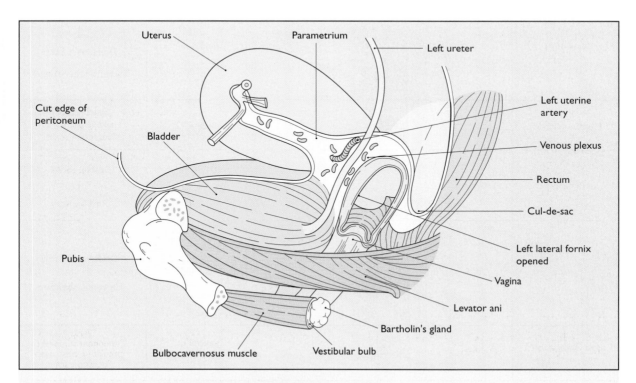

Fig. 44.7 Relationship of the parametrium to the vagina and other pelvic organs.

wall of the vagina, which is especially well developed at the lower end of the vagina, and which communicates with the vesical, pudendal and haemorrhoidal venous plexuses.

The lymphatic drainage of the lower third of the vagina is to the inferior gluteal nodes, near the ischial spine. Lymphatics also link with those of the upper vagina. The lymphatic drainage from the upper two-thirds of the vagina passes to the internal iliac, the obturator and the sacral nodes.

The uterus

The uterus is a thick-walled, hollow, muscular organ, shaped like a pear, its apex forming the cervix, which projects into the vaginal vault (Fig. 44.10). It is located in the middle of the true pelvis, lying between the bladder and the rectum. It is flattened from before backwards, and its muscular anterior and posterior walls bulge into the cavity, the walls thus being in apposition. Viewed from the front, the cavity has a triangular shape. It communicates with the peritoneal cavity via the Fallopian tubes (or oviducts) above, and with the exterior via the vaginal tube below. The uterus

varies in size, being largest during the reproductive years and in women who have had children. The 'average' uterus of a nulliparous woman, measures about 9cm in length, 6cm in width at its widest part and 4cm from before backwards, and weighs 40–60g. The wall is 1–2cm thick, and hence the length of the cavity measures about 7cm. All these dimensions are increased by about 1.5cm in women who have borne children.

STRUCTURE

Externally the uterus is covered with peritoneum on the anterior and posterior aspects, and this forms the serosal layer. Deep to the serosal layer is the muscle layer, the myometrium, which is composed of three interdigitating layers of muscle. The outer, mainly longitudinal, layer and the inner, mainly circular, layer are poorly developed, and the bulk of the myometrium is formed from the middle layer, which is composed of obliquely interdigitating strands of muscle. Deep to the myometrium is the endometrium, which is a soft layer of variable thickness made up of tubular glands, which dip into a stroma of cells held in a fine

			Vaginal		
	Oestrogen	Epithelium	Glycogen	pH	Flora
New born	+		+	Acid 4–5	Sterile ↓ Doderlein's bacilli Secretion abundant
Month-old child	–		+	Alkaline >7	Sparse, coccal and varied flora. Secretion scant
Puberty	Appears		– → +	Alkaline ↓ Acid	Sparse, coccal ↓ Rich bacillary
Mature	+ +		+	Acid 4–5	Doderlein's bacilli Secretion abundant
Post menopause	+ → –		–	Neutral or alkaline 6 to >7	Varied Dependent on level of circulating oestrogen Secretion scant

Fig. 44.8 Cyclic changes in the vagina related to age.

meshwork of connective tissue. A well-developed vasculature is derived from the myometrial vessels.

The uterus is made up of a *body*, or *corpus*, *isthmus* and a *cervix* (Fig. 44.11). The body is further divided into the area which lies above the insertion of the oviducts, and which is called the *fundus*. The area where the oviducts join the uterus on each side is termed the *cornu*. The body (including the fundus) comprises the greater portion of the organ, and is formed of thick bundles of muscle. The isthmus is a constricted, annular area, about 0.5cm wide, which lies between the corpus and the cervix. The proportion of muscle begins to diminish in the isthmus, and connective tissue appears in increasing amounts. The constriction at the upper end of the isthmus is called the *anatomical internal os*, and the line at the lower end of the isthmus, where the endometrium changes into columnar cervical epithelium, is termed the *histological internal os*.

On the surface of the uterus, the anatomical internal os is marked by the reflection of the peritoneum which covers the uterus, onto the superior surface of the bladder.

The *cervix* is fusiform or cylindrical in shape, and measures about 3cm from above downwards, half projecting into the vagina. The proportion of muscle tissue decreases rapidly in the cervix, and in its midportion only 10% of its bulk is made of muscle, the rest being connective tissue. The supravaginal portion of the cervix is surrounded by pelvic fascia, termed the parametrium, except, posteriorly, where it is covered with the peritoneum of the uterorectal pouch. The vaginal portion of the cervix is cone-shaped and projects into the vagina (see Fig. 44.11). It is covered with stratified squamous epithelium, which joins the columnar epithelium of the cervical canal at or near the external os. The cervical canal is spindle-shaped, and connects the cavity of the uterus to the vaginal cavity (see Fig. 44.11).

Vaginal arterial supply

Right ureter

Internal iliac artery

Uterine artery

Vaginal artery

Anterior azygous vaginal artery

Vaginal lymphatic drainage

Sacral nodes

Internal iliac nodes

Obturator nodes

Inferior gluteal nodes

Fig. 44.9 The vaginal arterial blood supply and lymphatic drainage systems. Note that the uterus is angled forward at about 90° to the vagina, and appears foreshortened.

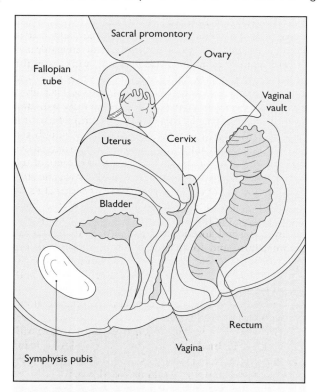

Fig. 44.10 The uterus from the side showing the anatomical relations.

The mucous membrane lining the canal is thrown up into anterior and posterior folds, from which circular folds radiate to give the appearance of a tree-trunk and branches. The folds are given the name *arbor vitae uteri*. The epithelium dips into the underlying stroma in a complicated system of clefts and crypts. The endocervical epithelium consists of columnar cells which secrete mucus, but the quality and quantity of this are under the control of the sex hormones.

RELATIONS

The uterus normally lies bent forwards at an angle of 90° to the direction of the vagina, but is freely mobile, rotating about a fulcrum at the level of the supravaginal cervix. Anteriorly, the uterus is separated from the bladder by the vesico-uterine pouch, and posteriorly, is in contact with coils of bowel and the omentum. The anterior and posterior surfaces are covered with peritoneum, but its narrow lateral surfaces are in direct contact with the broad ligament and, below, with the connective tissue, venous plexuses, arteries, nerves and the ureter, which make up the substance of the parametrium. The peritoneum, which covers the anterior and posterior walls, joins at the lateral margins of the uterus to form the two leaves of the *broad ligaments*; and these two sheets of peritoneum remain in close proximity, except where they diverge to accommodate the round ligament (more accurately, the round muscle) and the infundibulopelvic ligament. The broad ligament extends from the lateral uterine border to the pelvic wall.

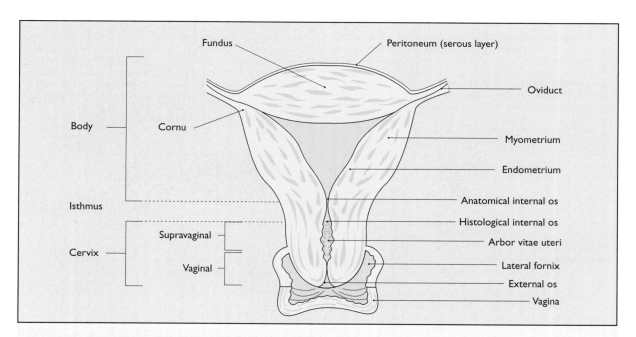

Fig. 44.11 Coronal section of the uterus showing the cavity and the cornual areas.

Its upper border is formed by the peritoneum covering the oviduct, and below, it merges, anteriorly, with the peritoneum of the pelvic floor and, posteriorly, with the peritoneum covering the recto-uterine shelf and the uterosacral ligaments (*Fig. 44.12*).

UTERINE SUPPORTS

These are discussed more fully in Chapter 39, Uterovaginal displacements, damage and prolapse, and a summary is presented here. The uterus is supported from below by the muscular vagina and the fibres of the levator ani muscles which interdigitate with the middle third of the muscular vaginal sheath. An additional support of great significance is the collection of connective tissue, muscular-walled blood vessels and areolar tissue, which forms a fan-shaped sheet on each side of the supravaginal cervix, and stretches from the fascia lining the pelvic wall to join the fibromuscular cervix. This fan-shaped sheet is condensed posteriorly to form the *uterosacral ligaments*, and medially to form the *cardinal ligament*, or the *transverse cervical ligament* (*Fig. 44.13*). Anteriorly, the fascia sweeps forward down the anterior wall of the vagina beneath the bladder base. This condensation is called the pubocervical fascia. Laterally, the broad ligament has a steadying effect on the uterus, whilst the round ligaments play some part – although a minor one – in keeping the uterus in an anteverted position.

VASCULAR CONNECTIONS

The uterus is supplied by the uterine arteries, which arise from the internal iliac artery. Each vessel runs forwards and inwards in the base of the broad ligament, and crosses the ureter above it and at right angles to it ('water *under* the bridge'), 1cm lateral to the supravaginal cervix. Each gives off a descending branch which anastomoses with the ascending branches of the vaginal artery, and which supplies the lower cervix; and a circular branch to supply the upper cervix. The main trunk changes direction and passes upwards, coiled and tortuous, between the layers of the broad ligament adjacent to the lateral uterine wall, and supplies branches to the myometrium at intervals. It ends by anastomosing with the ovarian artery (*Fig. 44.14*). Each branch supplying the uterus divides in the outer muscular layer, to send anterior and posterior branches to the myometrium, and to anastomose with those from the opposite side. These arteries give off branches at right angles, which penetrate and supply the myometrium, and, entering the endometrium, form the basal arteries.

The veins of the uterus accompany the uterine artery and form pampiniform plexuses of great complexity, particularly in the parametrium where they communicate with the veins of the bladder. The pampiniform plexus drains into the uterine vein and the ovarian vein, and has communications with the vertebral plexus of veins.

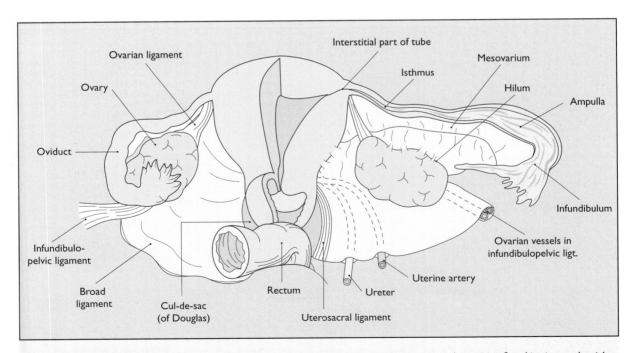

Fig. 44.12 The female pelvic organs viewed from behind. On the left the oviduct and ovary are in the position found in vivo; on the right dissection has been made.

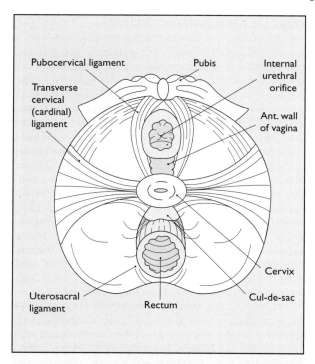

Fig. 44.13 *The 'ligaments' of the cervix.*

LYMPHATIC DRAINAGE

The lymphatic drainage of the uterus consists of three communicating networks: the deepest network lies in the endometrium, the second lies in the substance of the myometrium and the superficial network is subperitoneal. The networks form collecting trunks, which pass from the corpus between the layers of the broad ligament along with the ovarian lymphatics. These trunks then pass through the infundibulopelvic fold, and ascend, on the posterior abdominal wall, to join the nodes of the para-aortic group. A few channels pass along the round ligament to the superficial femoral nodes. The lowest two trunks communicate with the collecting trunks from the cervix, which pass through the base of the broad ligament to an inconstant node lateral to the parametrial node, to the nodes along the internal iliac arteries (the internal iliac or hypogastric nodes), and to the obturator nodes anteriorly. A few channels pass backwards along the uterosacral ligaments to the sacral nodes (*Fig. 44.15*).

NERVE SUPPLY

The nerve supply of the uterus is described on page 68.

The oviduct

The oviducts, or Fallopian tubes, are two small muscular tubes, one on each side, which extend for about 10cm from the uterine cornua towards the pelvic wall, forming the upper border of the broad ligaments. The outer half of each

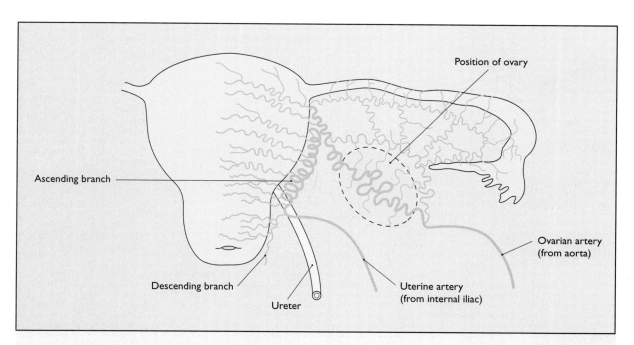

Fig. 44.14 *The blood supply of the uterus, oviduct and ovary.*

oviduct lies in contact with the ovary, curving over its superior surface to end in the abdominal ostium. Since the tube is hollow, a direct connection exists between the peritoneal cavity and the uterus. The mucous membrane lining of the tube is thrown up into folds which almost obliterate the lumen, and which are prolonged through the abdominal ostium to form the fimbriae of the tube. The oviduct can be divided into four parts. The *infundibulum* is the outermost portion of the tube. It includes the trumpet-shaped abdominal ostium, and lies in close proximity to the ovary. The *ampulla* is the longest segment of the oviduct, is normally rather tortuous, and has a relatively thin dilatable wall. The *isthmus* is a straight, narrow, relatively thick-walled segment, and the *interstitial* portion is the short, narrow portion within the uterine wall. The size of the lumen decreases from the infundibular to the interstitial portion, where it is only about 1mm in diameter, whilst the complexity of the folds in the mucous membrane increases from the interstitial to the infundibular portions (*Fig. 44.16*).

The mucous membrane is lined with epithelial cells, about half of which are mucus-secreting and half ciliated. The mucus secreted into the lumen is propelled towards the uterus by the action of the cilia and by peristaltic movements of the musculature of the tube. The mucus is rich in protein, and may provide nourishment for the fertilized ovum during its passage down the oviduct.

The ovary

The two ovaries are the homologues of the testes, and are ovoid-shaped organs. Each ovary normally lies in a shallow peritoneal fossa adjacent to the lateral pelvic wall, with its long axis in a vertical plane, but its position is influenced by movements of the uterus and broad ligament (*Fig. 44.17*). The ovaries have an irregular surface, are pinkish-grey in colour, and vary in size in different women, and at different times of the cycle. In the infant, the ovary is a delicate, elongated structure, with a smooth, glistening surface. The ovary of a neonate contains little stroma and mainly consists of primary follicles. As infancy and childhood progress, increasing numbers of follicles degenerate, and there is a progressive increase in stromal content, up to puberty. During puberty the ovary enlarges, and in the reproductive period it averages 3.5cm in length, 2cm in breadth and 1cm in thickness, and weighs about 7g. Postmenopausally, the ovary undergoes rapid regressive changes, becoming wrinkled, white in colour and less than half the size it was in the reproductive era. Each ovary is attached to the posterior leaf of the broad ligament by a fold of peritoneum called the mesovarium, through which pass the ovarian vessels and nerves (see *Fig. 44.12*). The peritoneum stops where the mesovarium

Fig. 44.15 *The lymphatic drainage of the female genital organs. For clarity, the lymphatic channels have been omitted and are indicated by arrows.*

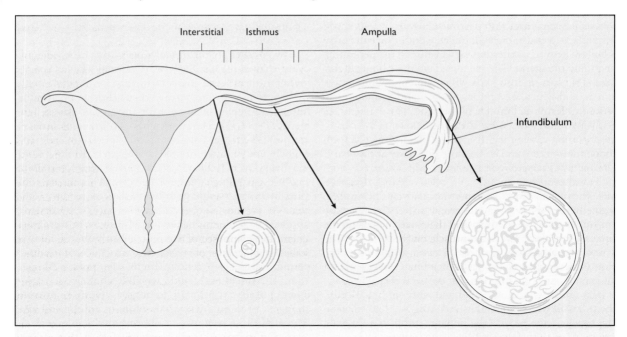

Fig. 44.16 The oviduct, showing the structure of the mucosal layer.

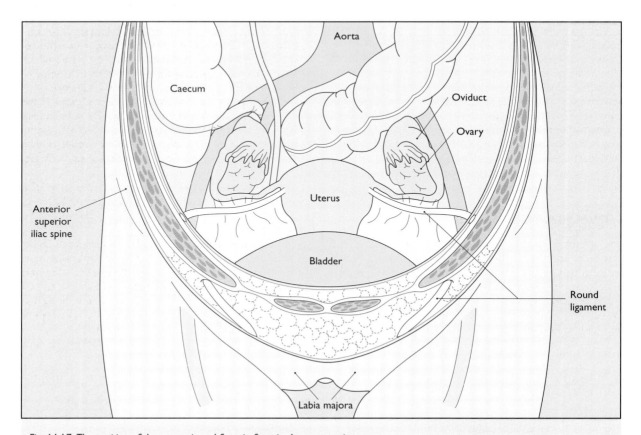

Fig. 44.17 The position of the ovary, viewed from in front in the erect patient.

joins the ovary, and this part of the ovary is called the hilum. The remainder of the ovarian cortex is covered by a single layer of low columnar epithelium under which is a layer of connective tissue, called the tunica albuginea. This layer increases in density with increasing age.

VASCULAR CONNECTIONS AND NERVE SUPPLY OF OVARY AND OVIDUCT

The arterial, venous and lymphatic connections of both ovary and oviduct are similar, and the two organs are often referred to as the *adnexae;* or uterine appendages.

The *arterial* supply is from the long, slender, ovarian artery, a branch of the abdominal aorta, which arises immediately below the renal artery and crosses the inferior vena cava, the ureter and the psoas muscle on the right side, and the left psoas muscle on the left side. The vessel crosses the external iliac artery at the pelvic brim, runs between the two layers of the infundibulopelvic fold and enters the broad ligament. Within the broad ligament it runs 0.5cm below the tube, and gives off branches to the ovary via the mesovarium, and to the oviduct between the layers of the broad ligament. It ends by joining the terminal branch of the uterine artery to form an arterial arcade. The *venous drainage* is into a pampiniform plexus, and then to the ovarian veins. The right ovarian vein joins the inferior vena cava, and the left ovarian vein usually enters the left renal vein.

The *lymphatics* of each adnexa drain to the para-aortic nodes, and there is some evidence of communicating trunks to the contralateral ovary via the subperitoneal lymphatic plexus of the fundus of the uterus.

The *nerve supply* of the ovary is very well developed, and arises from a sympathetic plexus which surrounds the ovarian vessels in the infundibulopelvic ligament. Its fibres derive from branches of the aortic and renal plexuses. Sensory nerves follow the arteries and are relayed in the spinal cord at the level of the tenth aortic segment. This well-developed nerve supply accounts for the extreme sensitivity of the ovary to squeezing.

Anatomy of the urinary tract

The urethral meatus lies in the anterior part of the vestibule, and the urethra runs upwards and backwards for 4cm to join the bladder base at an angle. It is intimately connected with the anterior vaginal wall, and a series of small crypts open into its posterior surface in the lowest third. These crypts are known as Skene's tubules and lie between the lateral urethral wall and the vagina.

They are homologues of the male prostate, and may become the site of chronic infection.

The bladder is a muscular organ with a considerable capacity for distension. The base is relatively flat, lies parallel with the axis of the vagina, and contains the internal urinary meatus and the orifices of the ureters (*Fig. 44.18*). The triangular area between these three openings constitutes the trigone. The dome, or fundus, of the bladder varies in shape and position depending upon the degree of distension. It is lined by transitional epithelium, and external to this is the muscular layer. The involuntary muscle which forms the bladder can be divided into two parts, that forming the fundus, which is poorly supplied by autonomic nerves, and that forming the base (the detrusor muscle), which is richly supplied by autonomic nerves. The female urethra is a muscular tube, composed of two muscle layers. It is about 4cm long. The inner layer of muscle is longitudinal and is a direct continuation of the inner longitudinal layer of the detrusor muscle. It is embedded in dense collagen. The outer layer, which is a continuation of the outer layer of the detrusor muscle, is composed of semicircular fibres, which never form a complete ring around the urethra. They loop around the urethra, at various degrees of obliquity, turning back to reach the bladder. Collectively they form a thick muscle layer, which encircles the urethra, to form a sphincter.

Elastic tissue, collagen fibres and fascial attachments are intermingled with the involuntary semicircular fibres of the urethral muscle, and with the striated, voluntary fibres surrounding the mid-third of the urethra. This complex combination gives the urethra an 'inherent tone', or intraurethral pressure, which is greatest at the mid-third of its length and which is important in maintaining urinary continence.

The voluntary muscle surrounding the mid-third of the urethra is part of the levator ani muscle (the puborectalis muscle), and its contraction cuts off micturition voluntarily. It also contracts to prevent urine leakage in response to the stress of coughing, bearing down, sneezing or heavy lifting. It therefore acts as an external sphincter.

The external sphincter is under the control of the pudendal nerve, whilst the involuntary musculature is mainly under the autonomic control of the parasympathetic (cholinergic) nerves.

How does the urethra resist sudden increases in abdominal pressure? It is now known that as well as contraction of the voluntary external sphincter, the raised abdominal pressure is transmitted not only to the bladder but also to the proximal urethra, thus increasing the intraurethral pressure as well as the intravesical pressure. This concept is important in understanding stress incontinence.

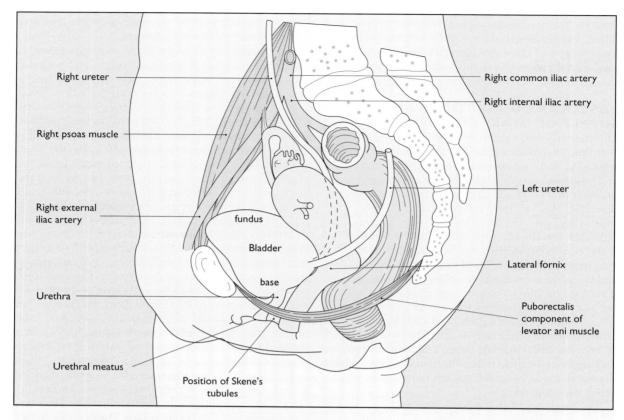

Fig. 44.18 *The relations of the urinary tract within the pelvis.*

The ureters pass from the renal pelves, behind the peritoneum, lying on the psoas muscle, to enter the true pelvis anterior to the sacro-iliac joint. They are separated from the joint by the ligaments of the joint, the psoas muscle and the common iliac vessels, and enter the pelvis in front of the common iliac artery at its bifurcation into the external and internal branches. Inside the true pelvis, each ureter turns downward and runs on the medial side of the internal iliac artery. In the parametrium, as it courses forward to the bladder, it is crossed by the uterine artery, and lies 1cm lateral to the supravaginal cervix and 1cm above the lateral fornix. It passes obliquely through the bladder wall on the posterior aspect of its base, and the ureteric orifices mark the posterior points of the trigone of the bladder (*Fig. 44.19*). The ureter is lined with transitional epithelium, and the main coats of its wall consist of involuntary muscle which constantly moves as peristaltic waves pass along it. The obliquity with which the ureter enters the bladder acts as a valve preventing reflux of urine when the bladder is full.

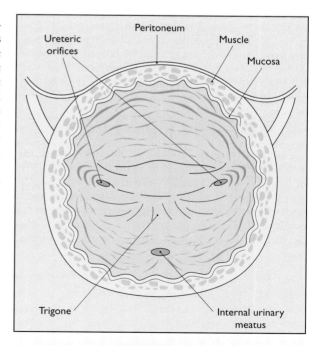

Fig. 44.19 *The trigone of the bladder.*

Index

BIBLIOGRAPHY

Today with the availability of computer-generated search programmes, I believe that students asked to explore a topic in greater depth are better served if they use these programmes, as references given in a textbook are often out of date. However, the list of books which follows, which are usually available in medical libraries, may help students and interns access more information about a topic quickly.

Obstetrics

Chalmers I, Enkin M, Keirse MJNC. *Effective care in Pregnancy and Childbirth*, 2nd ed. Oxford: Oxford University Press; 1996.
Subsequent data updated regularly and provided on disc as the Cochrane Library.

Chamberlain G, ed. Turnbull's *Obstetrics*, 2nd ed. London: Churchill Livingstone; 1995.
This excellent British text book is comprehensive, well written and deals with the current issues in obstetrics. However, this edition was compiled in 1994 and is dated. Recommended with reservations.

Cunningham FG, ed. Williams' *Obstetrics*, 19th ed. New York: Appleton Lang; 1993.

Enkin M, Keirse MJNC, Chalmers I. *A Guide to Effective Care in Pregnancy and Childbirth*. Oxford: Oxford University Press; 1989.
This is a summarized version of the Chalmers reference book.

De Swiet M, Chamberlain G. *Basic Science in Obstetrics and Gynaecology*, 2nd ed. Edinburgh: Churchill Livingstone; 1992.

Gabbe SG, Niebel JR, Simpson JL. *Obstetrics, Normal and Problem Pregnancies*, 3rd ed. New York: Churchill Livingstone; 1996.
This multi-authored text book is 1300 pages long and deals comprehensively with most aspects of obstetrics. In general it is easy to read, although some of the chapters contain a bewildering amount of information, which may confuse the reader. Strongly recommended as a reference book for students and a text for those in training to become obstetricians and gynaecologists.

Gynaecology

Anderson J, ed. *Gynaecological Imaging*. London: Churchill Livingstone; 1997.
This excellent and comprehensive reference book has 66 contributing authors and covers the field of gynaecological imagining. The text is readable and the images excellent.

Berek JS, ed. Novak's *Gynaecology*, 12th ed. Baltimore: Williams and Wilkins; 1996.
This American multi-author book contains a good deal of detail, but because of the several authors tends to be repetitive. As many American obstetricians and gynaecologists are increasingly responsible for women's preventive and primary health care, including family planning and psychiatric problems, several chapters are devoted to this topic. The gynaecological sections are comprehensive. There are extensive bibliographies for each chapter. The book is not didactic, offering the student the opportunity to evaluate disparate research findings. Recommended as a reference book.

Shaw RW, Soutter WP, Stanton SL. *Gynaecology*, 2nd ed. London: Churchill Livingstone; 1997.
A standard British text book which emphasizes clinical management including minimally invasive techniques. A useful reference book

Woodruff JD. *Atlas of Gynaecological Pathology*. New York: Raven Press; 1993.

Chapters 5 and 8
Hytten H, Chamberlain G. *Clinical Physiology in Obstetrics*, 2nd ed. Oxford: Blackwell Scientific; 1990.

Chapter 9
Browning P. Pain *Relief and Anaesthesia in Childbirth*. Melbourne: Ashwood Medical Library; 1994.

Chapter 15
Redman C, Walker I. *Pre-eclampsia – the Facts*. Oxford: Oxford University Press; 1992.

Chapters 16–18
De Swiet M, ed. *Medical Disorders in Obstetric Practice*, 3rd ed. Oxford: Blackwell; 1995.

Chapter 22
Berkowitz RS, Goldstein DP. *Chorionic Tumors*. *New England Journal of Medicine*. 1996;335:1740–8.

Chapter 27
Robertson NCR, ed. *Textbook of Neonatology*, 2nd ed. Edinburgh: Churchill Livingstone; 1992.

Chapter 29
Lewis VB, Magos AL. *Endometrial Ablation*. Edinburgh: Churchill Livingstone, 1993.

Chapter 32
Drife JO, Baird DT, eds. *Contraception*. Edinburgh: Churchill Livingstone, 1993.

Filshie M, Guillebaud J, eds. *Contraception: Science and Practice*. London: Butterworths; 1989.

Chapter 33
Inster V, Lunenfeld B, eds. *Infertility: Male and Female*, 2nd ed. Edinburgh: Churchill Livingstone; 1993.

Llewellyn-Jones D. *Getting Pregnant*. New York: Bantam–Double Day; 1991.

Chapter 34
Berger GS, Westrom LV. *Pelvic Inflammatory Disease*. New York: Raven Press; 1992.

Chapter 38
Coppleston M, ed. *Gynaecology Oncology – Fundamental Principles and Practice*, 2nd ed. Edinburgh: Churchill Livingstone; 1991.

Chapter 40
Sutherst JR, Fraser MI, Richmond RS, Haylen BR. *An Introduction to Gynaecological Urology*. London: Butterworths; 1991.

Chapter 41
Baum M. *Breast Cancer – the Facts*, 2nd ed. Oxford: Oxford University Press; 1993.

Chapter 42
Carpenter SE, Rock JA. *Pediatric and Adolescent Gynaecology*. New York: Raven; 1992.

Chapter 43
Burger HG, ed. *Clinical Endocrinology and Metabolism*. London: Baillière Tindall; 1993.

Llewellyn-Jones D, Abraham S. *Everywoman's Middle Years*, 2nd ed. Melbourne: Ashwood Medical; 1996.